Refugee Health Care

Aniyizhai Annamalai
Editor

Refugee Health Care

An Essential Medical Guide

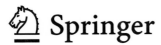 Springer

Editor
Aniyizhai Annamalai, M.D.
Yale University School of Medicine
New Haven, CT, USA

ISBN 978-1-4939-0270-5   ISBN 978-1-4939-0271-2 (eBook)
DOI 10.1007/978-1-4939-0271-2
Springer New York Heidelberg Dordrecht London

Library of Congress Control Number: 2014930743

Springer is part of Springer Science+Business Media (www.springer.com)

*For my mother, Nageswari Annamalai,
for her absolute support at every step
in my journey as a doctor.*

Preface

The field of refugee health has grown tremendously in recent years. Refugees are a heterogeneous group as they originate from different parts of the world and each refugee's path to resettlement is different. Consequently, risk factors for illness are not uniform among all refugee populations. However, there are some unifying features.

Refugees come from parts of the world where illness demographics are often different from those of the countries they resettle in. Certain infectious diseases and nutritional deficiencies are more common in some countries of origin. Some refugee populations have a cardiovascular risk profile comparable to that of the Western world. Chronic pain and other physical symptoms are prevalent in many refugees. By definition, they have all experienced some form of persecution, and psychiatric illness is often a significant part of their presentation. Social factors including access to health care greatly impact the level of preventive care refugees have received. Finally, refugees are a diversely multicultural group, and provision of culturally sensitive health care is of paramount importance.

This book provides an overview of refugee health. There is greater emphasis on health issues relevant at screening and in the first few months of resettlement. Within refugee health, screening is the area with the most evidence-based information. Clinical issues such as aging and end-of-life care in refugees are less well studied and are not addressed in this book. Infectious diseases prevalent in other parts of the world but rarely encountered in existing refugee populations are not discussed. Chronic disease in refugees is a developing area, and clinical management of chronic physical and mental illness is discussed. Given the high burden of mental health problems and its impact on self-sufficiency and successful acculturation, there is an entire section devoted to discussion of mental illness in refugees. Recommendations for behavioral health screening in primary care settings are provided. While integrated physical and mental health care is optimal for refugees, there is no single health care delivery model, and a detailed discussion of different models is beyond the scope of this book.

Many health care providers encounter refugees in their practice, and there is an increasing need for them to familiarize themselves with health issues specific to refugees. Primary care practitioners are usually the first point of contact for refugees within the US health care system when they are seen for a screening medical examination soon after arrival in the country.

The book is intended as a reference for these primary care practitioners as well as mental health providers who care for refugees. As in many areas of medicine, knowledge base is expanding rapidly and recommendations are constantly updated. Top experts in the field have gathered together the latest evidence-based information and presented it in a concise and clinically useful format.

Academic institutions have begun to include topics on refugee health in their curriculum as trainees are frequently called upon to provide care for refugees. This book will be a useful reference for this curriculum. Refugee health is also part of global health, and this book will be useful in global health curricula for medical and public health students.

Refugees are a uniquely vulnerable population. With appropriate support, many refugees can and do succeed in their new society. Providing appropriate physical and mental health care can go a long way in helping refugees in their journey to a healthy and productive life. Many providers want to care for refugees but lack the necessary knowledge and resources. My hope is that this book will be useful to fill this gap.

New Haven, CT, USA   Aniyizhai Annamalai

Acknowledgements

I want to thank Springer Science+Business Media for inviting me to write this timely and much needed book. I am very grateful to all the contributors who are experts in the field of refugee health and have been willing and gracious in helping bring this book together. I thank them and the community of refugee health care providers from whom I have learned much. I sincerely appreciate all the hard work of the Yale resident volunteers without whom we could not serve refugees in our community. Finally, I thank my family—my father and sister for their support and encouragement and my husband for comfort and a hot meal whenever I returned late from refugee clinic.

Contents

Part III   Mental Health

Part IV   Special Groups

Contributors

Jennifer Adelson-Mitty, M.D., M.P.H. Department of Infectious Diseases, Beth Israel Deaconess Medical Center, Harvard Medical School, Boston, MA, USA

Aniyizhai Annamalai, M.D. Yale University School of Medicine, New Haven, CT, USA

Kaya Belknap College of Medicine - Phoenix, University of Arizona, Phoenix, AZ, USA

Andrew T. Boyd, M.D. Médecins Sans Frontières, New York, NY, USA

Yale Internal Medicine Residency, New Haven, CT, USA

Peter Cronkright, M.D. Department of Medicine, Upstate Medical University, Syracuse, NY, USA

Beth Farmer, M.S.W. International Counseling and Community Services Program, Lutheran Community Services Northwest, SeaTac, WA, USA

Geetha Fink, M.D., M.P.H. Obstetrics and Gynecology, Phoenix Integrated Residency in Obstetrics and Gynecology, Phoenix, AZ, USA

Paul L. Geltman, M.D., M.P.H. Department of Pediatrics, Cambridge Health Alliance and Harvard Medical School, Cambridge, MA, USA

Refugee and Immigrant Health Program, Massachusetts Department of Public Health, Jamaica Plain, MA, USA

Amber Gray, M.P.H., M.A. New Mexico Department of Health, Santa Fe, NM, USA

Kelly Hebrank, B.A. IRIS—Integrated Refugee & Immigrant Services, New Haven, CT, USA

Tara Helm, M.P.H., B.S.N. Family Nurse Practitioner Program, Frontier Nursing University, Hyden, KY, USA

Michael Hollifield, M.D. Program for Traumatic Stress, VA Long Beach, Long Beach, CA, USA

Pacific Institute for Research and Evaluation, Albuquerque, NM, USA

Sachin Jain, M.D., M.P.H. Department of Infectious Diseases, Beth Israel Deaconess Medical Center, Harvard Medical School, Boston, MA, USA

Crista E. Johnson-Agbakwu, M.D., M.Sc., F.A.C.O.G. Obstetrics & Gynecology, Maricopa Integrated Health System, Phoenix, AZ, USA

Kristina Krohn, M.D. Department of Internal Medicine and Pediatrics, University of Minnesota, Minneapolis, MN, USA

Asha M.J. Madhar, M.D. General Internal Medicine, Hennepin Country Medical Center, University of Minnesota, Minneapolis, MN, USA

Katherine C. McKenzie, M.D. Department of Medicine, Yale School of Medicine, New Haven, CT, USA

Anne E.P. Frosch, M.D., M.P.H. Division of Infectious Diseases and International Medicine, Department of Medicine, University of Minnesota, Minneapolis, MN, USA

Maya Prabhu, M.D., L.L.B. Law and Psychiatry Division, Department of Psychiatry, Yale School of Medicine, New Haven, CT, USA

Douglas J. Pryce, M.D. General Internal Medicine, Hennepin Country Medical Center, University of Minnesota, Minneapolis, MN, USA

Mara Rabin, M.D. Utah Health and Human Rights, Salt Lake City, UT, USA

Astha K. Ramaiya, M.Sc. Department of Internal Medicine, SUNY Upstate Medical University, Syracuse, NY, USA

Susan Heffner Rhema, L.C.S.W., A.B.D. Kent School, University of Louisville, Louisville, KY, USA

Erika Schumacher, M.D., F.A.A.P. Pediatrics, Yale University, New Haven, CT, USA

Sural Shah, M.D. Internal Medicine and Pediatrics, Children's Hospital of Philadelphia, Hospital of the University of Pennsylvania, Philadelphia, PA, USA

Meera Siddharth, M.D., F.A.A.P. Primary Care, Karabots Primary Care Centre, Children's Hospital of Philadelphia, Philadelphia, PA, USA

William Stauffer, M.D., M.S.P.H., CTropMed, F.A.S.T.M.H. Division of Infectious Diseases and International Medicine, Department of Medicine, University of Minnesota, Minneapolis, MN, USA

Sasha Verbillis-Kolp, M.S.W. Lutheran Community Services Northwest, Portland, OR, USA

James Wallace, M.D., M.S.P.H. Department of Medicine, University of Minnesota Medical Center, Minneapolis, MN, USA

Cynthia Willard, M.D., M.P.H. Department of Community and Family Medicine, Keck School of Medicine, Chapcare Health Center, University of Southern California, Pasadena, CA, USA

Katherine Yun, M.D. Pediatrics, Perelman School of Medicine & The Children's Hospital of Philadelphia, University of Pennsylvania, Philadelphia, PA, USA

Paula Zimbrean, M.D. Department of Psychiatry, Yale University, New Haven, CT, USA

Part I
Introduction and Overview

Chapter 1
Introduction to Refugees

Kelly Hebrank

Who Are Refugees?

They are not likely to be mentioned in a State of the Union address or in other public speeches.

They are usually not referenced in the debate about immigration reform.

They are rarely included in a school curriculum.

But they should be.

Every year, up to 75,000 refugees enter the United States as documented immigrants. They have fled horrible persecution, repressive governments, or death threats. They are invited to the United States to start their lives over, continuing the country's long-standing tradition of welcoming persecuted people.

But often, their stories are lost among the statistics of the nearly 40 million foreign-born people who live in the United States [1].

Historical Context

As long as there have been wars, persecution, and political instability, there have been refugees. However, the two World Wars in the first half of the twentieth century left millions of people forcibly displaced or deported from their homes, necessitating the collaboration of the international community in drafting guidelines and laws related to their status, treatment, and protection. In July 1951, the United Nations

K. Hebrank, B.A. (✉)
IRIS—Integrated Refugee & Immigrant Services,
235 Nicoll Street, 2nd Floor, New Haven, CT 06511, USA
e-mail: khebrank@irisct.org

A. Annamalai (ed.), *Refugee Health Care: An Essential Medical Guide*,
DOI 10.1007/978-1-4939-0271-2_1, © Springer Science+Business Media New York 2014

convened a diplomatic conference in Geneva to "revise and consolidate previous international agreements" related to refugee travel and protection, and the legal obligations of states, based on principles affirmed in the Universal Declaration of Human Rights. This 1951 Convention relating to the Status of Refugees defined a refugee as someone who, "owing to well-founded fear of being persecuted for reasons of race, religion, nationality, membership of a particular social group or political opinion, is outside the country of his nationality and is unable or, owing to such fear, is unwilling to avail himself of the protection of that country" [2].

This definition initially applied only to people displaced "as a result of events occurring before 1 January 1951," and some signatories further limited the scope of the definition to refugees from Europe. In 1967, acknowledging that "new refugee situations have arisen since the Convention was adopted," a Protocol Relating to the Status of Refugees was signed, which removes the geographical and time limits of the original 1951 Convention.

Global Burden

It is staggering to consider the number of refugees and displaced people in the world today. The United Nations reports that at the end of 2010, there were over 43 million people in the world uprooted because of conflict or persecution [3].

Of these, over 15.3 million are refugees, who—in accordance with the 1951 Convention definition—are outside the country of their nationality. The United Nations High Commissioner for Refugees (UNHCR), established in 1950 to lead and coordinate international action to protect refugees, includes 10.55 million refugees in its "population of concern" [4], and 4.82 million Palestinian refugees fall under the responsibility of another UN agency, the United Nations Relief and Works Agency for Palestine Refugees (UNRWA). Almost 27.5 million people—known as internally displaced persons (IDPs)—have also been forced to flee their homes, but remain within the borders of their home countries [3].

Refugee assistance has changed dramatically since it was first organized over 60 years ago, with the mission of aiding European refugees from World War II. Today's refugees originate *from* countries throughout the world and seek asylum—temporary or permanent—*in* countries throughout the world.

According to estimates, in 2010, refugees from Afghanistan represented 29 % of the global refugee population or 3.05 million of the 10.55 million persons under UNHCR's responsibility. Iraq was the second largest country of origin of refugees (1.7 million), followed by Somalia (770,000), the Democratic Republic of the Congo (477,000), and Myanmar, formerly Burma (416,000) [5].

Pakistan hosted the highest number of refugees at the end of 2010, totaling 1.9 million. Other major countries of asylum included the Islamic Republic of Iran (1.1 million), the Syrian Arab Republic (1 million; Government estimate), Germany (594,000), Jordan (451,000; Government estimate), and Kenya (403,000) [5].

With each new conflict, these numbers can change dramatically. By March 2013, more than 1.1 million refugees from Syria were being assisted in neighboring countries such as Jordan, Lebanon, and Turkey [6]. Approximately 100,000 Syrian residents fleeing violence there have taken refuge in northern Iraq [7], even as Iraq continues to produce its own refugees.

Long-Term Solutions

People who work in refugee resettlement are often asked, "Are you resettling refugees from [insert here the political crisis currently in the media]?"

And the answer, sadly, is usually "No."

Resettlement—a nation's government inviting refugees to move to its country, access rights given to nationals, and obtain permanent residency leading to citizenship [8]—is usually a last resort and an option for very few. Each year, less than 1 % of the world's refugees will be offered resettlement in a third country. For a comprehensive look at the history, challenges, and benefits of resettlement on a global scale, see UNHCR report by Piper et al. [9].

Before resettlement, other durable solutions are considered. UNHCR first pursues the possibility of voluntary repatriation, a refugee returning to his or her country of origin if it became safe. Another option is local integration, a refugee remaining in the country to which he or she has fled and integrating into the local community.

For a small percentage of the world's refugees for whom the above options are not viable, resettlement becomes a possibility.

Currently, 26 countries have indicated a willingness to resettle refugees, but many of the programs are nascent and very limited in scope.

In fact, just three countries—the United States, Canada, and Australia—welcome 90 % of resettled refugees [10]. The United States alone resettles more refugees than all other countries combined.

Oftentimes, the decision of which refugees to admit is heavily influenced by political, economic, and social factors [9]. Unlike many other countries, the United States does not discriminate in its acceptance of cases based on a refugee's likely ability to integrate. While other nations may reserve resettlement for refugees deemed to have high "integration potential"—based on their age, education, work experience, and language skills—the United States accepts refugees regardless of their socioeconomic status, employment history, medical history, or family composition [9]. Therefore, a refugee resettlement agency in the United States is as likely to serve a single mother from Somalia with five children as it is to serve a highly skilled engineer from Iraq and his schoolteacher wife. It may welcome as many refugees with chronic or serious health problems as it does healthy refugees. Cases may be a single individual or a family of ten. This practice ensures that the most vulnerable refugees have access to protection and resettlement in the United States.

United States Resettlement Process

Most refugees who are considered for resettlement in the United States are referred to the federal government by UNHCR, but in some cases a United States Embassy makes the referral. The Department of State's Bureau of Population, Refugees, and Migration (PRM) oversees refugee assistance, including resettlement. PRM funds and manages nine Resettlement Support Centers (RSCs) throughout the world, which process refugee applications for resettlement in the United States. In some regions, refugees must physically present themselves to an RSC in order to receive assistance, but in other areas, RSC staff conduct "circuit rides" through vast territories to serve refugees in remote locations. After meeting with RSC staff, refugees are interviewed by officers from the United States Citizenship and Immigration Services (USCIS, within the Department of Homeland Security) to determine if they will be granted resettlement. The Department of Homeland Security conducts thorough background checks to ensure the refugees will not pose a threat to security. Refugees receive a health screening (known as the overseas health assessment) to identify conditions that might make them a public health risk; refugees with active infectious diseases would need to complete treatment prior to gaining admission to the United States. Approved refugees are then ready to travel to the United States—at their own expense, thanks to an interest-free loan from the International Organization for Migration.

The length of this process varies based on a refugee's location and other factors, but the average time it takes for a refugee referred by UNHCR to actually arrive in the United States is from 12 to 15 months [11]. However, most refugees have waited years—and some for more than a decade—just to access the resettlement process and reach the point of a UNHCR referral. UNHCR estimates that at the end of 2010, 7.2 million refugees were in a protracted refugee situation—meaning that 25,000 or more refugees of the same nationality had been in exile for 5 years or longer in a given asylum country [12].

Each year, the President, in consultation with Congress, sets the numerical goals for refugee admissions during the upcoming fiscal year. This Presidential Determination is a ceiling rather than a floor and includes the total maximum number of refugees the United States will resettle in the coming year (70,000 in FY14), as well as a breakdown by geographic region.

Over the past 5 years, refugee admissions have ranged from 56,424 to 74,654 individuals per year. In FY12, although the ceiling was set at 76,000, just 58,238 refugees were admitted to the United States (see Fig. 1.1). The states that resettled the most refugees were Texas (5,925 individuals), California (5,177), Michigan (3,601), New York (3,528), Pennsylvania (2,810), and Georgia (2,520) [13]. Figure 1.2 shows refugee admissions across states in FY12.

In FY12, three nationalities accounted for 71 % of all refugee admissions: Bhutan (15,070 individuals), Burma (14,160), and Iraq (12,163). The remaining 29 % came from a total of 63 countries [14].

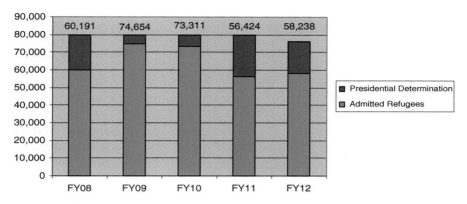

Fig. 1.1 Refugee admissions in the last 5 years. Refugees admitted to the US FY08–FY12 (data from Refugee Processing Center [14])

In the United States, refugees are assisted through a unique public–private partnership. At the federal level, the Department of State and the Department of Health and Human Services (HHS) work together to welcome refugees, by providing basic needs support and services to help them integrate into their new communities and become economically self-sufficient. The federal government contracts with nine national nongovernmental agencies; each has a network of affiliates (not-for-profit organizations) across the country—about 350 in total—which carry out the work of resettlement. There are resettlement agencies in nearly all 50 states. Large metropolitan areas, such as Houston, Minneapolis, and Atlanta, are often home to multiple resettlement agencies. If a refugee approved for resettlement in the United States knows someone already in the country—a relative or close friend—they can often be resettled in the same city. Without this connection, called a United States tie, the refugee would be randomly assigned to a city and resettlement organization that has the capability to serve refugees of their nationality and language group.

Because they have already had to share their persecution story numerous times—first to be granted refugee status by UNHCR, then to United States government officials—once refugees arrive in the United States, the resettlement agency focuses on helping them move forward and start life over.

Each affiliate organization adheres to the same federal regulations and must provide the same basic services delineated in a Cooperative Agreement signed yearly with PRM. The initial resettlement period, called the Reception and Placement (R&P) program, is for 30–90 days after arrival, during which the agency must provide housing, food, clothing, and other basic needs; enrollment in benefits such as food stamps, medical insurance, and social security cards; help accessing health care, English class, and employment services; and cultural orientation including instruction on United States laws and customs. One federal requirement stands out among the others, a reminder of the importance of offering hospitality to refugees:

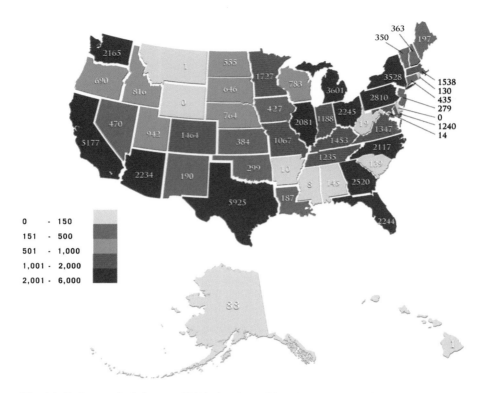

Fig. 1.2 Refugee arrivals by state, FY12 (October 1, 2011–September 30, 2012)

when refugees arrive to their new home, the resettlement agency must provide them with a hot, culturally appropriate meal [15].

Funding to affiliate agencies is on a per capita basis; for each refugee resettled, the affiliate receives $1,925 (as of FY14), $1,125 of which is to be given to or spent on behalf of the refugee for basic needs and $800 of which is for the agency's expenses including program staff and operating expenses. This government funding is not meant to cover the total cost of resettlement; each affiliate must raise private funds to supplement and relies heavily on community members who volunteer their time and donate in-kind goods.

Many organizations operate additional programs and services funded by the Office of Refugee Resettlement (ORR, an office within HHS) and other government and private sources. Overall, financial assistance to refugees usually lasts no more than 6 months after arrival, although more limited services might be available for years after arrival. Regardless of the city in which a refugee resettles, an urgent priority is that he or she finds work quickly after arrival and becomes economically self-sufficient. Refugees are expected to apply for legal permanent residency after 1 year in the United States (commonly known as receiving a green card) and for citizenship after 5 years in the United States.

When they arrive, refugees are eligible for many of the safety net programs available to low-income United States citizens, including the Supplemental Nutrition Assistance Program (SNAP, commonly referred to as "food stamps"). A refugee family with children will likely be eligible for cash assistance through the Temporary Assistance for Needy Families (TANF) program and for medical insurance through Medicaid. Refugees determined ineligible for TANF and Medicaid may be eligible for Refugee Cash Assistance (RCA) and Refugee Medical Assistance (RMA) for up to 8 months from the date of arrival in the United States [16]. The Refugee Act of 1980 (which created the Office of Refugee Resettlement and formalized the federal refugee resettlement program) allows for the federal government to reimburse states for RCA and RMA for up to 3 years after a refugee's arrival in the United States [17]; unfortunately, over the years funding for this program has reduced steadily, to the current provision of only 8 months of benefits.

Refugees and the Health Care System

Having Medicaid coverage does not necessarily make it easy for refugees to access medical care. Refugees face many barriers in accessing care, including lack of English language ability, cultural differences in approaches to health, and unfamiliarity with the American health care system. The federal government recognizes the importance of caring for the health needs of refugees and mandates that refugee resettlement agencies help clients receive a comprehensive health exam, initiated within 30 days of arrival. The purpose of this domestic health assessment is to ensure follow-up of any serious conditions identified during the overseas medical examination, identify conditions of public health importance, and diagnose and treat health conditions that may adversely affect resettlement. Each state, however, implements these guidelines differently—often based on the public health capacity of the state—so the scope and organization of health assessments vary widely from state to state [18]. Some states have public health departments that provide this initial screening; in states that do not, the resettlement agency must find a community health center or other health-care provider who will screen and treat refugees.

In many states, it is difficult to find appointments for refugees at health clinics that accept Medicaid and consistently provide interpretation services. In these situations, the resettlement agency might need to make special arrangements with a health-care provider. Since refugees may lose their Medicaid coverage after just 8 months in the United States, it is essential for them to receive not only primary care but also specialty care and any procedures or surgeries they need, within this time frame. Refugees are eligible for Affordable Care Act (ACA) benefits and this may increase refugees' access to health insurance in the coming years.

A refugee's ability to access health care and address their health needs is one factor in his or her ability to successfully become self-sufficient in their new homes.

The work of refugee resettlement is both big—helping a refugee learn English, find work, and support themselves in a new country—and nuanced, such as teaching someone the difference between prescription and over-the-counter medication, how to discern between official mail and junk solicitations, and why they should not pick flowers from their neighbor's front yard.

Though the United States currently welcomes fewer than one-half the refugees it did in decades past, it is also important to remember that it provides more than half of the world's resettlement. Assisting these refugees in their path to self-sufficiency and citizenship requires the commitment of federal, state, and local governments, as well as the contributions of money, volunteer time, professional skills, and friendship of thousands of residents across the country.

References

1. Grieco EM, Acosta YD, de la Cruz GP, et al. The foreign-born population in the United States: 2010. U.S. Census Bureau. 2012. http://www.census.gov/prod/2012pubs/acs-19.pdf. Accessed Aug 2013.
2. 1951 Convention Related to the Status of Refugees. 2010. http://www.unhcr.org/3b66c2aa10.html. Accessed Aug 2013.
3. UNHCR Global Trends 2010: 60 years and still counting. UNHCR. http://www.unhcr.org/cgi-bin/texis/vtx/home/opendocPDFViewer.html?docid=4dfa11499&query=4.82%20million. Accessed Aug 2013.
4. History of UNHCR. UNHCR. http://www.unhcr.org/pages/49c3646cbc.html. Accessed Aug 2013.
5. UNHCR statistical yearbook 2010. 10th ed. Trends in displacement, protection and solutions: ten years of statistics. http://www.unhcr.org/4ef9c8d10.html. Accessed Aug 2013.
6. Beals G, Fleming M. Escaping Syria in the dead of night: UNHCR chief visits Jordan border. UNHCR. 2013. http://www.unhcr.org/5141eade6.html. Accessed Aug 2013.
7. Syria regional response plan: January to June 2013. UNHCR. http://www.unhcr.org/cgi-bin/texis/vtx/home/opendocPDFViewer.html?docid=5139fccf9&query=syrian%20refugees%20in%20iraq%202013. Accessed Aug 2013.
8. UNHCR resettlement handbook. UNHCR Web site. 2011. http://www.unhcr.org/4a2ccf4c6.html. Accessed Aug 2013.
9. Piper M, Power P, Thom G. New issues in refugee research. Research Paper No. 253. Refugee resettlement: 2012 and beyond. 2013. http://www.unhcr.org/510bd3979.html. Accessed Aug 2013.
10. Frequently asked questions about resettlement. UNHCR. 2012. http://www.unhcr.org/4ac0873d6.html. Accessed Aug 2013.
11. Refugee admissions. U.S. Department of State. http://www.state.gov/j/prm/ra/index.htm. Accessed Aug 2013.
12. UNHCR resettlement handbook. UNHCR. 2011. http://www.unhcr.org/4a2ccf4c6.html. July 2011. Accessed Aug 2013.
13. Arrivals by destination city by nationality by FY. Refugee Processing Center http://www.wrapsnet.org/Reports/AdmissionsArrivals/tabid/211/Default.aspx. Accessed Aug 2013.
14. FY 2011 Reception and Placement Basic Terms of the Cooperative Agreement Between the Government of the United States of America and the (Name of Organization) 8.c.4.c.1. U.S. Department of State. http://www.state.gov/j/prm/releases/sample/181172.htm. Accessed Aug 2013.

15. About cash & medical assistance. Office of Refugee Resettlement. http://www.acf.hhs.gov/programs/orr/programs/cma/about. Accessed Aug 2013.
16. The Refugee Act. Office of Refugee Resettlement. 2012. http://www.acf.hhs.gov/programs/orr/resource/the-refugee-act. Accessed Aug 2013.
17. Health assessment. Refugee Health Technical Assistance Center. http://www.refugeehealthta.org/physical-mental-health/health-assessments/. Accessed Aug 2013.
18. Refugee Admissions report. Refugee Processing Center. http://www.wrapsnet.org/Reports/AdmissionsArrivals/tabid/211/Default.aspx. Accessed Aug 2013.

Chapter 2
Culturally Appropriate Care

Aniyizhai Annamalai

Introduction to Cultural Competence

The Institute of Medicine (IOM) committee concluded in their 2002 report that minorities are less likely to receive necessary care even after controlling for demographic variables and those related to access to health care. The minority groups' attitudes toward health care and preferences for treatment do not explain this disparity. The following factors are thought to contribute to this disparity:

1. Operation of health care systems—linguistic barriers, fragmentation of health care systems, and location of services (e.g., minorities are less likely to access care at private clinics even when insured at the same level)
2. Factors during clinical encounters—provider bias against minorities, stereotyped beliefs held by providers, and greater clinical uncertainty during interaction with minority communities [1]

Given that health care provider factors contribute to health care disparities, education is an important tool in eliminating some of this disparity. There is often a disconnect between the desire to provide equal treatment and unintentional influence of ethnicity on clinical decisions. Cross-cultural differences exist in all encounters but are more obvious in the presence of language differences. Also, language barriers make resolution of cultural differences much harder.

Many definitions of cultural competence exist but the seminal work of Cross et al. in 1989 established a solid foundation in the field of health and human services. The core principles espoused in this work have formed the framework for later adaptations. Culture refers to integrated patterns of human behavior that include language, communications, actions, beliefs, and values. Cultural competence is a set of congruent behaviors, attitudes, and policies that come together in a

A. Annamalai, M.D. (✉)
Yale University School of Medicine, 34 Park Street, New Haven, CT 06519-1187, USA
e-mail: aniyizhai.annamalai@yale.edu

A. Annamalai (ed.), *Refugee Health Care: An Essential Medical Guide*,
DOI 10.1007/978-1-4939-0271-2_2, © Springer Science+Business Media New York 2014

system, agency, or among professionals and enable that system, agency, or those professions to work effectively in cross-cultural situations [2]. Cultural competence in health care describes the ability of systems to provide care to patients with diverse values, beliefs, and behaviors, including tailoring delivery to meet patients' social, cultural, and linguistic needs [3].

For individual providers, the basic cultural issues to be addressed are (1) their own identity and relationship to people from other communities, (2) communication skills and ability to work with interpreters and culture brokers, (3) an understanding of the influence of cultural background on illness and treatment, and (4) knowledge of specific communities that are in the provider's practice [4]. Ethnic matching of the provider and patient can result in better communication and promote safety and trust in the patient. Alternative concepts such as cultural responsiveness, cultural safety, and cultural humility have been proposed to stress respect and engagement in another's lifeworld rather than simply claim competence in the other's culture [5].

There are several different pedagogic methods to train providers in cultural competency. Some examples are prescribed readings, didactic presentations, case studies, individual and group reflective exercises, observed interviews, role-plays, and direct patient care. The United States Department of Health and Human Services in combination with other agencies provides an online resource for health care providers and organizations to assist in providing culturally competent services to multiethnic populations [6]. Some highlights of the training tips are provided below.

Tools for Enhancing Effectiveness of Cross-Cultural Patient-Provider Communication

1. *Cultural self-awareness*. Examine your own cultural beliefs and explore personal biases and assumptions about cultures that are not your own. As you learn about other cultures, examine how their belief systems integrate with or are in contrast to your own beliefs. One suggested exercise adapted from Senge et al. [7] is helpful in uncovering some tacit assumptions you may have. (A) Select a difficult clinical encounter you had with someone from a different culture. (B) Describe the encounter briefly in writing. (C) Make three columns and record the actual interaction between you and your patient in one column, record your unsaid thoughts and feelings during that time, and finally record what might have been the feelings of the patient during the encounter. Repeat this exercise when you encounter a new clinical situation that is difficult to handle.

   If there are certain cultural groups you encounter more often, it may help to familiarize yourself with their profile. The Cultural Orientation Resource Center publishes profiles of different refugee groups [8]. But remember that there are individual cultural variations, and being sensitive to verbal and nonverbal cues from patients is finally the key to a successful clinical encounter.

2. *Clinical practice.* Levin et al. describe a mnemonic ETHNIC as a guide to use during cross-cultural encounters [9]. (A) Explanation—Ask if patients have an opinion on the cause of their symptoms or if they have heard about their diagnosis from family, friends, or media. (B) Treatment—Ask if they have already tried other remedies and what kind of treatment they expect from you. (C) Healers—Ask if they believe in traditional healers and assess their faith in these alternative modes of treatment. (D) Negotiate—If the patient does not agree with your treatment, negotiate a plan that is clinically safe and acceptable to the patient. (E) Intervention—Determine the intervention by involving the patient in active problem solving. (F) Collaboration—Collaborate with family members and other community supports, as appropriate, to set realistic goals for any behavior change. Family involvement is especially relevant in special situations such as pregnancy, childcare, and end of life care.

Throughout this exchange, ask questions nonjudgmentally and listen carefully to the patient's replies as this can indicate willingness and ability to adhere to treatment.

Another tool widely used for cross-cultural communication is LEARN (Listen with understanding of the patient's perception of the problem; Explain your perception of the problem; Acknowledge and discuss differences and similarities; Recommend treatment; Negotiate agreement) [10].

3. *Nonverbal communication* [11]. Follow the patient's lead in any physical contact. Comfort levels for touching and personal space can vary across cultures. Do not force patients to have eye contact with you if they avoid it. Use hand or other physical gestures with caution as they can have different meanings in other cultures. Facial expression of pain and other symptoms can vary between cultures and should not be used as the sole indicator of symptom severity.

Applying Cultural Competence in Refugee Care

Refugees come from many different places around the world, and their response to trauma, migration stressors, and resettlement difficulties can vary widely based on their cultural background as well as personal traits of vulnerability or resilience. The place of origin affects not only exposure to endemic diseases but also health care experiences. Culture can influence many aspects of health—types of symptoms that are manifested, reactions to these symptoms, explanations of illness, approach to treatment, beliefs about medications and other forms of treatment, relationship of patients to their families, and attitude toward physicians and other providers.

Psychosocial distress often manifests as physical symptoms, and this is especially true in refugee populations. Primary care providers should be aware of this when evaluating refugees. There are also somatic syndromes that are applicable to specific ethnic and cultural groups. These cultural syndromes are described in traumatized refugees and may represent a manifestation of posttraumatic stress. These issues are described in more detail in later chapters.

Refugees may follow traditional forms of healing and be skeptical of allopathic medications as effective treatment for their illnesses. Refugees from urban settings are likely to have exposure to allopathic treatments in addition to other traditional forms. Questions about previous consultations with a physician or healer from their own or other communities can uncover health concerns that can affect adherence and treatment response. Some refugees are rooted to their prior medical treatments, and it is then difficult to convince them of alternative evidence-based treatments.

Refugees often have close family members left behind, sometimes in dangerous circumstances. Families are often fragmented and do not always arrive in the new country together. Close attention should be paid to the family system and social network during the refugee's treatment in a primary care setting. Family members who have also migrated with the patient may accompany them to their medical visits. Rather than excluding them because of privacy, involving them in treatment decisions can be an important step to building trust and a source of valuable information. Rules of confidentiality and disclosure should be applied in a way that respects cultural context. For adolescents, interventions should be framed in ways that avoid alienating family members or aggravating intergenerational conflicts [12].

Working with Interpreters

Effective communication requires use of interpreters when there is a language barrier between the refugee patient and the provider. The importance of this is recognized in Title VI of the Civil Rights Act of 1964, which mandates that any health care agency that receives federal assistance must provide adequate interpreter services. The International Medical Interpreters Association (IMIA) provides information on this and other issues related to interpreting services. Readers can refer to their educational resource on standards for medical interpreters at www.imiaweb.org.

Even if the refugee has some English language proficiency, it may not be sufficient to express concerns, describe symptoms, and discuss treatment. Failure to use interpreters is an important barrier to accessing services for refugees. Professional interpreters should be used to facilitate communication. Qualified medical interpreters should know the basics of human anatomy and physiology and meaning of medical terms and be able to translate complex medical terminology to simple language. Ideally, they are familiar with common health beliefs of both cultures and can translate not only language but also cultural concepts. They have been taught to appropriately handle their role in the clinical encounter as a third person so that a triadic relationship is not promoted.

Interpreting service can be either in-person or via the telephone. The type of interpreter service used is dependent on local availability and provider and patient preferences. Advantages and disadvantages of live and telephonic interpreters are outlined in Table 2.1 [13].

It is not recommended to use untrained clinic staff unless professional interpreters are inaccessible. Except in urgent situations where there is no alternative, family members should not be used as interpreters.

Table 2.1 In-person versus telephonic interpretation

Type of interpreter service	Advantages	Disadvantages
In-person interpreter	The interpreter is able to assist with nonverbal cues of the patient Communication is not dependent on technology and not disrupted by external noises Written translation of instructions for the patient can be requested if the interpreter is present	The patient may not want to discuss sensitive information with a third person present The patient may not want an interpreter of the opposite gender In a small community, the interpreter may even be someone familiar to the patient raising confidentiality issues
Telephone interpreter	The patient might be more comfortable talking about sensitive information The gender of the interpreter is less important when he/she is not in the room There is less potential for a triadic relationship with a remote interpreter	Nonverbal responses are not communicated to the interpreter Quality of the communication is heavily dependent on quality of the telephone connection

Effective collaboration with interpreters requires knowledge and specific skills. Time in a primary care visit is often limited, and using interpreters, at a minimum, doubles the time required for the interview. However, given that effective communication is so crucial in a successful patient-provider encounter, providers should make every attempt to adhere to standard guidelines for using interpreters. Some guidelines are provided below [11]:

- Explain goals of the interview to the interpreter and review his/her role.
- Ascertain if the interpreter's social position is likely to interfere with his/her professional relationship with the refugee.
- Explain any special elements such as a mental health assessment, if planned.
- As much as possible, arrange for the provider and patient to face each other.
- Allow the interpreter to introduce his/her role to the patient and ascertain the patient's consent.
- Address the patient directly during the interview and observe the patient's expressions when he/she talks, rather than looking at the interpreter.
- Speak only a few sentences at a time so the interpreter is able to translate.
- If responses are ambiguous, clarify the meaning with the interpreter and if necessary, repeat to the patient to determine if information was communicated correctly.
- It is highly recommended that the patient repeat the treatment plan to verify understanding; if feasible, written instructions should be provided via the interpreter.
- After the interview, ask the interpreter for feedback on the interview process.

Conclusion

Refugees come from very traumatic environments and face difficulties adjusting to the new host country. These factors, in addition to linguistic and cultural differences, make the issues of cultural competence especially relevant for this population. Readers are encouraged to avail themselves of the resources listed in this chapter when providing health care for refugees.

References

1. Unequal treatment: what healthcare providers need to know about racial and ethnic disparities in healthcare; Institute of Medicine. http://www.iom.edu/Reports/2002/Unequal-Treatment-Confronting-Racial-and-Ethnic-Disparities-in-Health-Care.aspx. Accessed Aug 2013.
2. Cross T, Bazron B, Dennis K, et al. Towards a culturally competent system of care, vol. I. Washington, DC: Georgetown University Child Development Center, CASSP Technical Assistance Center; 1989.
3. Betancourt J, Green A, Carrillo E, et al. Cultural competence in health care: emerging frameworks and practical approaches. New York: The Commonwealth Fund; 2002.
4. Kirmayer LJ, Fung K, Rousseau C et al. Guidelines for training in cultural psychiatry. Canadian Psychiatric Association. http://publications.cpa-apc.org/browse/documents/69. Accessed Aug 2013.
5. Kirmayer LJ. Rethinking cultural competence. Transcult Psychiatry. 2012;49(2):149–64.
6. The Providers Guide to Quality and Culture; Department of Health and Human Services. http://erc.msh.org/mainpage.cfm?file=1.0.htm&module=provider&language=English&ggroup=&mgroup=. Accessed Aug 2013.
7. Senge PM, Ross RB, Smith BJ, et al. The fifth discipline field book: strategies and tools for building a learning organization. 1st ed. New York: Broadway Books; 1994.
8. Cultural Orientation Resource Center. http://www.culturalorientation.net/. Accessed Aug 2013.
9. Levin SJ, Like RC, Gottlieb JE. Appendix: useful clinical interviewing mnemonics. Patient Care(Special Issue: Caring for Diverse Populations: Breaking Down Barriers); 2000:189.
10. Berlin EA, Fowkes WS. A teaching framework for cross-cultural healthcare. West J Med. 1983;139(6):934–8.
11. Morris D. Body talk: the meaning of human gestures. 1st ed. New York: Crown Trade Paperbacks; 1995.
12. Kirmayer LJ, Narasiah L, Munoz M, et al. Canadian Collaboration for Immigrant and Refugee Health (CCIRH). Common mental health problems in immigrants and refugees: general approach in primary care. CMAJ. 2011;183(12):E959–67.
13. Brown CE, Stronach M (Massachusetts Medical Interpreters Association). Working with interpreters to improve health outcomes: trained interpreters save lives—an interactive workshop. North American Refugee Healthcare Conference. 2012.

Chapter 3
Overview of Domestic Screening

Aniyizhai Annamalai and Paul L. Geltman

Overview of Refugee Screening Guidelines

This chapter provides a brief overview of recommendations for the initial screening of refugees newly arrived in the United States. These recommendations are based on guidelines published by Centers for Disease Control and Prevention (CDC) and include a general outline on performing a history and physical examination and obtaining relevant laboratory tests [1]. Details of screening and management of specific diseases follow in subsequent chapters.

Overseas Medical Examination

In accordance with Title IV, Chapter 2 of the Immigration and Nationality Act [2], all refugees accepted to resettle into the United States are required to undergo a medical examination before they enter the country. Panel physicians appointed by the US consulate, who follow the technical instructions provided by the Division of Global Migration and Quarantine (DGMQ) of CDC, conduct the examination. The examination is designed to identify individuals with health conditions that are either grounds for inadmissibility into the country or are significant and need notification of

A. Annamalai, M.D. (✉)
Yale University School of Medicine, Park Street 34, New Haven, CT 06519-1187, USA
e-mail: aniyizhai.annamalai@yale.edu

P.L. Geltman, M.D., M.P.H.
Assistant Professor of Pediatrics, Department of Pediatrics, Cambridge Health Alliance and Harvard Medical School, 305 South Street, Cambridge, MA 02130, USA

Refugee and Immigrant Health Program, Massachusetts Department of Public Health, Jamaica Plain, MA, USA
e-mail: paul.geltman@state.ma.us

A. Annamalai (ed.), *Refugee Health Care: An Essential Medical Guide*,
DOI 10.1007/978-1-4939-0271-2_3, © Springer Science+Business Media New York 2014

consular authorities. In recent years, the majority of overseas medical examinations have been performed by the International Organization for Migration, an international agency based in Switzerland.

The laws and regulations governing refugee resettlement define health conditions designated as "Class A" to include communicable diseases of public health significance, drug abuse, and mental or physical health conditions with harmful behaviors. Refugees with Class A conditions are denied entry into the United States unless treatment is completed and there is no further risk to the public health. The list of infectious Class A conditions includes active infectious tuberculosis, lepromatous leprosy, untreated syphilis, and other sexually transmitted diseases (chancroid, gonorrhea, granuloma inguinale, lymphogranuloma venereum). When no longer infectious, refugees with Class A conditions may be reclassified as Class B or receive a waiver allowing travel to the United States and including specification for follow-up in the United States. Other health conditions, at the discretion of the overseas panel physician, may be designated as "Class B" if they are deemed to confer significant disability or deviation from normal functioning. Refugees with Class B conditions usually require follow-up evaluation and treatment soon after arrival in the United States. Examples of Class B conditions are noninfectious tuberculosis and the tuberculoid form of leprosy. It should be noted, however, that the government designates holders of other visa categories also as eligible for domestic refugee services. These people frequently will not have received overseas health screening; examples include Haitian and Cuban entrants and recipients of political asylum. A detailed listing of the federal laws and regulations governing overseas medical screening and the definitions of Class A and B conditions can be found on the CDC website [3].

During the overseas medical exam, panel physicians perform a history and physical examination. The screening for applicants 15 years of age and older will also include a test for syphilis and a chest radiograph to screen for tuberculosis. Children aged 2–14 years will have only either a tuberculin skin test or gamma-interferon release assay to test for tuberculosis, but no test for syphilis. Further evaluation for tuberculosis will depend on the results of these initial tests and risk factors such as known HIV disease and/or exposures to an individual with active, infectious tuberculosis. Refugees may also be administered prophylactic treatment for locally endemic diseases. In particular, the CDC has an extensive program for presumptive treatment of soil-transmitted intestinal helminths (with single-dose albendazole), strongyloidiasis (with ivermectin), and schistosomiasis (with praziquantel). In addition to these, in Sub-Saharan Africa, the regimen includes use of artemether–lumefantrine for malaria. The presumptive treatment program has now been implemented in Sub-Saharan Africa for all four conditions, in East Asia for intestinal helminths and strongyloidiasis, and in the Middle East for helminths only. Details of the program as of Dec 2013 can be found on the CDC website [4].

Domestic Medical Examination

A screening medical examination is recommended by CDC after arrival, and this is strongly encouraged by the Office of Refugee Resettlement (ORR). This exam is important for several reasons. Of primary importance is the imperative to ensure that refugees start their new lives in the United States in good health. Addressing immediate health concerns can be especially valuable for refugees who may not have had access to adequate medical care. Refugees come from varied backgrounds and circumstances. Prior medical care received by individuals can be widely different. Many refugees have not received routine, preventive medical care before arriving in the United States, and the initial visit should be an opportunity to provide education on preventive health care. The initial encounter can also help the newly arrived refugee develop trust in the provider and the medical system. Familiarizing the refugee with local health care delivery systems is important for continued care. In addition, the domestic health screening continues the public health rationale behind screening by looking for conditions that may have consequences for public health such as latent tuberculosis and chronic hepatitis B virus infection.

Models of Care

Care coordination for a newly arrived refugee can be challenging. The results of the overseas medical exam are transmitted to the local health provider, through the state health department. At present, for arriving refugees, the information is transmitted via the CDC's Electronic Disease Notification (EDN) system or in paper form by the referring local resettlement agency or the refugee himself/herself. When refugees with complex medical problems are anticipated, active communication between local medical providers, local resettlement agencies, and public health departments before the refugee's arrival is necessary to plan for appropriate care.

The Bureau of Population, Refugees, and Migration (PRM), US Department of State, sets a goal of 30 days from arrival for linkage with a health care provider. The Office of Refugee Resettlement (ORR), part of the Administration for Children and Families, Department of Health and Human Services, is the federal agency responsible for providing resettlement and placement services. ORR requires medical services be arranged for by the local resettlement agency within 90 days of arrival as a condition of funding the agency.

There is no single model for domestic health assessments of refugees. Refugee resettlement agencies often serve a crucial facilitative role in helping the refugee enter the system very quickly after arrival in the United States. States may contract with a network of community providers. In most cases, state programs utilize clinics at county and local health departments or private, not-for-profit clinics such as those at federally qualified community health centers and academic medical centers. A more limited number of states rely on a mix of funding streams, including the above federal sources as well as state funds.

Each states' system for domestic screening usually depends on the funding stream utilized to support it. Funding for the domestic refugee exam comes from different sources [5]. ORR provides refugee medical assistance (RMA) and other public health discretionary grants that may also be used to support medical screening and preventive services. By regulation, all refugees are eligible for cash and medical assistance (Medicaid) for up to 8 months after arrival in the United States. For those not categorically eligible for Medicaid, the RMA funding stream supports their coverage. Some states rely on their Medicaid programs to reimburse medical practitioners who perform the domestic health assessment. Other states, through agreements negotiated with ORR, will instead use RMA funding to reimburse directly for all components of their domestic health screening program through special programs administered by their public health departments. The Affordable Care Act (ACA) may enable more refugees to be eligible for Medicaid or refugees may be able to purchase an affordable insurance plan in the new health care marketplace.

Components of Domestic Medical Exam

During the domestic medical exam, all overseas documentation should be reviewed. It can provide corroborative data on the refugee's health status. It also contains information on screening tests, immunizations, and prophylactic treatment.

History

It should be made clear to the refugee that the process of history and physical examination is for the benefit of the refugee's health. In addition, it is important to educate the refugee that the health assessment will start them on the process of meeting immunization requirements for school enrollment, adjustment of legal status (i.e., applying for legal permanent residence, a.k.a. a "green card"), and some employment. It is important that the refugee understand that the assessment is otherwise unrelated to the immigration legal process and no one will be returned to their home country because of diagnosis or treatment of a medical condition.

As in any new patient evaluation, a detailed history should include any current symptoms, currently active medical conditions, past medical problems, surgeries, medications, allergies, and family history of heritable conditions. Current symptoms may indicate underlying infectious disease such as tuberculosis or malaria. Specific examples of symptoms are fever, weight loss, night sweats, pulmonary complaints, abdominal pain, diarrhea, and skin lesions. Sexual history should be obtained in a culturally sensitive manner to screen for risk of sexually transmitted diseases (STDs), although historically the prevalence of STDs in refugees is quite low [6].

The initial visit also serves as an important opportunity to begin to address chronic conditions such as diabetes, hypertension, and somatic complaints such as low back pain and headache that have not been treated before or, if treated, may not have received proper evaluation and ongoing care. Accurate past medical history may be difficult to obtain as the notion of what conditions are considered significant can vary in refugee populations when compared to western norms; therefore, specific questions on hospitalizations, medications, and other forms of treatments should be asked. Medication history should include use of traditional herbal substances that may contain toxic ingredients such as lead and arsenic. This is particularly relevant for refugee children who have a substantially increased prevalence of elevated blood lead levels compared to US-born children [7]. Vaccination history should be obtained, though this is often not useful in adults who typically do not have records of their childhood vaccinations. Only valid, written documentation of vaccines that adhere to US or World Health Organization schedules should be accepted. Anecdotal reports of diseases (particularly measles) or immunizations should not be considered valid proof of immunity to vaccine-preventable diseases, with the exception of chicken pox.

The social history is usually more detailed for refugees. Their travel and asylum history should be reviewed as many refugees have passed through at least one intermediate country in their journey from their country of origin to the United States. Where a refugee has lived and what they experienced along the way may be the most important predictors of their health status. Some refugees have lived for many years in a country of temporary asylum before permanent resettlement. This information helps assess for environmental exposures, nutritional deficiencies due to living in refugee camps, and occupational risks in addition to physical and mental trauma including torture and other exposure to violence. Also, the refugee's recent history of multiple upheavals and losses can provide clues to psychological problems. Appropriate ways to assess for trauma and torture are provided in Chap. 14.

The refugee's current social situation is very important for assessing the risk of psychological problems arising from resettlement stressors. Educational level, work history, language fluency, current support network, family structure, and employment potential are all factors in determining risk of poor adjustment to a new society.

Lastly, the substance use history should include, in addition to tobacco and alcohol, the use of traditional recreational substances such as betel nut (used in Asia) and khat (used in Africa) that can have unrecognized toxic potential.

Physical Examination

As in any new patient evaluation, a complete and thorough physical exam should be performed on all refugees. Whenever possible, requests for examiners of the same gender should be honored. As with the history, the purpose of the exam should be explained at the outset. For many refugees, this may be the first time a complete physical exam is being done. It is not uncommon to detect previously undiagnosed hypertension in a refugee on the initial medical visit. The exam should include screening for vision, hearing, and oral and dental abnormalities. Previously undiagnosed abnormalities in these areas are common in newly arrived refugees, and oral health problems, in particular, are among the most prevalent diagnoses in refugee health screening [8, 9]. An external genital exam can offer important information on practices such as female genital cutting; however, in most instances, it may not be appropriate at the initial screening visit. This is especially true when the patient has a history of sexual abuse or such examination violates cultural norms of gender interaction and religion. In some cultures, genital and pelvic examinations of young unmarried women are considered inappropriate, and in these cases, their wishes should be respected. Many men and women from other cultures also will prefer having a clinician from the same gender to perform genital examinations. (Screening for STDs and HIV can be accomplished without genital examination through the use of urine-amplified DNA probes for gonorrhea and chlamydia, serum testing for syphilis, and salivary or serum testing for HIV.)

Skin exam is important to identify both localized and systemic diseases as well as evidence of physical trauma. It can also reveal traditional healing techniques, such as burns, cutting, and coining that may indicate past disease. Cardiac auscultation may reveal undiagnosed congenital heart disease or rheumatic heart disease that is more common in developing countries. Other important components of the exam are a careful respiratory examination, an abdominal examination for assessment of hepatic and splenic enlargement, a musculoskeletal exam for assessment of physical trauma and injuries, and a full lymph node exam. An assessment of the patient's mental status may indicate a need for further psychiatric evaluation.

A complete history and physical examination can identify important acute and chronic health issues that may need to be addressed or triaged at the initial medical visit. When performed thoroughly and with cultural competence, it can engender the development of trust and comfort with the provider and the local health care delivery services. Development of trust is perhaps the most important role of the health assessment.

Laboratory Tests

A complete blood count (CBC) with five-cell differential is recommended for all refugees. The prevalence of anemia is high among refugee populations [10] and can result from multiple etiologies, but usually nutritional. Iron deficiency is often the cause of microcytic anemia, which can also be from chronic blood loss due to hookworm infection and gastric ulcers. Some recent refugee populations appear to have a somewhat high prevalence of *Helicobacter pylori* infection that can lead to ulcer formation and blood loss. Other nutritional deficiencies such as vitamin B12 can also be the cause for macrocytic anemia and has been frequently noted in Bhutanese refugees [11]. It is important to recognize, however, that B12 deficiency can cause important neuropsychiatric and other symptoms without evidence of macrocytosis or anemia [12]. Thalassemias may also cause anemia and are seen more frequently in recent refugee arrivals from South Asia and the Middle East [13]. When patients have an alpha or beta thalassemia trait, they have no active symptoms and a mild microcytic anemia detected on the CBC is the only clinical sign. A very low mean corpuscular volume (microcytosis) in the setting of high absolute number of red blood cells and normal red cell distribution width (RDW) is strongly associated with thalassemia traits. In contrast, an elevated RDW may still suggest concurrent iron deficiency. Sickle cell anemia and trait is seen in people of African origin, and hemoglobin E disease is seen in parts of South Asia and the Middle East [14]. Glucose-6-phosphate-dehydrogenase deficiency, which is commonly seen in

Southeast Asians [13], is of particular importance in refugees as certain oxidizing medications used for malaria such as primaquine can lead to hemolysis.

Thrombocytopenia can be seen in conditions that cause hypersplenism in malaria or schistosomiasis, both of which are more endemic in Sub-Saharan Africa [15]. Isolated hypersplenism in an otherwise asymptomatic patient from Sub-Saharan Africa is suggestive of tropical splenomegaly syndrome due to chronic infection with falciparum malaria. Clinicians should have a high suspicion for current or recent infection in a newly arrived refugee with eosinophilia, though other causes also have to be considered.

A urinalysis can be used to screen for hematuria caused by *Schistosoma haematobium*, which is prevalent in refugees from Sub-Saharan Africa [15]. It is also useful for picking up undiagnosed glucosuria and proteinuria.

There is no evidence for cost-effectiveness of routine testing of serum chemistries, mainly glucose, transaminases, blood urea nitrogen, and creatinine. However, providers may consider ordering these tests to facilitate the transition to primary care for refugees with evidence of renal or hepatic abnormalities. As noted, liver or renal disease may rarely be indicative of chronic parasitic infections, malaria, or extrapulmonary tuberculosis. Renal disease can also detect complications of diabetes and hypertension in refugees with these conditions. In addition, a hemoglobin A1c level may be appropriate for helping to triage a refugee with known or newly diagnosed diabetes.

Research has documented high prevalence of nutritional deficiencies in refugees. Recent concerns have centered around vitamins B12 (in Nepali Bhutanese) [11] and D (in all refugee populations) [16]. Clinicians should consider a test for B12 level in Bhutanese or other refugees with macrocytosis or symptoms suggestive of deficiency. For vitamin D, all refugees should be started on repletion treatment for 8–12 weeks, after which a level may be checked.

Cardiovascular risk assessment by screening for diabetes and hyperlipidemia and cancer screening is recommended according to the US preventive task force guidelines. Higher suspicion should be maintained for malignancies that are more common in developing countries such as esophageal and liver cancers. Preventive screening does not have to be done at the initial visit for all refugees, but the screening visit can be used as a starting point for this discussion, especially if the refugee's source of future health care is uncertain.

Pregnancy testing should be done for all reproductive-age females especially prior to administration of live viral vaccines and if any pharmacological treatment is planned. While pregnancy testing is not mandatory for vaccinating females of child-bearing years, most adult medical practitioners would prefer to have a documented test. Given the importance of these vaccines, as demonstrated by the case of congenital rubella in an African refugee born in New Hampshire, pregnancy testing should be encouraged if it facilitates immunization of young women [17].

Other important screening includes testing for hepatitis B surface antigen and antibodies as well as tuberculosis. Screening for these as well as HIV and other sexually transmitted diseases, intestinal parasitic infections, immunity to vaccine-preventable diseases, and lead testing in children are discussed in later chapters.

Table 3.1 provides a summary of screening recommendations.

Table 3.1 Screening examination

History
Review predeparture information
Obtain information on past and current social circumstances
Focus on symptoms indicating highly prevalent infectious diseases
Screen for mental health problems
Ask about use of herbal medicine and traditional treatments
Physical exam
Routine exam including vital signs
Pay special attention to hepatosplenomegaly, lymph node enlargement, skin lesions, past genital procedures, and dental and vision exam
Laboratory evaluation
CBC with five-cell differential
Interferon gamma assay or tuberculin skin testing
Hepatitis B serologies
HIV 1 and 2 antibodies
Lead in children
Vaccine titers
Stool parasite testing as indicated
Urine chlamydia and gonorrhea
Optional tests based on risk factors
Urinalysis
Vitamin B12
Vitamin D
Hepatitis C antibody
Complete metabolic profile
HbA1c
Fasting lipid profile

References

1. Centers for Disease Control. http://www.cdc.gov/immigrantrefugeehealth/guidelines/domestic/domestic-guidelines.html
2. U.S. Citizenship and Immigration Services. http://www.uscis.gov/portal/site/uscis/menuitem.f6da51a2342135be7e9d7a10e0dc91a0/?vgnextoid=fa7e539dc4bed010VgnVCM1000000ecd190aRCRD&vgnextchannel=fa7e539dc4bed010VgnVCM1000000ecd190aRCRD&CH=act
3. Centers for Disease Control. http://www.cdc.gov/immigrantrefugeehealth/laws-regulations.html
4. Centers for Disease Control. http://www.cdc.gov/immigrantrefugeehealth/guidelines/overseas/interventions.html
5. Geltman PL, Cochran J. A private-sector preferred provider network model for public health screening of newly resettled refugees. Am J Public Health. 2005;95(2):196–9.
6. Stauffer WM, Painter J, Mamo B, et al. Sexually transmitted infections in newly arrived refugees: is routine screening for *Neisseria gonorrhoeae* and *Chlamydia trachomatis* infection indicated? Am J Trop Med Hyg. 2012;86(2):292–5.
7. Geltman PL, Brown MJ, Cochran J. Lead poisoning among refugee children resettled in Massachusetts, 1995 to 1999. Pediatrics. 2001;108(1):158–62.

8. Yun K, Hebrank K, Graber LK, et al. High prevalence of chronic non-communicable conditions among adult refugees: implications for practice and policy. J Community Health. 2012;37(5): 1110–8. doi:10.1007/s10900-012-9552-1.
9. Cote S, Geltman P, Nunn M, et al. Dental caries of refugee children compared with US children. Pediatrics. 2004;114:e733–40.
10. Geltman PL, Dookeran NM, Battaglia T, et al. Chronic disease and its risk factors among refugees and asylees in Massachusetts, 2001–2005. Prev Chronic Dis. 2010;7(3):A51. Epub 2010 Apr 15.
11. Centers for Disease Control and Prevention. Vitamin B12 deficiency in resettled Bhutanese refugees-United States, 2008–2011. MMWR Morb Mortal Wkly Rep. 2011;60(11):343–6.
12. Lindenbaum J, Healton EB, Savage DG, et al. Neuropsychiatric disorders caused by cobalamin deficiency in the absence of anemia or macrocytosis. N Engl J Med. 1988;318(26):1720–8.
13. Jeng MR, Vichinsky E. Hematologic problems in immigrants from Southeast Asia. Hematol Oncol Clin North Am. 2004;18:1405–22.
14. Theodorsson E, Birgens H, Hagve TA. Haemoglobinopathies and glucose-6-phosphate dehydrogenase deficiency in a Scandinavian perspective. Scand J Clin Lab Invest. 2007;67:3–10.
15. Posey DL, Blackburn BG, Weinberg M, et al. High prevalence and presumptive treatment of schistosomiasis and strongyloidiasis among African refugees. Clin Infect Dis. 2007;45(10): 1210–5.
16. Penrose K, Hunter Adams J, Nguyen T, et al. Vitamin D deficiency among newly resettled refugees in Massachusetts. J Immigr Minor Health. 2012;14(6):941–8.
17. Plotinsky RN, Talbot EA, Kellenberg JE, et al. Congenital rubella syndrome in a child born to Liberian refugees: clinical and public health perspectives. Clin Pediatr (Phila). 2007;46(4): 349–55.

Part II
Primary Care

Chapter 4
Immunizations and Refugees

Erika Schumacher

Introduction

Access to immunization against vaccine-preventable disease is a prime determinant of the health of refugee populations. It is the role of clinicians conducting the refugee domestic health assessment to accurately interpret vaccine histories and to "… prevent the importation of infectious diseases and other conditions of public health significance into the US…" [1]. Thus, the challenge of determining when and whom to vaccinate goes hand-in-hand with the need to identify individuals who are carriers of vaccine-preventable disease.

Refugees are one of the few groups of immigrants to USA who are not required to have any vaccinations prior to arrival. Refugees are infrequently up-to-date with age appropriate vaccinations as recommended by Advisory Committee on Immunization Practices (ACIP) [2]. Thanks to the efforts of the World Health Organization (WHO) Extended Program on Immunization, many more children over the last 30 years have received a full series of measles, diphtheria, pertussis, tetanus, polio, and Bacillus Calmette–Guerin vaccine than their elders [3]. Mumps, rubella, varicella, *Haemophilus influenzae*, and *Streptococcus pneumoniae* are not included in the program, thus most refugees arriving from developing countries will not be immune to these entities unless they have contracted the disease itself (families of higher socioeconomic status and those from certain states in the Middle East or elsewhere such as Cuba may be exceptions, depending on their access to more developed systems of health care).

It is mandated that at the time of applying for adjustment of status from legal temporary resident to legal permanent resident (1 year or more after arrival), a refugee must be fully vaccinated in accordance with recommendations of the ACIP. For a refugee, the adjustment of status application includes Form I-693, which includes

E. Schumacher, M.D., F.A.A.P. (✉)
Pediatrics, Yale University, 333 Cedar Street, New Haven, CT 06510, USA
e-mail: erika.schumacher@yale.edu

A. Annamalai (ed.), *Refugee Health Care: An Essential Medical Guide*,
DOI 10.1007/978-1-4939-0271-2_4, © Springer Science+Business Media New York 2014

the vaccination assessment performed by a civil surgeon or designated health department in the USA. Information about the requirements for successful "green card" application can be found here: http://www.cdc.gov/immigrantrefugeehealth/exams/ti/civil/vaccination-civil-technical-instructions.html.

Approach to Determining Immunity and Need for Vaccination

Vaccine records are reviewed and documented in the pre-departure health assessment overseas, although families often bring records from their native or host country or camp as well. Vaccination histories should generally be considered valid if immunizations were received in a manner that corresponds to the intervals and age restrictions of the current ACIP schedule. Written records only should be considered, although verbal reports should be acknowledged by the domestic practitioner and addressed with serologic testing as appropriate (discussed below). It should be noted that vaccines administered outside the US are often delivered with alternate components and labeled with unfamiliar nomenclature. Clinicians should make use of resources located on the CDC website (http://www.cdc.gov/immigrantrefugeehealth/guidelines/domestic/immunizations-guidelines.html) and local interpreter services to help translate records as accurately and thoroughly as possible. There are several other online resources to help decode such records, the best of which come from the Immunization Action Coalition (http://www.immunize.org), a nonprofit organization funded in part by the CDC [4].

For some pediatricians, this approach of accepting written records as valid may conflict with long-promoted recommendations in the field of adoption medicine to ignore international immunization records and "start from scratch." Children adopted from orphanages, especially through for-profit channels, are theoretically at higher risk than other immigrant groups for forged immunization records or inaccurate record-keeping, in an attempt to facilitate the adoption process. Regardless, in refugee medicine it is always true that a healthy dose of skepticism—and a frank conversation with parents—about the validity of the vaccine record is warranted in every case. Despite the standard channels through which refugee families receive their overseas medical evaluation (by a physician selected and monitored by the US Department of State), occasionally, pre-departure immunization records are compiled through verbal or other invalid sources and supported by insufficient written documentation.

Once vaccine records have been interpreted, it is worth keeping in mind that adults and children alike can still be susceptible to vaccine-preventable disease at the time of arrival on foreign shores because of a combination of under-immunization, failed immunization, or waning immunity. Failed immunization results either from disruption of the "cold chain" of vaccine transportation and storage at controlled temperatures, improper administration of vaccine, or inappropriate dosing intervals which preclude proper immune response. Waning immunity is a large problem in adults, but also affects children who have been subject to years of malnutrition and comorbid disease. Also, we are learning more about the natural history of vaccine-induced immunity, which is shorter-lived than previously thought in the case of many common diseases such as hepatitis B [5] and mumps [6].

Laboratory assessment of relevant antibody levels is always a safe approach to determining vaccine catch-up schedules when vaccine records are incomplete or immunity is questioned. This approach should be considered especially when families insist on a history of vaccination for which they do not have medical documentation. A cost–benefit analysis should be undertaken before deciding if drawing titers is the more appropriate course of action as compared to restarting the vaccine series, taking into account direct costs to the medical system, the number of follow-up visits required for each approach, and the likelihood of patient return to clinic for appropriate follow-up. The author encourages every institution to perform such a cost analysis for each age group of refugee patients treated. The Office of Refugee Resettlement (ORR) does publish some data on the subject, which can be found under "CPT Codes for Refugee Medical Assistance" at http://www.acf.hhs.gov/programs/orr/resource/medical-screening-protocol-for-newly-arriving-refugees [7]. Guidance from CDC on vaccination versus serologic testing for diseases can be found at www.cdc.gov/mmwr/preview/mmwrhtml/rr5515a1.htm#tab12.

The CDC is in the process of developing a useful tool entitled "Refugee Health Profiles," found on their Immigrant and Refugee Health site (http://www.cdc.gov/immigrantrefugeehealth/). The profiles are compiled with information gathered by the WHO, International Organization for Migration (IOM), the Office of the United Nations High Commission for Refugees (UNHCR), US Department of State, and other sources, in order to guide domestic health assessors with population-specific data. The epidemiologic information provided on the topic of vaccine-preventable disease can serve as an excellent point of reference for clinicians during the process of evaluating overseas immunization records and determining appropriate screening. Refugee camp-specific data, while helpful, are generally difficult to track down for the average clinician, although the CDC provides some data here: http://www.cdc.gov/immigrantrefugeehealth/pdf/immunizations-schedule-us-bound-refugees.pdf.

Other Considerations

It is important for clinicians to be aware of state vaccination requirements for entrance into public school. If titers are checked, those values must be provided to the school. The patient may be denied entrance until one dose of each vaccine has been given or immunity demonstrated. The desire to get refugee children into school must be weighed with the natural tendency to limit the number of vaccines given during any single visit, although there is no set maximum number of injections per visit.

Absolute and relative contraindications to routine immunizations need to be reviewed prior to vaccination and can be found on the Immunization Action Coalition website at http://www.immunize.org/catg.d/p3072a.pdf. The following conditions are not contraindications for the administration of a vaccine: mild to

Table 4.1 Summary of immunization recommendations for refugees

	Recommended approach if no documentation of prior vaccination	Adults	Children
Measles, mumps, rubella	Vaccinate or serotest	At least one dose	Two dose series
Diphtheria, pertussis, tetanus	Vaccinate	One dose *TdaP* followed by two doses Td	Age appropriate DTaP/Tdap series
Polio	Vaccinate or serotest	Three dose series	Three dose series
Varicella	Serotest	Two dose series	Two dose series
Hepatitis B	Serotest if from intermediate or highly endemic area, vaccinate otherwise	Three dose series	Three dose series
Hepatitis A	Serotest	Two dose series	Two dose series
HPV	Vaccinate	Two dose series <26 years of age	Two dose series >11 years of age
Meningococcus	Vaccinate with MCV4	Only if medically indicated	Two dose series 11–18 years of age
Influenza	Vaccinate	Yearly	Yearly >6 months

moderate local reactions to a previous dose of vaccine, mild acute illness (e.g., upper respiratory infection, diarrhea, fever), breastfeeding, antimicrobial therapy, or coincident tuberculin skin testing [8]. Pregnancy is not a contraindication to the administration of Td/Tdap, inactivated influenza, or hepatitis B vaccine.

Vaccine Information Sheets (VIS) are required to be provided to all patients receiving vaccines, in their own language if at all possible. VIS sheets can be found in over 40 different languages on the Immunization Action Coalition Website.

Specific vaccine preventable diseases are discussed below. See also Table 4.1 for an overview of recommendations. It is critically important that providers understand the intricacies of the CDC vaccine catch-up schedule, as reprinted in Appendix B.

Measles, Mumps, and Rubella

Data show that the MMR vaccine is highly effective against both measles (100 % protection after two doses) and rubella (more than 95 % protection after single dose), with antibodies persisting for at least 15 years [9]. The effectiveness of the mumps vaccine is significantly inferior and may depend on the vaccine strain used and time since vaccination; as evidenced by the 2009 mumps outbreak in the northeastern US, effectiveness of the mumps vaccine is estimated to be as low as 64 % after one dose and 79 % after two doses [10].

There is lack of data on cost–benefit of vaccination versus serologic testing for measles, mumps, and rubella. Seroprevalence studies routinely show that a large proportion (15–25 %) of migrant adults is susceptible to rubella [11]. A 2002 study looking at seroprevalence of antibodies to measles and rubella in newly arrived refugee children aged 0–20 showed that only 82 % had antibodies to measles and 82 % to rubella [12]. Immigrant and refugee families account for the majority of cases of congenital rubella syndrome in North America [13].

It is recommended that adult refugees born after 1957 without clear documentation or evidence of immunization receive at least one dose of MMR [14]. All women of childbearing age should be assessed for immunity to rubella, and immunized appropriately. Children should receive a two-dose series of MMR in accordance with the ACIP-recommended schedule, with one dose administered between 12 and 15 months and the second between 4 and 6 years. Catch-up dosing should be performed on all school-aged and teenage children, allowing for a minimum 4-week interval between the first and second dose.

MMR and other live-virus vaccines should be avoided in those with known severe immunodeficiency or those who are pregnant. Importantly, since January 4, 2010 refugees and immigrants are no longer tested for HIV before entry to the US. Therefore it is highly encouraged that practitioners complete HIV testing prior to administering any live-virus vaccines during the post-arrival health assessment. Also, MMR vaccine and the Tuberculin Skin Test (TST) must be administered simultaneously OR 4 weeks apart, given theoretical suppression of tuberculin reactivity by the measles vaccination temporarily. Thus, as patients may have been administered an MMR vaccine close to their departure date, especially when arriving from Kenya, Thailand, and Malaysia, vigilance is required.

Tetanus, Diphtheria, and Acellular Pertussis

Compared with the MMR vaccine, there is a relative paucity of data on the seroprevalence of tetanus, diphtheria, and pertussis in refugee populations in North America. It is well documented, however, that even in individuals properly vaccinated with a primary series of tetanus and diphtheria, immunity wanes significantly with time (although antibodies to tetanus persist longer than those to diphtheria after the primary series; 25 versus 10 years, respectively) [15]. Data suggest that a single booster of both at age 65 years does not confer sufficient immunity in older individuals [15].

The ACIP recommends administration of a primary series of diphtheria and tetanus toxoids and acellular pertussis vaccine in the first year of life, followed by doses of these vaccines at 15–18 months of age and 4–6 years of age. A booster of adult-formulation diphtheria and tetanus toxoids should be administered beginning at 11 years of age and every 10 years thereafter. It is recommended that adult refugees without documentation of prior vaccination receive a primary dose of tetanus-diphtheria-pertussis (Tdap), followed by two doses of tetanus-diphtheria (Td) [2], and pediatric patients be caught up per the standard catch-up schedule.

Laboratory evidence of immunity to tetanus, diphtheria, or pertussis is *not* considered as meeting criteria for successful completion of a Form I-693, for those persons

seeking adjustment of status to permanent resident status in USA (http://www.cdc.
gov/immigrantrefugeehealth/exams/ti/civil/vaccination-civil-technical-instructions.
html#assessment) [8]. It is, thus, recommended that all patients without proper documentation are vaccinated upon arrival.

It may be noted that the CDC schedule for tetanus, diphtheria, and pertussis immunization has a gap in guidance regarding tetanus, diphtheria, and pertussis immunization between the ages of 7–10 years, as the two TdaP products Boostrix and Adacel
are licensed for age >10 years and 11–64 years respectively. The ACIP endorses use
of adult formulation of tetanus–diphtheria–pertussis vaccine followed by two doses
of tetanus–diphtheria vaccine for those children in the 7–10 age group who need a
primary or secondary series of vaccine. It should also be noted that Pentacel (DTaP-
IPV-HiB) can be used for the primary series in children <5 years of age, while
Pediarix (DTaP-IPV-HepB) can be used for the primary series in children <7 years of
age. Kinrix (DTaP-IPV) should only be used as the 4–6-year-old booster dose.

TdaP should be routinely administered to pregnant women during each pregnancy.

Polio

Seroprevalence studies in North American refugees are also lacking for polio. It is
reasonable to check polio titers prior to administering a three-dose series of Inactivated
Polio Vaccine (IPV), as is recommended for all refugees, including adults, without
laboratory evidence of immunity or record of vaccination. IPV should be administered
to children at 2, 4, and 6 months of age as per the ACIP, with a final dose administered
on or after the fourth birthday, with a catch-up schedule as per Appendix B. IPV is
contraindicated during pregnancy.

Hepatitis B

Since 2008, the CDC recommends testing for hepatitis B surface antigen (HbsAg)
for persons born in geographic regions with HBsAg prevalence of ≥2 % and
US-born persons not vaccinated as infants whose parents were born in geographic
regions with HBsAg prevalence of ≥8 % [16]. A map showing geographic distribution of chronic Hepatitis B infection can be found on the CDC website (http://
wwwnc.cdc.gov/travel/yellowbook/2012/chapter-3-infectious-diseases-related-to-
travel/hepatitis-b.htm) and is reproduced in Chap. 7.

In a meta-analysis published in 2012, a review of 110 studies representing more
than 209,000 migrant patients in the US showed a prevalence of hepatitis B infection of 7.2 %, and prior immunity from any cause in 39.7 % [17]. Migrants from
East Asia and sub-Saharan Africa were at highest risk for infection, and those from
Eastern Europe were found to be at medium risk [17].

Table 4.2 Interpretation of Hepatitis B serologic test results

HBsAg	Negative	Susceptible
Anti-HBc	Negative	
Anti-HBs	Negative	
HBsAg	Negative	Immune due to natural infection
Anti-HBc	Positive	
Anti-HBs	Positive	
HBsAg	Negative	Immune due to hepatitis B vaccination
Anti-HBc	Negative	
Anti-HBs	Positive	
HBsAg	Positive	Acutely infected
Anti-HBc	Positive	
IgM anti-HBc	Positive	
Anti-HBs	Negative	
HBsAg	Positive	Chronically infected
Anti-HBc	Positive	
IgM anti-HBc	Negative	
Anti-HBs	Negative	
HBsAg	Negative	Interpretation unclear; four possibilities:
Anti-HBc	Positive	1. Resolved infection (most common)
Anti-HBs	Negative	2. False-positive anti-HBc, thus susceptible
		3. "Low level" chronic infection
		4. Resolving acute infection

Source: CDC. Division of viral Hepatitis. Available at http://www.cdc.gov/hepatitis/hbv/pdfs/serologicchartv8.pdf [18]

The current ACIP recommendation is to vaccinate any individual without natural or immunization-induced immunity according to the ACIP schedule. Serologies should be interpreted as shown in Table 4.2 (see also Chap. 7). Of note, vaccine-induced immunity to hepatitis B wanes by adolescence, and thus, refugee teenagers who present for domestic health screening may not have a positive HBsAb despite completion of a full hepatitis B immunization series.

Varicella

Varicella immunization is not included in the WHO Extended Program on Immunization. For those refugees arriving from tropical areas of the world where Varicella strikes at a later age, it is also unlikely that younger individuals are immune to varicella through primary infection [19, 20]. Given the greater risk of severe, complicated disease in older individuals and pregnant women, proper screening and vaccine administration for nonimmune individuals is critical.

Varicella seroprevalence studies have demonstrated up to 50 % susceptibility rate for teenage refugees from tropical countries, and up to 10–15 % susceptibility in individuals aged 30–35 years [15]. In a study of 200 Somali refugees in Minnesota, 48 % of children less than 10 years were seronegative for varicella, and 6 % of women childbearing age (12–49) were seronegative [21]. Cost-effectiveness studies have concluded that performing serologies for varicella on all newly arrived refugees is cost-saving when compared with universal vaccination with a two-dose series, possibly with the exception of children under age 5 years [21, 22]. It is important to note that commercially available enzyme immunoassay tests are generally >95 % specific for varicella, although only 60–92 % sensitive in detecting antibodies after natural infection and even less so for vaccine-induced infection [23].

As per the CDC schedule found in the Appendices, two doses of varicella-containing vaccine are recommended for all people aged ≥12 months without evidence of immunity who do not have contraindications to the vaccine. The first dose should be administered at age 12–15 months and the second dose at 4–6 years of age. A second catch-up dose of varicella vaccination is recommended for children, adolescents, and adults who have received only one dose. The minimum interval between doses for children <13 years is 3 months, and those aged ≥13 years can be vaccinated after an interval of 4 weeks.

Varicella vaccine contains live, attenuated virus. Contraindications to vaccination with the varicella vaccine include pregnancy or intended pregnancy within 1 month of receiving the vaccine, active tuberculosis or other severe disease, and impaired cellular immune function. Those receiving low-dose prednisone (<2 mg/kg of body weight per day or <20 mg/day), those whose immunosuppressive therapy with steroids has been discontinued for 1 month and/or chemotherapy for 3 months, and those with impaired humoral immunity may be vaccinated. The ACIP recommends considering varicella vaccine for HIV-infected children aged ≥12 months who have CD4+ T-lymphocyte percentages of ≥15 %, and for HIV-infected older children and adults with CD4+ T-lymphocyte count ≥200 cells/mL [2].

Other

All other ACIP-recommended vaccinations, including hepatitis A, *Haemophilus influenzae* type b, Pneumococcus, human papillomavirus (HPV), and meningococcus, should be administered according to the standard schedule. The 2009 revision to the Technical Manual for Civil Surgeons saw several changes to the requirements for successful completion of the Form I-693, Vaccination Record. HPV and zoster are no longer required vaccinations, tetravalent meningococcal conjugate vaccine is required for all persons 11–18 years of age, and influenza vaccine is required for applicants 6 months through 18 years, as well as applicants 50 years of age and older [8].

Appendix A

Figure 1. Recommended immunization schedule for persons aged 0 through 18 years – 2013.
(FOR THOSE WHO FALL BEHIND OR START LATE, SEE THE CATCH-UP SCHEDULE [FIGURE 2]).

These recommendations must be read with the footnotes that follow. For those who fall behind or start late, provide catch-up vaccination at the earliest opportunity as indicated by the green bars in Figure 1. To determine minimum intervals between doses, see the catch-up schedule (Figure 2). School entry and adolescent vaccine age groups are in bold.

Vaccines	Birth	1 mo	2 mos	4 mos	6 mos	9 mos	12 mos	15 mos	18 mos	19–23 mos	2–3 yrs	4–6 yrs	7–10 yrs	11–12 yrs	13–15 yrs	16–18 yrs
Hepatitis B[1] (HepB)	←1st dose→	←—2nd dose—→			←——————————————— 3rd dose ———————————————→											
Rotavirus[2] (RV) RV-1 (2-dose series); RV-5 (3-dose series)			←1st dose→	←2nd dose→	See footnote 2											
Diphtheria, tetanus, & acellular pertussis[3] (DTaP: <7 yrs)			←1st dose→	←2nd dose→	←3rd dose→		←———— 4th dose ————→				←5th dose→				
Tetanus, diphtheria, & acellular pertussis[4] (Tdap: ≥7 yrs)														(Tdap)		
Haemophilus influenzae type b[5] (Hib)			←1st dose→	←2nd dose→	See footnote 5		←——— 3rd or 4th dose, see footnote 5 ———→									
Pneumococcal conjugate[6,6c] (PCV13)			←1st dose→	←2nd dose→	←3rd dose→		←———— 4th dose ————→									
Pneumococcal polysaccharide[6a,6c] (PPSV23)																
Inactivated Poliovirus[7] (IPV) (<18years)			←1st dose→	←2nd dose→	←——————————————— 3rd dose ———————————————→							←4th dose→				
Influenza[8] (IIV; LAIV) 2 doses for some: see footnote 8					Annual vaccination (IIV only)						Annual vaccination (IIV or LAIV)					
Measles, mumps, rubella[9] (MMR)							←——— 1st dose ———→					←2nd dose→				
Varicella[10] (VAR)							←——— 1st dose ———→					←2nd dose→				
Hepatitis A[11] (HepA)							←—— 2-dose series, see footnote 11 ——→									
Human papillomavirus[12] (HPV2: females only; HPV4: males and females)														(3-dose series)		
Meningococcal[13] (Hib-MenCY ≥ 6 weeks; MCV4-D≥9 mos; MCV4-CRM ≥ 2 yrs.)						see footnote 13								←1st dose→		booster

Range of recommended ages for all children	Range of recommended ages for catch-up immunization	Range of recommended ages for certain high-risk groups	Range of recommended ages during which catch-up is encouraged and for certain high-risk groups	Not routinely recommended

This schedule includes recommendations in effect as of January 1, 2013. Any dose not administered at the recommended age should be administered at a subsequent visit, when indicated and feasible. The use of a combination vaccine generally is preferred over separate injections of its equivalent component vaccines. Vaccination providers should consult the relevant Advisory Committee on Immunization Practices (ACIP) statement for detailed recommendations, available online at http://www.cdc.gov/vaccines/pubs/acip-list.htm. Clinically significant adverse events that follow vaccination should be reported to the Vaccine Adverse Event Reporting System (VAERS) online (http://www.vaers.hhs.gov) or by telephone (800-822-7967).Suspected cases of vaccine-preventable diseases should be reported to the state or local health department. Additional information, including precautions and contraindications for vaccination, is available from CDC online (http://www.cdc.gov/vaccines) or by telephone (800-CDC-INFO (800-232-4636)).

Appendix A (continued)

This schedule is approved by the Advisory Committee on Immunization Practices (http://www.cdc.gov/vaccines/acip/index.html), the American Academy of Pediatrics (http://www.aap.org), the American Academy of Family Physicians (http://www.aafp.org), and the American College of Obstetricians and Gynecologists (http://www.acog.org).

NOTE: The above recommendations must be read along with the footnotes of this schedule.

Footnotes — Recommended immunization schedule for persons aged 0 through 18 years—United States, 2013

For further guidance on the use of the vaccines mentioned below, see: http://www.cdc.gov/vaccines/pubs/acip-list.htm.

1. **Hepatitis B (HepB) vaccine. (Minimum age: birth)**
   Routine vaccination:
   At birth
   • Administer monovalent HepB vaccine to all newborns before hospital discharge.
   • For infants born to hepatitis B surface antigen (HBsAg)–positive mothers, administer HepB vaccine and 0.5 mL of hepatitis B immune globulin (HBIG) within 12 hours of birth. These infants should be tested for HBsAg and antibody to HBsAg (anti-HBs) 1 to 2 months after completion of the HepB series, at age 9 through 18 months (preferably at the next well-child visit).
   • If mother's HBsAg status is unknown, within 12 hours of birth administer HepB vaccine to all infants regardless of birth weight. For infants weighing <2,000 grams, administer HBIG in addition to HepB within 12 hours of birth. Determine mother's HBsAg status as soon as possible and, if she is HBsAg-positive, also administer HBIG for infants weighing ≥2,000 grams (no later than age 1 week).
   Doses following the birth dose
   • The second dose should be administered at age 1 or 2 months. Monovalent HepB vaccine should be used for doses administered before age 6 weeks.
   • Infants who did not receive a birth dose should receive 3 doses of a HepB-containing vaccine on a schedule of 0, 1 to 2 months, and 6 months starting as soon as feasible. See Figure 2.
   • The minimum interval between dose 1 and dose 2 is 4 weeks and between dose 2 and 3 is 8 weeks. The final (third or fourth) dose in the HepB vaccine series should be administered no earlier than age 24 weeks, and at least 16 weeks after the first dose.
   • Administration of a total of 4 doses of HepB vaccine is recommended when a combination vaccine containing HepB is administered after the birth dose.
   Catch-up vaccination:
   • Unvaccinated persons should complete a 3-dose series.
   • A 2-dose series (doses separated by at least 4 months) of adult formulation Recombivax HB is licensed for use in children aged 11 through 15 years.
   • For other catch-up issues, see Figure 2.

2. **Rotavirus (RV) vaccines. (Minimum age: 6 weeks for both RV-1 [Rotarix] and RV-5 [RotaTeq]).**
   Routine vaccination:
   • Administer a series of RV vaccine to all infants as follows:
     1. If RV-1 is used, administer a 2-dose series at ages 2 and 4 months of age.
     2. If RV-5 is used, administer a 3-dose series at ages 2, 4, and 6 months.
     3. If any dose in series was RV-5 or vaccine product is unknown for any dose in the series, a total of 3 doses of RV vaccine should be administered.
   Catch-up vaccination:
   • The maximum age for the first dose in the series is 14 weeks, 6 days.
   • Vaccination should not be initiated for infants aged 15 weeks 0 days or older.
   • The maximum age for the final dose in the series is 8 months, 0 days.
   • If RV-1 (Rotarix) is administered for the first and second doses, a third dose is not indicated.
   • For other catch-up issues, see Figure 2.

3. **Diphtheria and tetanus toxoids and acellular pertussis (DTaP) vaccine. (Minimum age: 6 weeks)**
   Routine vaccination:
   • Administer a 5-dose series of DTaP vaccine at ages 2, 4, 6, 15–18 months, and 4 through 6 years. The fourth dose may be administered as early as age 12 months, provided at least 6 months have elapsed since the third dose.
   Catch-up vaccination:
   • The fifth (booster) dose of DTaP vaccine is not necessary if the fourth dose was administered at age 4 years or older.
   • For other catch-up issues, see Figure 2.

4. **Tetanus and diphtheria toxoids and acellular pertussis (Tdap) vaccine. (Minimum age: 10 years for Boostrix, 11 years for Adacel).**
   Routine vaccination:
   • Administer 1 dose of Tdap vaccine to all adolescents aged 11 through 12 years.
   • Tdap can be administered regardless of the interval since the last tetanus and diphtheria toxoid-containing vaccine.
   • Administer one dose of Tdap vaccine to pregnant adolescents during each pregnancy (preferred during 27 through 36 weeks gestation) regardless of number of years from prior Td or Tdap vaccination.
   Catch-up vaccination:
   • Persons aged 7 through 10 years who are not fully immunized with the childhood DTaP vaccine series, should receive Tdap vaccine as the first dose in the catch-up series; if additional doses are needed, use Td vaccine. For these children, an adolescent Tdap vaccine should not be given.
   • Persons aged 11 through 18 years who have not received Tdap vaccine should receive a dose followed by tetanus and diphtheria toxoids (Td) booster doses every 10 years thereafter.
   • An inadvertent dose of DTaP vaccine administered to children aged 7 through 10 years can count as part of the catch-up series. This dose can count as the adolescent Tdap dose, or the child can later receive a Tdap booster dose at age 11–12 years.
   • For other catch-up issues, see Figure 2.

5. **Haemophilus influenzae type b (Hib) conjugate vaccine. (Minimum age: 6 weeks)**
   Routine vaccination:
   • Administer a Hib vaccine primary series and a booster dose to all infants. The primary series doses should be administered at 2, 4, and 6 months of age; however, if PRP-OMP (PedvaxHib or Comvax) is administered at 2 and 4 months of age, a dose at age 6 months is not indicated. One booster dose should be administered at age 12 through15 months.
   • Hiberix (PRP-T) should only be used for the booster (final) dose in children aged 12 months through 4 years, who have received at least 1 dose of Hib.
   Catch-up vaccination:
   • If dose 1 was administered at ages 12–14 months, administer booster (as final dose) at least 8 weeks after dose 1.
   • If the first 2 doses were PRP-OMP (PedvaxHIB or Comvax), and were administered at age 11 months or younger, the third (and final) dose should be administered at age 12 through 15 months and at least 8 weeks after the second dose.
   • If the first dose was administered at age 7 through 11 months, administer the second dose at least 4 weeks later and a final dose at age 12 through 15 months, regardless of Hib vaccine (PRP-T or PRP-OMP) used for first dose.
   • For unvaccinated children aged 15 months or older, administer only 1 dose.

Appendix A (continued)

For further guidance on the use of the vaccines mentioned below, see: http://www.cdc.gov/vaccines/pubs/acip-list.htm.

- For other catch-up issues, see Figure 2.

Vaccination of persons with high-risk conditions:

- Hib vaccine is not routinely recommended for patients older than 5 years of age. However one dose of Hib vaccine should be administered to unvaccinated or partially vaccinated persons aged 5 years or older who have leukemia, malignant neoplasms, anatomic or functional asplenia (including sickle cell disease), human immunodeficiency virus (HIV) infection, or other immunocompromising conditions.

6a. Pneumococcal conjugate vaccine (PCV). (Minimum age: 6 weeks)

Routine vaccination:

- Administer a series of PCV13 vaccine at ages 2, 4, 6 months with a booster at age 12 through 15 months.
- For children aged 14 through 59 months who have received an age-appropriate series of 7-valent PCV (PCV7), administer a single supplemental dose of 13-valent PCV (PCV13).

Catch-up vaccination:

- Administer 1 dose of PCV13 to all healthy children aged 24 through 59 months who are not completely vaccinated for their age.
- For other catch-up issues, see Figure 2.

Vaccination of persons with high-risk conditions:

- For children aged 24 through 71 months with certain underlying medical conditions (see footnote 6c), administer 1 dose of PCV13 if 3 doses of PCV were received previously, or administer 2 doses of PCV13 at least 8 weeks apart if fewer than 3 doses of PCV were received previously.
- A single dose of PCV13 may be administered to previously unvaccinated children aged 6 through 18 years who have anatomic or functional asplenia (including sickle cell disease), HIV infection or an immunocompromising condition, cochlear implant or cerebrospinal fluid leak. See MMWR 2010;59 (No. RR-11), available at http://www.cdc.gov/mmwr/pdf/rr/rr5911.pdf.
- Administer PPSV23 at least 8 weeks after the last dose of PCV to children aged 2 years or older with certain underlying medical conditions (see footnotes 6b and 6c).

6b. Pneumococcal polysaccharide vaccine (PPSV23). (Minimum age: 2 years)

Vaccination of persons with high-risk conditions:

- Administer PPSV23 at least 8 weeks after the last dose of PCV to children aged 2 years or older with certain underlying medical conditions (see footnote 6c). A single revaccination with PPSV should be administered after 5 years to children with anatomic or functional asplenia (including sickle cell disease) or an immunocompromising condition.

6c. Medical conditions for which PPSV23 is indicated in children aged 2 years and older and for which use of PCV13 is indicated in children aged 24 through 71 months:

- Immunocompetent children with chronic heart disease (particularly cyanotic congenital heart disease and cardiac failure); chronic lung disease (including asthma if treated with high-dose oral corticosteroid therapy), diabetes mellitus; cerebrospinal fluid leaks; or cochlear implant.
- Children with anatomic or functional asplenia (including sickle cell disease and other hemoglobinopathies, congenital or acquired asplenia, or splenic dysfunction);
- Children with immunocompromising conditions: HIV infection, chronic renal failure and nephrotic syndrome, diseases associated with treatment with immunosuppressive drugs or radiation therapy, including malignant neoplasms, leukemias, lymphomas and Hodgkin disease; or solid organ transplantation, congenital immunodeficiency.

7. Inactivated poliovirus vaccine (IPV). (Minimum age: 6 weeks)

Routine vaccination:

- Administer a series of IPV at ages 2, 4, 6–18 months, with a booster at age 4–6 years. The final dose in the series should be administered on or after the fourth birthday and at least 6 months after the previous dose.

Catch-up vaccination:

first at age 12 through 15 months (12 months if the child remains in an area where disease risk is high), and the second dose at least 4 weeks later.

- Administer 2 doses of MMR vaccine to children aged 12 months and older, before departure from the United States for international travel. The first dose should be administered on or after age 12 months and the second dose at least 4 weeks later.

Catch-up vaccination:

- Ensure that all school-aged children and adolescents have had 2 doses of MMR vaccine; the minimum interval between the 2 doses is 4 weeks.

10. Varicella (VAR) vaccine. (Minimum age: 12 months)

Routine vaccination:

- Administer the first dose of VAR vaccine at age 12 through 15 months, and the second dose at age 4 through 6 years. The second dose may be administered before age 4 years, provided at least 3 months have elapsed since the first dose. If the second dose was administered at least 4 weeks after the first dose, it can be accepted as valid.

Catch-up vaccination:

- Ensure that all persons aged 7 through 18 years without evidence of immunity (see MMWR 2007;56 [No. RR-4], available at http://www.cdc.gov/mmwr/pdf/rr/rr5604.pdf) have 2 doses of varicella vaccine. For children aged 7 through 12 years the recommended minimum interval between doses is 3 months (if the second dose was administered at least 4 weeks after the first dose, it can be accepted as valid); for persons aged 13 years and older, the minimum interval between doses is 4 weeks.

11. Hepatitis A vaccine (HepA). (Minimum age: 12 months)

Routine vaccination:

- Initiate the 2-dose HepA vaccine series for children aged 12 through 23 months; separate the 2 doses by 6 to 18 months.
- Children who have received 1 dose of HepA vaccine before age 24 months, should receive a second dose 6 to 18 months after the first dose.
- For any person aged 2 years and older who has not already received the HepA vaccine series, 2 doses of HepA vaccine separated by 6 to 18 months may be administered if immunity against hepatitis A virus infection is desired.

Catch-up vaccination:

- The minimum interval between the two doses is 6 months.

Special populations:

- Administer 2 doses of Hep A vaccine at least 6 months apart to previously unvaccinated persons who live in areas where vaccination programs target older children, or who are at increased risk for infection.

12. Human papillomavirus (HPV) vaccines. (HPV4 [Gardasil] and HPV2 [Cervarix]). (Minimum age: 9 years)

Routine vaccination:

- Administer a 3-dose series of HPV vaccine on a schedule of 0, 1-2, and 6 months to all adolescents aged 11-12 years. Either HPV4 or HPV2 may be used for females, and only HPV4 may be used for males.
- The vaccine series can be started beginning at age 9 years.
- Administer the second dose 1 to 2 months after the first dose and the third dose 6 months after the first dose (at least 24 weeks after the first dose).

Catch-up vaccination:

- Administer the vaccine series to females (either HPV2 or HPV4) and males (HPV4) at age 13 through 18 years if not previously vaccinated.
- Use recommended routine dosing intervals (see above) for vaccine series catch-up.

13. Meningococcal conjugate vaccines (MCV). (Minimum age: 6 weeks for Hib-MenCY, 9 months for Menactra [MCV4-D], 2 years for Menveo [MCV4-CRM]).

Appendix A (continued)

- In the first 6 months of life, minimum age and minimum intervals are only recommended if the person is at risk for imminent exposure to circulating poliovirus (i.e., travel to a polio-endemic region or during an outbreak).
- If 4 or more doses are administered before age 4 years, an additional dose should be administered at age 4 through 6 years.
- A fourth dose is not necessary if the third dose was administered at age 4 years or older and at least 6 months after the previous dose.
- If both OPV and IPV were administered as part of a series, a total of 4 doses should be administered, regardless of the child's current age.
- IPV is not routinely recommended for U.S. residents aged 18 years or older.
- For other catch-up issues, see Figure 2.

8. **Influenza vaccines. (Minimum age: 6 months for inactivated influenza vaccine [IIV]; 2 years for live, attenuated influenza vaccine [LAIV])**

Routine vaccination:
- Administer influenza vaccine annually to all children beginning at age 6 months. For most healthy, nonpregnant persons aged 2 through 49 years, either LAIV or IIV may be used. However, LAIV should NOT be administered to some persons, including 1) those with asthma, 2) children 2 through 4 years who had wheezing in the past 12 months, or 3) those who have any other underlying medical conditions that predispose them to influenza complications. For all other contraindications to use of LAIV see MMWR 2010;59 (No. RR-8), available at http://www.cdc.gov/mmwr/pdf/rr/rr5908.pdf.
- Administer 1 dose to persons aged 9 years and older.

For children aged 6 months through 8 years:
- For the 2012–13 season, administer 2 doses (separated by at least 4 weeks) to children who are receiving influenza vaccine for the first time. For additional guidance, follow dosing guidelines in the 2012 ACIP influenza vaccine recommendations, MMWR 2012;61:613–618, available at http://www.cdc.gov/mmwr/pdf/wk/mm6132.pdf.
- For the 2013–14 season, follow dosing guidelines in the 2013 ACIP influenza vaccine recommendations.

9. **Measles, mumps, and rubella (MMR) vaccine. (Minimum age: 12 months for routine vaccination)**

Routine vaccination:
- Administer the first dose of MMR vaccine at age 12 through 15 months, and the second dose at age 4 through 6 years. The second dose may be administered before age 4 years, provided at least 4 weeks have elapsed since the first dose.
- Administer 1 dose of MMR vaccine to infants aged 6 through 11 months before departure from the United States for international travel. These children should be revaccinated with 2 doses of MMR vaccine, the

Additional information
- For contraindications and precautions to use of a vaccine and for additional information regarding that vaccine, vaccination providers should consult the relevant ACIP statement available online at http://www.cdc.gov/vaccines/pubs/acip-list.htm.
- For the purposes of calculating intervals between doses, 4 weeks = 28 days. Intervals of 4 months or greater are determined by calendar months.
- Information on travel vaccine requirements and recommendations is available at http://wwwnc.cdc.gov/travel/page/vaccinations.htm.
- For vaccination of persons with primary and secondary immunodeficiencies, see Table 13, "Vaccination of persons with primary and secondary immunodeficiencies," in General Recommendations on Immunization (ACIP), available at http://www.cdc.gov/mmwr/preview/mmwrhtml/rr6002a1.htm; and American Academy of Pediatrics. Immunization in Special Clinical Circumstances. In: Pickering LK, Baker CJ, Kimberlin DW, Long SS eds. Red book: 2012 report of the Committee on Infectious Diseases. 29th ed. Elk Grove Village, IL: American Academy of Pediatrics.

Routine vaccination:
- Administer MCV4 vaccine at age 11–12 years, with a booster dose at age 16 years.
- Adolescents aged 11 through 18 years with human immunodeficiency virus (HIV) infection should receive a 2-dose primary series of MCV4, with at least 8 weeks between doses. See MMWR 2011;60:1018–1019 available at: http://www.cdc.gov/mmwr/pdf/wk/mm6030.pdf.
- For children aged 2 months through 10 years with high-risk conditions, see below.

Catch-up vaccination:
- Administer MCV4 vaccine at age 13 through 18 years if not previously vaccinated.
- If the first dose is administered at age 13 through 15 years, a booster dose should be administered at age 16 through 18 years with a minimum interval of at least 8 weeks between doses.
- If the first dose is administered at age 16 years or older, a booster dose is not needed.
- For other catch-up issues, see Figure 2.

Vaccination of persons with high-risk conditions:
- For children younger than 19 months of age with anatomic or functional asplenia (including sickle cell disease), administer an infant series of Hib-MenCY at 2, 4, 6, and 12-15 months.
- For children aged 2 through 18 months with persistent complement component deficiency, administer either an infant series of Hib-MenCY at 2, 4, 6, and 12 through 15 months or a 2-dose primary series of MCV4-D starting at 9 months, with at least 8 weeks between doses. For children aged 19 through 23 months with persistent complement component deficiency who have not received a complete series of Hib-MenCY or MCV4-D, administer 2 primary doses of MCV4-D at least 8 weeks apart.
- For children aged 24 months and older with persistent complement component deficiency or anatomic or functional asplenia (including sickle cell disease), who have not received a complete series of Hib-MenCY or MCV4-D, administer 2 primary doses of either MCV4-D or MCV4-CRM. If MCV4-D (Menactra) is administered to a child with asplenia (including sickle cell disease), do not administer MCV4-D until 2 years of age and at least 4 weeks after the completion of all PCV13 doses. See MMWR 2011;60:1391–2, available at http://www.cdc.gov/mmwr/pdf/wk/mm6040.pdf.
- For children aged 9 months and older who are residents of or travelers to countries in the African meningitis belt or to the Hajj, administer an age appropriate formulation and series of MCV4 for protection against serogroups A and W-135. Prior receipt of Hib-MenCY is not sufficient for children traveling to the meningitis belt or the Hajj. See MMWR 2011;60:1391–2, available at http://www.cdc.gov/mmwr/pdf/wk/mm6040.pdf.
- For children who are present during outbreaks caused by a vaccine serogroup, administer or complete an age and formulation-appropriate series of Hib-MenCY or MCV4.
- For booster doses among persons with high-risk conditions refer to http://www.cdc.gov/vaccines/pubs/acip-list.htm#mening.

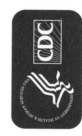

**U.S. Department of
Health and Human Services**
Centers for Disease
Control and Prevention

Appendix B

FIGURE 2. Catch-up immunization schedule for persons aged 4 months through 18 years who start late or who are more than 1 month behind —United States - 2013

The figure below provides catch-up schedules and minimum intervals between doses for children whose vaccinations have been delayed. A vaccine series does not need to be restarted, regardless of the time that has elapsed between doses. Use the section appropriate for the child's age. Always use this table in conjunction with Figure 1 and the footnotes that follow.

Vaccine	Minimum Age for Dose 1	Minimum Interval Between Doses			
		Dose 1 to dose 2	Dose 2 to dose 3	Dose 3 to dose 4	Dose 4 to dose 5
Persons aged 4 months through 6 years					
Hepatitis B[1]	Birth	4 weeks	8 weeks and at least 16 weeks after first dose; minimum age for the final dose is 24 weeks		
Rotavirus[2]	6 weeks	4 weeks	4 weeks[2]		
Diphtheria, tetanus, pertussis[3]	6 weeks	4 weeks	4 weeks	6 months	6 months[3]
Haemophilus influenzae type b[5]	6 weeks	4 weeks if first dose administered at younger than age 12 months / 8 weeks (as final dose) if first dose administered at age 12–14 months / No further doses needed if first dose administered at age 15 months or older	4 weeks[5] if current age is younger than 12 months / 8 weeks (as final dose)[5] if current age is 12 months or older and first dose administered at younger than age 12 months and second dose administered at younger than 15 months / No further doses needed if previous dose administered at age 15 months or older	8 weeks (as final dose) This dose only necessary for children aged 12 through 59 months who received 3 doses before age 12 months	
Pneumococcal[6]	6 weeks	4 weeks if first dose administered at younger than age 12 months / 8 weeks (as final dose for healthy children) if first dose administered at age 12 months or older or current age 24 through 59 months / No further doses needed for healthy children if first dose administered at age 24 months or older	4 weeks if current age is younger than 12 months / 8 weeks (as final dose for healthy children) if current age is 12 months or older / No further doses needed for healthy children if previous dose administered at age 24 months or older	8 weeks (as final dose) This dose only necessary for children aged 12 through 59 months who received 3 doses before age 12 months or for children at high risk who received 3 doses at any age	
Inactivated poliovirus[7]	6 weeks	4 weeks	4 weeks	6 months[7] minimum age 4 years for final dose	
Meningococcal[13]	6 weeks	8 weeks[13]	see footnote 13	see footnote 13	
Measles, mumps, rubella[9]	12 months	4 weeks			
Varicella[10]	12 months	3 months			
Hepatitis A[11]	12 months	6 months			
Persons aged 7 through 18 years					
Tetanus, diphtheria; tetanus,		4 weeks if first dose administered at younger than	6 months if first dose administered at younger than	6 months if first dose administered at	

Appendix B (continued)

		4 weeks	age 12 months / 6 months / if first dose administered at 12 months or older	younger than age 12 months
diphtheria, pertussis[4]	7 years	4 weeks		
Human papillomavirus[12]	9 years		Routine dosing intervals are recommended[12]	
Hepatitis A[11]	12 months		6 months	
Hepatitis B[1]	Birth	4 weeks	8 weeks (and at least 16 weeks after first dose)	
Inactivated poliovirus[7]	6 weeks	4 weeks	4 weeks[7]	6 months[7]
Meningococcal[13]	6 weeks	8 weeks[13]		
Measles, mumps, rubella[9]	12 months	4 weeks		
Varicella[10]	12 months	3 months if person is younger than age 13 years / 4 weeks if person is aged 13 years or older		

NOTE: The above recommendations must be read along with the footnotes of this schedule.

Footnotes — Recommended immunization schedule for persons aged 0 through 18 years—United States, 2013

For further guidance on the use of the vaccines mentioned below, see: http://www.cdc.gov/vaccines/pubs/acip-list.htm.

1. **Hepatitis B (HepB) vaccine. (Minimum age: birth)**
   Routine vaccination:
   At birth
   - Administer monovalent HepB vaccine to all newborns before hospital discharge.
   - For infants born to hepatitis B surface antigen (HBsAg)–positive mothers, administer HepB vaccine and 0.5 mL of hepatitis B immune globulin (HBIG) within 12 hours of birth. These infants should be tested for HBsAg and antibody to HBsAg (anti-HBs) 1 to 2 months after completion of the HepB series, at age 9 through 18 months (preferably at the next well-child visit).
   - If mother's HBsAg status is unknown, within 12 hours of birth administer HepB vaccine to all infants regardless of birth weight. For infants weighing <2,000 grams, administer HBIG in addition to HepB within 12 hours of birth. Determine the mother's HBsAg status as soon as possible and, if she is HBsAg-positive, also administer HBIG for infants weighing ≥2,000 grams (no later than age 1 week).
   Doses following the birth dose
   - The second dose should be administered at age 1 or 2 months. Monovalent HepB vaccine should be used for doses administered before age 6 weeks.
   - Infants who did not receive a birth dose should receive 3 doses of a HepB-containing vaccine on a schedule of 0, 1 to 2 months, and 6 months starting as soon as feasible. See Figure 2.
   - The minimum interval between dose 1 and dose 2 is 4 weeks and between dose 2 and 3 is 8 weeks. The final (third or fourth) dose in the HepB vaccine series should be administered no earlier than age 24 weeks, and at least 16 weeks after the first dose.
   - Administration of a total of 4 doses of HepB vaccine is recommended when a combination vaccine containing HepB is administered after the birth dose.
   Catch-up vaccination:
   - Unvaccinated persons should complete a 3-dose series.
   - A 2-dose series (doses separated by at least 4 months) of adult formulation Recombivax HB is licensed for use in children aged 11 through 15 years.
   - For other catch-up issues, see Figure 2.

2. **Rotavirus (RV) vaccines. (Minimum age: 6 weeks for both RV-1 [Rotarix] and RV-5 [RotaTeq]).**
   Routine vaccination:
   - Administer a series of RV vaccine to all infants as follows:
     1. If RV-1 is used, administer a 2-dose series at 2 and 4 months of age.
     2. If RV-5 is used, administer a 3-dose series at ages 2, 4, and 6 months.
     3. If any dose in series was RV-5 or vaccine product is unknown for any dose in the series, a total of 3 doses of RV vaccine should be administered.
   Catch-up vaccination:
   - The maximum age for the first dose in the series is 14 weeks, 6 days.
   - Vaccination should not be initiated for infants aged 15 weeks 0 days or older.
   - The maximum age for the final dose in the series is 8 months, 0 days.
   - If RV-1 (Rotarix) is administered for the first and second doses, a third dose is not indicated.
   - For other catch-up issues, see Figure 2.

3. **Diphtheria and tetanus toxoids and acellular pertussis (DTaP) vaccine. (Minimum age: 6 weeks)**
   Routine vaccination:
   - Administer a 5-dose series of DTaP vaccine at ages 2, 4, 6, 15–18 months, and 4 through 6 years. The fourth dose may be administered as early as age 12 months, provided at least 6 months have elapsed since the third dose.
   Catch-up vaccination:
   - The fifth (booster) dose of DTaP vaccine is not necessary if the fourth dose was administered at age 4 years or older.
   - For other catch-up issues, see Figure 2.

4. **Tetanus and diphtheria toxoids and acellular pertussis (Tdap) vaccine. (Minimum age: 10 years for Boostrix, 11 years for Adacel).**
   Routine vaccination:
   - Administer 1 dose of Tdap vaccine to all adolescents aged 11 through 12 years.
   - Tdap can be administered regardless of the interval since the last tetanus and diphtheria toxoid-containing vaccine.

Appendix B (continued)

For further guidance on the use of the vaccines mentioned below, see: http://www.cdc.gov/vaccines/pubs/acip-list.htm.

- Administer one dose of Tdap vaccine to pregnant adolescents during each pregnancy (preferred during 27 through 36 weeks gestation) regardless of number of years from prior Td or Tdap vaccination.

Catch-up vaccination:
- Persons aged 7 through 10 years who are not fully immunized with the childhood DTaP vaccine series, should receive Tdap vaccine as the first dose in the catch-up series; if additional doses are needed, use Td vaccine. For these children, an adolescent Tdap vaccine should not be given.
- Persons aged 11 through 18 years who have not received Tdap vaccine should receive a dose followed by tetanus and diphtheria toxoids (Td) booster doses every 10 years thereafter.
- An inadvertent dose of DTaP vaccine administered to children aged 7 through 10 years can count as part of the catch-up series. This dose can count as the adolescent Tdap dose, or the child can later receive a Tdap booster dose at age 11–12 years.
- For other catch-up issues, see Figure 2.

5. **Haemophilus influenzae type b (Hib) conjugate vaccine. (Minimum age: 6 weeks)**
Routine vaccination:
- Administer a Hib vaccine primary series and a booster dose to all infants. The primary series doses should be administered at 2, 4, and 6 months of age; however, if PRP-OMP (PedvaxHib or Comvax) is administered at 2 and 4 months of age, a dose at age 6 months is not indicated. One booster dose should be administered at age 12 through 15 months.
- Hiberix (PRP-T) should only be used for the booster (final) dose in children aged 12 months through 4 years, who have received at least 1 dose of Hib.

Catch-up vaccination:
- If dose 1 was administered at ages 12–14 months, administer booster (as final dose) at least 8 weeks after dose 1.
- If the first 2 doses were PRP-OMP (PedvaxHIB or Comvax), and were administered at age 11 months or younger, the third (and final) dose should be administered at age 12 through 15 months and at least 8 weeks after the second dose.
- If the first dose was administered at age 7 through 11 months, administer the second dose at least 4 weeks later and a final dose at age 12 through 15 months, regardless of Hib vaccine (PRP-T or PRP-OMP) used for first dose.
- For unvaccinated children aged 15 months or older, administer only 1 dose.
- For other catch-up issues, see Figure 2.

Vaccination of persons with high-risk conditions:
- Hib vaccine is not routinely recommended for patients older than 5 years of age. However one dose of Hib vaccine should be administered to unvaccinated or partially vaccinated persons aged 5 years or older who have leukemia, malignant neoplasms, anatomic or functional asplenia (including sickle cell disease), human immunodeficiency virus (HIV) infection, or other immunocompromising conditions.

6a. **Pneumococcal conjugate vaccine (PCV). (Minimum age: 6 weeks)**
Routine vaccination:
- Administer a series of PCV13 vaccine at ages 2, 4, 6 months with a booster at age 12 through 15 months.
- For children aged 14 through 59 months who have received an age-appropriate series of 7-valent PCV (PCV7), administer a single supplemental dose of 13-valent PCV (PCV13).

Catch-up vaccination:
- Administer 1 dose of PCV13 to all healthy children aged 24 through 59 months who are not completely vaccinated for their age.
- For other catch-up issues, see Figure 2.

Vaccination of persons with high-risk conditions:
- For children aged 24 through 71 months with certain underlying medical conditions (see footnote 6c), administer 1 dose of PCV13 if 3 doses of PCV were received previously, or administer 2 doses of PCV13 at least 8 weeks apart if fewer than 3 doses of PCV were received previously.
- A single dose of PCV13 may be administered to previously unvaccinated children aged 6 through 18 years who have anatomic or functional asplenia (including sickle cell disease), HIV infection or an immunocompromising condition, cochlear implant or cerebrospinal fluid leak. See MMWR 2010;59 (No. RR-11), available at http://www.cdc.gov/mmwr/pdf/rr/rr5911.pdf.
- Administer PPSV23 at least 8 weeks after the last dose of PCV to children aged 2 years or older with certain

- Administer 1 dose to persons aged 9 years and older.
For children aged 6 months through 8 years:
- For the 2012–13 season, administer 2 doses (separated by at least 4 weeks) to children who are receiving influenza vaccine for the first time. For additional guidance, follow dosing guidelines in the 2012 ACIP influenza vaccine recommendations, MMWR 2012;61:613–618, available at http://www.cdc.gov/mmwr/pdf/wk/mm6132.pdf.
- For the 2013–14 season, follow dosing guidelines in the 2013 ACIP influenza vaccine recommendations.

9. **Measles, mumps, and rubella (MMR) vaccine. (Minimum age: 12 months for routine vaccination)**
Routine vaccination:
- Administer the first dose of MMR vaccine at age 12 through 15 months, and the second dose at age 4 through 6 years. The second dose may be administered before age 4 years, provided at least 4 weeks have elapsed since the first dose.
- Administer 1 dose of MMR vaccine to infants aged 6 through 11 months before departure from the United States for international travel. These children should be revaccinated with 2 doses of MMR vaccine, the first at age 12 through 15 months (12 months if the child remains in an area where disease risk is high), and the second dose at least 4 weeks later.
- Administer 2 doses of MMR vaccine to children aged 12 months and older, before departure from the United States for international travel. The first dose should be administered on or after age 12 months and the second dose at least 4 weeks later.

Catch-up vaccination:
- Ensure that all school-aged children and adolescents have had 2 doses of MMR vaccine; the minimum interval between the 2 doses is 4 weeks.

10. **Varicella (VAR) vaccine. (Minimum age: 12 months)**
Routine vaccination:
- Administer the first dose of VAR vaccine at age 12 through 15 months, and the second dose at age 4 through 6 years. The second dose may be administered before age 4 years, provided at least 3 months have elapsed since the first dose. If the second dose was administered at least 4 weeks after the first dose, it can be accepted as valid.

Catch-up vaccination:
- Ensure that all persons aged 7 through 18 years without evidence of immunity (see MMWR 2007;56 [No. RR-4], available at http://www.cdc.gov/mmwr/pdf/rr/rr5604.pdf) have 2 doses of varicella vaccine. For children aged 7 through 12 years the recommended minimum interval between doses is 3 months (if the second dose was administered at least 4 weeks after the first dose, it can be accepted as valid); for persons aged 13 years and older, the minimum interval between doses is 4 weeks.

11. **Hepatitis A vaccine (HepA). (Minimum age: 12 months)**
Routine vaccination:
- Initiate the 2-dose HepA vaccine series for children aged 12 through 23 months; separate the 2 doses by 6 to 18 months.
- Children who have received 1 dose of HepA vaccine before age 24 months, should receive a second dose 6 to 18 months after the first dose.
- For any person aged 2 years and older who has not already received the HepA vaccine series, 2 doses of HepA vaccine separated by 6 to 18 months may be administered if immunity against hepatitis A virus infection is desired.

Catch-up vaccination:
- The minimum interval between the two doses is 6 months.

Special populations:
- Administer 2 doses of Hep A vaccine at least 6 months apart to previously unvaccinated persons who live in areas where vaccination programs target older children, or who are at increased risk for infection.

12. **Human papillomavirus (HPV) vaccines. (HPV4 [Gardasil] and HPV2 [Cervarix]). (Minimum age: 9 years)**
Routine vaccination:
- Administer a 3-dose series of HPV vaccine on a schedule of 0, 1-2, and 6 months to all adolescents aged 11-12 years. Either HPV4 or HPV2 may be used for females, and only HPV4 may be used for males.
- The vaccine series can be started beginning at age 9 years.
- Administer the second dose 1 to 2 months after the <u>first</u> dose and the third dose 6 months after the <u>first</u> dose (at least 24 weeks after the first dose).

Appendix B (continued)

underlying medical conditions (see footnotes 6b and 6c).

6b. Pneumococcal polysaccharide vaccine (PPSV23). (Minimum age: 2 years)

Vaccination of persons with high-risk conditions:

- Administer PPSV23 at least 8 weeks after the last dose of PCV to children aged 2 years or older with certain underlying medical conditions (see footnote 6c). A single revaccination with PPSV should be administered after 5 years to children with anatomic or functional asplenia (including sickle cell disease) or an immunocompromising condition.

6c. Medical conditions for which PPSV23 is indicated in children aged 2 years and older and for which use of PCV13 is indicated in children aged 24 through 71 months:

- Immunocompetent children with chronic heart disease (particularly cyanotic congenital heart disease and cardiac failure); chronic lung disease (including asthma if treated with high-dose oral corticosteroid therapy), diabetes mellitus; cerebrospinal fluid leaks; or cochlear implant.
- Children with anatomic or functional asplenia (including sickle cell disease and other hemoglobinopathies, congenital or acquired asplenia, or splenic dysfunction).
- Children with immunocompromising conditions: HIV infection, chronic renal failure and nephrotic syndrome, diseases associated with treatment with immunosuppressive drugs or radiation therapy, including malignant neoplasms, leukemias, lymphomas and Hodgkin disease; or solid organ transplantation, congenital immunodeficiency.

7. Inactivated poliovirus vaccine (IPV). (Minimum age: 6 weeks)

Routine vaccination:

- Administer a series of IPV at ages 2, 4, 6–18 months, with a booster dose at age 4–6 years. The final dose in the series should be administered on or after the fourth birthday and at least 6 months after the previous dose.

Catch-up vaccination:

- In the first 6 months of life, minimum age and minimum intervals are only recommended if the person is at risk for imminent exposure to circulating poliovirus (i.e., travel to a polio-endemic region or during an outbreak).
- If 4 or more doses are administered before age 4 years, an additional dose should be administered at age 4 through 6 years.
- A fourth dose is not necessary if the third dose was administered at age 4 years or older and at least 6 months after the previous dose.
- If both OPV and IPV were administered as part of a series, a total of 4 doses should be administered, regardless of the child's current age.
- IPV is not routinely recommended for U.S. residents aged 18 years or older.
- For other catch-up issues, see Figure 2.

8. Influenza vaccines. (Minimum age: 6 months for inactivated influenza vaccine [IIV]; 2 years for live, attenuated influenza vaccine [LAIV])

Routine vaccination:

- Administer influenza vaccine annually to all children beginning at age 6 months. For most healthy, nonpregnant persons aged 2 through 49 years, either LAIV or IIV may be used. However, LAIV should NOT be administered to some persons, including 1) those with asthma, 2) children 2 through 4 years who had wheezing in the past 12 months, or 3) those who have any other underlying medical conditions that predispose them to influenza complications. For all other contraindications to use of LAIV see MMWR 2010; 59 (No. RR-8), available at http://www.cdc.gov/mmwr/pdf/rr/rr5908.pdf.

Additional Information

- For contraindications and precautions to use of a vaccine and for additional information regarding that vaccine, vaccination providers should consult the relevant ACIP statement available online at http://www.cdc.gov/vaccines/pubs/acip-list.htm.
- For the purposes of calculating intervals between doses, 4 weeks = 28 days. Intervals of 4 months or greater are determined by calendar months.
- Information on travel vaccine requirements and recommendations is available at http://wwwnc.cdc.gov/travel/page/vaccinations.htm.
- For vaccination of persons with primary and secondary immunodeficiencies, see Table 13, "Vaccination of persons with primary and secondary immunodeficiencies," in General Recommendations on Immunization (ACIP), available at http://www.cdc.gov/mmwr/preview/mmwrhtml/rr6002a1.htm; and American Academy of Pediatrics. Immunization in Special Clinical Circumstances. In: Pickering LK, Baker CJ, Kimberlin DW, Long SS eds. Red book: 2012 report of the Committee on Infectious Diseases. 29th ed. Elk Grove Village, IL: American Academy of Pediatrics.

Catch-up vaccination:

- Administer the vaccine series to females (either HPV2 or HPV4) and males (HPV4) at age 13 through 18 years if not previously vaccinated.
- Use recommended routine dosing intervals (see above) for vaccine series catch-up.

13. Meningococcal conjugate vaccines (MCV). (Minimum age: 6 weeks for Hib-MenCY, 9 months for Menactra [MCV4-D], 2 years for Menveo [MCV4-CRM]).

Routine vaccination:

- Administer MCV4 vaccine at age 11–12 years, with a booster dose at age 16 years.
- Adolescents aged 11 through 18 years with human immunodeficiency virus (HIV) infection should receive a 2-dose primary series of MCV4, with at least 8 weeks between doses. See MMWR 2011;60:1018–1019 available at http://www.cdc.gov/mmwr/pdf/wk/mm6030.pdf.
- For children aged 2 months through 10 years with high-risk conditions, see below.

Catch-up vaccination:

- Administer MCV4 vaccine at age 13 through 18 years if not previously vaccinated.
- If the first dose is administered at age 13 through 15 years, a booster dose should be administered at age 16 through 18 years with a minimum interval of at least 8 weeks between doses.
- If the first dose is administered at age 16 years or older, a booster dose is not needed.
- For other catch-up issues, see Figure 2.

Vaccination of persons with high-risk conditions:

- For children younger than 19 months of age with anatomic or functional asplenia (including sickle cell disease), administer an infant series of Hib-MenCY at 2, 4, 6, and 12-15 months.
- For children aged 2 through 18 months with persistent complement component deficiency, administer either an infant series of Hib-MenCY at 2, 4, 6, and 12 through 15 months or a 2-dose primary series of MCV4-D starting at 9 months, with at least 8 weeks between doses. For children aged 19 through 23 months with persistent complement component deficiency who have not received a complete series of Hib-MenCY or MCV4-D, administer 2 primary doses of MCV4-D at least 8 weeks apart.
- For children aged 24 months and older with persistent complement component deficiency or anatomic or functional asplenia (including sickle cell disease), who have not received a complete series of Hib-MenCY or MCV4-D, administer 2 primary doses of either MCV4-D or MCV4-CRM. If MCV4-D (Menactra) is administered to a child with asplenia (including sickle cell disease), do not administer MCV4-D until 2 years of age and at least 4 weeks after the completion of all PCV13 doses. See MMWR 2011;60:1391–2, available at http://www.cdc.gov/mmwr/pdf/wk/mm6040.pdf.
- For children aged 9 months and older who are residents of or travelers to countries in the African meningitis belt or to the Hajj, administer an age appropriate formulation and series of MCV4 for protection against serogroups A and W-135. Prior receipt of Hib-MenCY is not sufficient for children traveling to the meningitis belt or the Hajj. See MMWR 2011;60:1391–2, available at http://www.cdc.gov/mmwr/pdf/wk/mm6040.pdf.
- For children who are present during outbreaks caused by a vaccine serogroup, administer or complete an age and formulation-appropriate series of Hib-MenCY or MCV4.
- For booster doses among persons with high-risk conditions refer to http://www.cdc.gov/vaccines/pubs/acip-list.htm#mening.

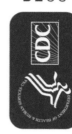

U.S. Department of Health and Human Services
Centers for Disease Control and Prevention

http://www.cdc.gov/vaccines/schedules/hcp/index.html

Appendix C

Recommended Adult Immunization Schedule—United States - 2013

Note: These recommendations must be read with the footnotes that follow containing number of doses, intervals between doses, and other important information.

VACCINE ▼ AGE GROUP ▶	19-21 years	22-26 years	27-49 years	50-59 years	60-64 years	≥ 65 years
Influenza [2,*]	1 dose annually					
Tetanus, diphtheria, pertussis (Td/Tdap) [3,*]	Substitute 1-time dose of Tdap for Td booster; then boost with Td every 10 yrs					
Varicella [4,*]	2 doses					
Human papillomavirus (HPV) Female [5,*]	3 doses	3 doses				
Human papillomavirus (HPV) Male [5,*]	3 doses	3 doses				
Zoster [6]					1 dose	1 dose
Measles, mumps, rubella (MMR) [7,*]	1 or 2 doses					
Pneumococcal polysaccharide (PPSV23) [8,9]	1 or 2 doses					1 dose
Pneumococcal 13-valent conjugate (PCV13) [10,*]	1 dose					
Meningococcal [11,*]	1 or more doses					
Hepatitis A [12,*]	2 doses					
Hepatitis B [13,*]	3 doses					

*Covered by the Vaccine Injury Compensation Program

Legend:
- For all persons in this category who meet the age requirements and who lack documentation of vaccination or have no evidence of previous infection; zoster vaccine recommended regardless of prior episode of zoster
- Recommended if some other risk factor is present (e.g., on the basis of medical, occupational, lifestyle, or other indication)
- No recommendation

Report all clinically significant postvaccination reactions to the Vaccine Adverse Event Reporting System (VAERS). Reporting forms and instructions on filing a VAERS report are available at www.vaers.hhs.gov or by telephone, 800-822-7967.

Information on how to file a Vaccine Injury Compensation Program claim is available at www.hrsa.gov/vaccinecompensation or by telephone, 800-338-2382. To file a claim for vaccine injury, contact the U.S. Court of Federal Claims, 717 Madison Place, N.W., Washington, D.C. 20005; telephone, 202-357-6400.

Additional information about the vaccines in this schedule, extent of available data, and contraindications for vaccination is also available at www.cdc.gov/vaccines or from the CDC-INFO Contact Center at 800-CDC-INFO (800-232-4636) in English and Spanish, 8:00 a.m.- 8:00 p.m. Eastern Time, Monday - Friday, excluding holidays.

Use of trade names and commercial sources is for identification only and does not imply endorsement by the U.S. Department of Health and Human Services.

The recommendations in this schedule were approved by the Centers for Disease Control and Prevention's (CDC) Advisory Committee on Immunization Practices (ACIP), the American Academy of Family Physicians (AAFP), the American College of Physicians (ACP), American College of Obstetricians and Gynecologists (ACOG) and American College of Nurse-Midwives (ACNM).

Appendix C (continued)

VACCINE ▼ INDICATION ►	Pregnancy	Immunocompromising conditions (excluding human immunodeficiency virus [HIV])[1,4,6,7,10,13]	HIV infection CD4+ T lymphocyte count[4,6,7,10,14,15] <200 cells/µL	HIV infection CD4+ T lymphocyte count ≥200 cells/µL	Men who have sex with men (MSM)	Heart disease, chronic lung disease, chronic alcoholism	Asplenia (including elective splenectomy and persistent complement component deficiencies)[10,14]	Chronic liver disease	Kidney failure, end-stage renal disease, receipt of hemodialysis	Diabetes	Healthcare personnel
Influenza[2,*]	1 dose IIV annually	1 dose IIV annually	1 dose IIV annually	1 dose IIV annually	1 dose IIV or LAIV annually	1 dose IIV annually	1 dose IIV annually	1 dose IIV annually	1 dose IIV annually	1 dose IIV annually	1 dose IIV or LAIV annually
Tetanus, diphtheria, pertussis (Td/Tdap)[3,*]	1 dose Tdap each pregnancy	Substitute 1-time dose of Tdap for Td booster; then boost with Td every 10 yrs									
Varicella[4,*]		Contraindicated	Contraindicated	2 doses							
Human papillomavirus (HPV) Female[5,*]		3 doses through age 26 yrs	3 doses through age 26 yrs			3 doses through age 26 yrs					
Human papillomavirus (HPV) Male[5,*]		3 doses through age 26 yrs	3 doses through age 26 yrs		3 doses through age 26 yrs	3 doses through age 21 yrs					
Zoster[6]		Contraindicated	Contraindicated			1 dose					
Measles, mumps, rubella (MMR)[7,*]		Contraindicated	Contraindicated			1 or 2 doses					
Pneumococcal polysaccharide (PPSV23)[8,9]						1 or 2 doses					
Pneumococcal 13-valent conjugate (PCV13)[10,*]						1 dose					
Meningococcal[11,*]						1 or more doses					
Hepatitis A[12,*]						2 doses					
Hepatitis B[13,*]						3 doses					

*Covered by the Vaccine Injury Compensation Program

For all persons in this category who meet the age requirements and who lack documentation of vaccination or have no evidence of previous infection; zoster vaccine recommended regardless of prior episode of zoster

Recommended if some other risk factor is present (e.g., on the basis of medical, occupational, lifestyle, or other indications)

No recommendation

These schedules indicate the recommended age groups and medical indications for which administration of currently licensed vaccines is commonly indicated for adults ages 19 years and older, as of January 1, 2013. For all vaccines being recommended on the Adult Immunization Schedule: a vaccine series does not need to be restarted, regardless of the time that has elapsed between doses. Licensed combination vaccines may be used whenever any components of the combination are indicated and when the vaccine's other components are not contraindicated. For detailed recommendations on all vaccines, including those used primarily for travelers or that are issued during the year, consult the manufacturers' package inserts and the complete statements from the Advisory Committee on Immunization Practices (www.cdc.gov/vaccines/pubs/acip-list.htm). Use of trade names and commercial sources is for identification only and does not imply endorsement by the U.S. Department of Health and Human Services.

U.S. Department of
Health and Human Services
Centers for Disease
Control and Prevention

Appendix C (continued)

Footnotes — Recommended Immunization Schedule for Adults Aged 19 Years and Older—United States, 2013

1. Additional Information

- Additional guidance for the use of the vaccines described in this supplement is available at http://www.cdc.gov/vaccines/pubs/acip-list.htm.
- Information on vaccination recommendations when vaccination status is unknown and other general immunization information can be found in the General Recommendations on Immunization at http://www.cdc.gov/mmwr/preview/mmwrhtml/rr6002a1.htm.
- Information on travel vaccine requirements and recommendations (e.g., for hepatitis A and B, meningococcal, and other vaccines) are available at http://wwwnc.cdc.gov/travel/page/vaccinations.htm.

2. Influenza vaccination

- Annual vaccination against influenza is recommended for all persons aged 6 months and older.
- Persons aged 6 months and older, including pregnant women, can receive the inactivated influenza vaccine (IIV).
- Healthy, nonpregnant persons aged 2–49 years without high-risk medical conditions can receive either intranasally administered live, attenuated influenza vaccine (LAIV) (FluMist), or IIV. Health-care personnel who care for severely immunocompromised persons (i.e., those who require care in a protected environment) should receive IIV rather than LAIV.
- The intramuscularly or intradermally administered IIV are options for adults aged 18–64 years.
- Adults aged 65 years and older can receive the standard dose IIV or the high-dose IIV (Fluzone High-Dose).

3. Tetanus, diphtheria, and acellular pertussis (Td/Tdap) vaccination

- Administer one dose of Tdap vaccine to pregnant women during each pregnancy (preferred during 27–36 weeks' gestation), regardless of number of years since prior Td or Tdap vaccination.
- Administer Tdap to all adults who have not previously received Tdap or for whom vaccine status is unknown. Tdap can be administered regardless of interval since the most recent tetanus or diphtheria-toxoid containing vaccine.
- Adults with an unknown or incomplete history of completing a 3-dose primary vaccination series with Td-containing vaccines should begin or complete a primary vaccination series including a Tdap dose.
- For unvaccinated adults, administer the first 2 doses at least 4 weeks apart and the third dose 6–12 months after the second.
- For incompletely vaccinated (i.e., less than 3 doses) adults, administer remaining doses.
- Refer to the Advisory Committee on Immunization Practices (ACIP) statement for recommendations for administering Td/Tdap as prophylaxis in wound management (see footnote #1).

4. Varicella vaccination

- All adults without evidence of immunity to varicella (as defined below) should receive 2 doses of single-antigen varicella vaccine or a second dose if they have received only 1 dose.
- Special consideration for vaccination should be given to those who have close contact with persons at high risk for severe disease (e.g., health-care personnel and family contacts of persons with immunocompromising conditions) or are at high risk for exposure or transmission (e.g., teachers; child care employees; residents and staff members of institutional settings, including correctional institutions; college students; military personnel; adolescents and adults living in households with children; nonpregnant women of childbearing age; and international travelers).
- Pregnant women should be assessed for evidence of varicella immunity. Women who do not have evidence of immunity should receive the first dose of varicella vaccine upon completion or termination of pregnancy and before discharge from the health-care facility. The second dose should be administered 4–8 weeks after the first dose.
- Evidence of immunity to varicella in adults includes any of the following:
  — documentation of 2 doses of varicella vaccine at least 4 weeks apart;
  — U.S.-born before 1980 except health-care personnel and pregnant women;
  — history of varicella based on diagnosis or verification of varicella disease by a health-care provider;
  — history of herpes zoster based on diagnosis or verification of herpes zoster disease by a health-care provider; or
  — laboratory evidence of immunity or laboratory confirmation of disease.

5. Human papillomavirus (HPV) vaccination

- Two vaccines are licensed for use in females, bivalent HPV vaccine (HPV2) and quadrivalent HPV vaccine (HPV4), and one HPV vaccine for use in males (HPV4).
- For females, either HPV4 or HPV2 is recommended in a 3-dose series for routine vaccination at age 11 or 12 years, and for those aged 13 through 26 years, if not previously vaccinated.
- For males, HPV4 is recommended in a 3-dose series for routine vaccination at age 11 or 12 years, and for those aged 13 through 21 years,

— adults younger than age 65 years with chronic lung disease (including chronic obstructive pulmonary disease, emphysema, and asthma); chronic cardiovascular diseases; diabetes mellitus; chronic renal failure; nephrotic syndrome; chronic liver disease (including cirrhosis); alcoholism; cochlear implants; cerebrospinal fluid leaks; immunocompromising conditions; and functional or anatomic asplenia (e.g., sickle cell disease and other hemoglobinopathies, congenital or acquired asplenia, splenic dysfunction, or splenectomy [if elective splenectomy is planned, vaccinate at least 2 weeks before surgery]);
— residents of nursing homes or long-term care facilities; and
— adults who smoke cigarettes.

- Persons with immunocompromising conditions and other selected conditions are recommended to receive PCV13 and PPSV23 vaccines. See footnote #10 for information on timing of PCV13 and PPSV23 vaccinations.
- Persons with symptomatic or symptomatic HIV infection should be vaccinated as soon as possible after their diagnosis.
- When cancer chemotherapy or other immunosuppressive therapy is being considered, the interval between vaccination and initiation of immunosuppressive therapy should be at least 2 weeks. Vaccination during chemotherapy or radiation therapy should be avoided.
- Routine use of PPSV23 is not recommended for American Indians/Alaska Natives or other persons younger than age 65 years unless they have underlying medical conditions that are PPSV23 indications. However, public health authorities may consider recommending PPSV23 for American Indians/Alaska Natives who are living in areas where the risk for invasive pneumococcal disease is increased.
- When indicated, PPSV23 should be administered to patients who are uncertain of their vaccination status and there is no record of previous vaccination. When PCV13 is also indicated, a dose of PCV13 should be given first (see footnote #10).

9. Revaccination with PPSV23

- One-time revaccination 5 years after the first dose is recommended for persons aged 19 through 64 years with chronic renal failure or nephrotic syndrome; functional or anatomic asplenia (e.g., sickle cell disease or splenectomy); and for persons with immunocompromising conditions.
- Persons who received 1 or 2 doses of PPSV23 before age 65 years for any indication should receive another dose of the vaccine at age 65 years or later if at least 5 years have passed since their previous dose.
- No further doses are needed for persons vaccinated with PPSV23 at or after age 65 years.

10. Pneumococcal conjugate 13-valent vaccination (PCV13)

- Adults aged 19 years or older with immunocompromising conditions (including chronic renal failure and nephrotic syndrome), functional or anatomic asplenia, CSF leaks or cochlear implants, and who have not previously received PCV13 or PPSV23 should receive a single dose of PCV13 followed by a dose of PPSV23 at least 8 weeks later.
- Adults aged 19 years or older with the aforementioned conditions who have previously received one or more doses of PPSV23 should receive a dose of PCV13 one or more years after the last PPSV23 dose was received. For those that require additional doses of PPSV23, the first such dose should be given no sooner than 8 weeks after PCV13 and at least 5 years since the most recent dose of PPSV23.
- When indicated, PCV13 should be administered to patients who are uncertain of their vaccination status history and there is no record of previous vaccination.
- Although PCV13 is licensed by the Food and Drug Administration (FDA) for use among and can be administered to persons aged 50 years and older, ACIP recommends PCV13 for adults aged 19 years and older with the specific medical conditions noted above.

11. Meningococcal vaccination

- Administer 2 doses of meningococcal conjugate vaccine quadrivalent (MCV4) at least 2 months apart to adults with functional asplenia or persistent complement component deficiencies.
- HIV-infected persons who are vaccinated also should receive 2 doses.
- Administer a single dose of meningococcal vaccine to microbiologists routinely exposed to isolates of Neisseria meningitidis, military recruits, and persons who travel to or live in countries in which meningococcal disease is hyperendemic or epidemic.
- First-year college students up through age 21 years who are living in residence halls should be vaccinated if they have not received a dose on or after their 16th birthday.
- MCV4 is preferred for adults with any of the preceding indications who are aged 55 years and younger; meningococcal polysaccharide vaccine (MPSV4) is preferred for adults aged 56 years and older.
- Revaccination with MCV4 every 5 years is recommended for adults previously vaccinated with MCV4 or MPSV4 who remain at increased risk for infection (e.g., adults with anatomic or functional asplenia or persistent complement component deficiencies).

12. Hepatitis A vaccination

- Vaccinate any person seeking protection from hepatitis A virus (HAV) infection and persons with any of the following indications:

Appendix C (continued)

— men who have sex with men and persons who use injection or noninjection illicit drugs;

— persons working with HAV-infected primates or with HAV in a research laboratory setting;

— persons with chronic liver disease and persons who receive clotting factor concentrates;

— persons travelling to or working in countries that have high or intermediate endemicity of hepatitis A; and

— unvaccinated persons who anticipate close personal contact (e.g., household or regular babysitting) with an international adoptee during the first 60 days after arrival in the United States from a country with high or intermediate endemicity. (See footnote #1 for more information on travel recommendations). The first dose of the 2-dose hepatitis A vaccine series should be administered as soon as adoption is planned, ideally 2 or more weeks before the arrival of the adoptee.

• Single-antigen vaccine formulations should be administered in a 2-dose schedule at either 0 and 6–12 months (Havrix), or 0 and 6–18 months (Vaqta). If the combined hepatitis A and hepatitis B vaccine (Twinrix) is used, administer 3 doses at 0, 1, and 6 months; alternatively, a 4-dose schedule may be used, administered on days 0, 7, and 21–30, followed by a booster dose at month 12.

13. **Hepatitis B vaccination**

• Vaccinate persons with any of the following indications and any person seeking protection from hepatitis B virus (HBV) infection:

— sexually active persons who are not in a long-term, mutually monogamous relationship (e.g., persons with more than one sex partner during the previous 6 months); persons seeking evaluation or treatment for a sexually transmitted disease (STD); current or recent injection-drug users; and men who have sex with men;

— health-care personnel and public-safety workers who are potentially exposed to blood or other infectious body fluids;

— persons with diabetes younger than age 60 years as soon as feasible after diagnosis; persons with diabetes who are age 60 years or older at the discretion of the treating clinician based on increased need for assisted blood glucose monitoring in long-term care facilities, likelihood of acquiring hepatitis B infection, its complications or chronic sequelae, and likelihood of immune response to vaccination;

— persons with end-stage renal disease, including patients receiving hemodialysis; persons with HIV infection; and persons with chronic liver disease;

— household contacts and sex partners of hepatitis B surface antigen-positive persons; clients and staff members of institutions for persons with developmental disabilities; and international travelers to countries with high or intermediate prevalence of chronic HBV infection; and

— all adults in the following settings: STD treatment facilities; HIV testing and treatment facilities; facilities providing drug-abuse treatment and prevention services; health-care settings targeting services to injection-drug users or men who have sex with men; correctional facilities; end-stage renal disease programs and facilities for chronic hemodialysis patients; and institutions and nonresidential daycare facilities for persons with developmental disabilities.

• Administer missing doses to complete a 3-dose series of hepatitis B vaccine to those persons not vaccinated or not completely vaccinated. The second dose should be administered 1 month after the first dose; the third dose should be given at least 2 months after the second dose (and at least 4 months after the first dose). If the combined hepatitis A and hepatitis B vaccine (Twinrix) is used, give 3 doses at 0, 1, and 6 months; alternatively, a 4-dose Twinrix schedule, administered on days 0, 7, and 21–30 followed by a booster dose at month 12 may be used.

• Adult patients receiving hemodialysis or with other immunocompromising conditions should receive 1 dose of 40 μg/mL (Recombivax HB) administered on a 3-dose schedule at 0, 1, and 6 months or 2 doses of 20 μg/mL (Engerix-B) administered simultaneously on a 4-dose schedule at 0, 1, 2, and 6 months.

14. **Selected conditions for which Haemophilus influenzae type b (Hib) vaccine may be used**

• 1 dose of Hib vaccine should be considered for persons who have sickle cell disease, leukemia, or HIV infection, or who have anatomic or functional asplenia if they have not previously received Hib vaccine.

15. **Immunocompromising conditions**

• Inactivated vaccines generally are acceptable (e.g., pneumococcal, meningococcal, and influenza [inactivated influenza vaccine]), and live vaccines generally are avoided in persons with immune deficiencies or immunocompromising conditions. Information on specific conditions is available at http://www.cdc.gov/vaccines/pubs/acip-list.htm.

If not previously vaccinated. Males aged 22 through 26 years may be vaccinated.

• HPV4 is recommended for men who have sex with men (MSM) through age 26 years for those who did not get any or all doses when they were younger.

• Vaccination is recommended for immunocompromised persons (including those with HIV infection) through age 26 years for those who did not get any or all doses when they were younger.

• A complete series for either HPV4 or HPV2 consists of 3 doses. The second dose should be administered 1–2 months after the first dose; the third dose should be administered 6 months after the first dose (at least 24 weeks after the first dose).

• HPV vaccines are not recommended for use in pregnant women. However, pregnancy testing is not needed before vaccination. If a woman is found to be pregnant after initiating the vaccination series, no intervention is needed; the remainder of the 3-dose series should be delayed until completion of pregnancy.

• Although HPV vaccination is not specifically recommended for health-care personnel (HCP) based on their occupation, HCP should receive the HPV vaccine as is recommended (see above).

6. **Zoster vaccination**

• A single dose of zoster vaccine is recommended for adults aged 60 years and older regardless of whether they report a prior episode of herpes zoster. Although the vaccine is licensed by the Food and Drug Administration (FDA) for use among and can be administered to persons aged 50 years and older, ACIP recommends that vaccination begin at age 60 years.

• Persons aged 60 years and older with chronic medical conditions may be vaccinated unless their condition constitutes a contraindication, such as pregnancy or severe immunodeficiency.

• Although zoster vaccination is not specifically recommended for HCP, they should receive the vaccine if they are in the recommended age group.

7. **Measles, mumps, rubella (MMR) vaccination**

• Adults born before 1957 generally are considered immune to measles and mumps. All adults born in 1957 or later should have documentation of 1 or more doses of MMR vaccine unless they have a medical contraindication to the vaccine, or laboratory evidence of immunity to each of the three diseases. Documentation of provider-diagnosed disease is not considered acceptable evidence of immunity for measles, mumps, or rubella.

Measles component:

• A routine second dose of MMR vaccine, administered a minimum of 28 days after the first dose, is recommended for adults who

— are students in postsecondary educational institutions;

— work in a health-care facility; or

— plan to travel internationally.

• Persons who received inactivated (killed) measles vaccine or measles vaccine of unknown type during 1963–1967 should be revaccinated with 2 doses of MMR vaccine.

Mumps component:

• A routine second dose of MMR vaccine, administered a minimum of 28 days after the first dose, is recommended for adults who

— are students in a postsecondary educational institution;

— work in a health-care facility; or

— plan to travel internationally.

• Persons vaccinated before 1979 with either killed mumps vaccine or mumps vaccine of unknown type who are at high risk for mumps infection (e.g., persons who are working in a health-care facility) should be considered for revaccination with 2 doses of MMR vaccine.

Rubella component:

• For women of childbearing age, regardless of birth year, rubella immunity should be determined. If there is no evidence of immunity, women who are not pregnant should be vaccinated. Pregnant women who do not have evidence of immunity should receive MMR vaccine upon completion or termination of pregnancy and before discharge from the health-care facility.

HCP born before 1957:

• For unvaccinated health-care personnel born before 1957 who lack laboratory evidence of measles, mumps, and/or rubella immunity or laboratory confirmation of disease, health-care facilities should consider vaccinating personnel with 2 doses of MMR vaccine for measles and mumps and/or 1 dose of MMR vaccine for rubella.

8. **Pneumococcal polysaccharide (PPSV23) vaccination**

• Vaccinate all persons with the following indications:

— all adults aged 65 years and older;

http://www.cdc.gov/vaccines/schedules/hcp/index.html

References

1. Immigrant, Refugee and Migrant Health Branch. About refugees. CDC. 2012. http://www.cdc. gov/immigrantrefugeehealth/about-refugees.html. Accessed Jul 2013.
2. Advisory Committee on Immunization Practices (ACIP). CDC. 2012. http://www.cdc.gov/ vaccines/acip/index.html. Accessed Jul 2013.
3. WHO vaccine-preventable diseases: monitoring system, 2004 global summary. WHO. Geneva: World Health Organization; 2004. Accessed Jul 2013.
4. Immunization Action Coalition. 2013. http://www.immunize.org. Accessed Aug 2013.
5. Wu T, Lin H, Wang L. Chronic hepatitis B infection in adolescents who received primary infantile vaccination. Hepatology. 2013;57:37–45.
6. Ogbuanu I, Kutty P, Hudson J, et al. Impact of a third dose of measles-mumps-rubella vaccine on a mumps outbreak. Pediatrics. 2012;130(6):e1567–74.
7. CPT Codes for Refugee Medical Assistance. Office for Refugee Resettlement. 2012. http:// www.acf.hhs.gov/programs/orr/resource/medical-screening-protocol-for-newly-arriving-refugees. Accessed Aug 2013.
8. Technical instructions for vaccination for civil surgeons. CDC. 2009. http://www.cdc.gov/ immigrantrefugeehealth/exams/ti/civil/vaccination-civil-technical-instructions.html#changes. Accessed Jul 2013.
9. Plotkin S, Orenstein W, Offit P. Vaccines. 5th ed. London: Saunders Elsevier; 2008.
10. Quinlisk M. Mumps control today. J Infect Dis. 2010;202:655–6.
11. Greenaway C, Dongier P, Boivin J, et al. Susceptibility to measles, mumps, and rubella in newly arrived adult immigrants and refugees. Ann Intern Med. 2007;146:20–4.
12. Barnett E, Christiansen D, Figueira M. Seroprevalence of measles, rubella, and varicella in refugees. Clin Infect Dis. 2002;35(4):403–8.
13. Danovaro-Holliday M, LeBaron C, Allensworth C, et al. A large rubella outbreak with spread from the workplace to community. JAMA. 2000;284:2733–9.
14. Epidemiology and prevention of vaccine-preventable diseases (The Pink Book). May 2012. http://www.cdc.gov/vaccines/pubs/pinkbook/downloads/meas.pdf.
15. Pottie K, Greenaway C, Feightner J, et al. Evidence-based clinical guidelines for immigrants and refugees. CMAJ. 2011;183(12):E824–925.
16. Recommendations for routine testing and follow-up for chronic hepatitis B virus (HBV) infection. CDC. 2012. http://www.cdc.gov/hepatitis/hbv/PDFs/ChronicHepBTestingFlwUp.pdf. Accessed Aug 2013.
17. Rossi C, Shrier I, Marshall L, et al. Seroprevalence of chronic hepatitis B virus infection and prior immunity in immigrants and refugees: a systematic review and meta-analysis. PLoS One. 2012;7(9):e44611.
18. Interpretation of hepatitis B serologic test results. CDC. 2012. http://www.cdc.gov/hepatitis/ HBV/PDFs/SerologicChartv8.pdf. Accessed Aug 2013.
19. Lee B. Review of varicella zoster seroepidemiology in India and Southeast Asia. Trop Med Int Health. 1998;3:886–90.
20. Garnett G, Cox M, Bundy D, et al. The age of infection with varicella virus in St Lucia, West Indies. Epidemiol Infect. 1993;110:361–72.
21. Nysse L, Pinksy N, Bratberg J, et al. Seroprevalence of antibodies to varicella zoster virus among Somali refugees. Mayo Clin Proc. 2007;82:175–80.
22. Figueira M, Christiansen D, Barnett E. Cost-effectiveness of serotesting compared with universal immunization for varicella in refugee children from six geographic regions. J Travel Med. 2003;10:203–7.
23. Breuer J, Schmid D, Gershon A. Use and limitations of varicella-zoster virus-specific serological testing to evaluate breakthrough disease in vaccines and to screen for susceptibility to varicella. J Infect Dis. 2008;197 Suppl 2:S147–51.

Chapter 5
Tuberculosis

Andrew T. Boyd

Introduction

Tuberculosis (TB) remains a worldwide threat to global health. Despite the existence of a multidrug treatment regimen known to cure 90 % of cases, there were 9 million new cases of tuberculosis and 1.4 million deaths from the disease in 2011 [1]. An infectious disease caused by the bacillus *Mycobacterium tuberculosis*, it is transmitted by inhalation of aerosolized droplets containing the bacillus and can affect the lungs or many other sites in the body. Recognition of cases of tuberculosis is difficult, since most people carrying tuberculosis do not develop active disease but instead have *latent tuberculosis infection* (LTBI); recognition, however, is important because reactivation of latent infection leads to transmission of the bacteria.

Pathogenesis

Primary tuberculosis infection occurs when inhaled bacilli enter the lungs, where they are ingested by alveolar macrophages. The mycobacteria-laden macrophages can then penetrate the alveolar wall to enter the circulation and the lymphatic system, allowing lymphocytic sensitization to mycobacterial antigens. At that point, in most patients, the lymphocytes and macrophages form granulomas around the mycobacteria in sites where it has settled, effectively "walling off" the mycobacteria. The mycobacteria, though still viable, enter into a quiescent or latent phase in order to survive in these sites, which usually consist of lung tissue, but can also include

A.T. Boyd, M.D. (✉)
Médecins Sans Frontières, 333, Seventh Avenue, Second Floor, New York, NY 10001, USA

Yale Internal Medicine Residency, New Haven, CT, USA
e-mail: andrewthomasboyd@gmail.com

A. Annamalai (ed.), *Refugee Health Care: An Essential Medical Guide*,
DOI 10.1007/978-1-4939-0271-2_5, © Springer Science+Business Media New York 2014

lymph nodes, bones, and other organs. It should be noted that in immunosuppressed, HIV-positive patients, this containment does not occur, and the mycobacteria circulate further, leading to the failure of multiple organ systems and death [2].

In the setting of a normal immune system, the mycobacteria remain in a latent phase, and the patient is said to have *latent tuberculosis infection* (*LTBI*). In about 10 % of cases of LTBI, however, the latency of the mycobacteria is disturbed and the infection again becomes active, resulting in a clinical entity known as *reactivation tuberculosis*. Those cases in which reactivation occurs are difficult to predict, though risk factors include several medical conditions, including HIV/AIDS, chronic steroid use, chemotherapy, post-organ transplant, use of TNF-alpha inhibitors, diabetes mellitus, lymphoma/leukemia, and end-stage renal disease [3]. Because a prior latent state is required for reactivation, and because reactivation is required for infectious transmission of the bacteria, treating LTBI as a means to prevent active tuberculosis disease has become a priority for US public health officials [3].

Due to the high morbidity burden of tuberculosis, worsened in the setting of the HIV pandemic, the World Health Organization declared TB a global health emergency in 1993, and since then, substantial progress has been made in controlling the disease. Specifically, incident cases of TB have fallen from 150 cases per 100,000 people in 1990 to 125 cases per 100,000 people in 2011. More impressively, the mortality rate from TB has fallen 41 % during the same time period [1].

Tuberculosis control in the United States has been yet more successful. The incident active TB case rate was 3.4 cases per 100,000 people in 2011, which represented a 6.4 % drop from the rate in 2010 as well as the lowest incident rate recorded since national reporting began in 1953 [4]. It should be noted, however, that the rate of incident cases of active tuberculosis (both new infections and reactivation of latent infection) among foreign-born people in the United States was 12 times that of native-born people [4].

Overseas Screening for TB

Federal law requires that anyone applying for refugee status in the United States receive a predeparture, overseas medical evaluation. The content of the medical evaluation is dictated by the Centers for Disease Control and Prevention's Division of Global Migration and Quarantine. In general, the purpose of the medical examination is to identify applicants with diseases or conditions that, by federal law, either exclude them from entering the United States or require documented treatment before entering the United States. In the specific case of tuberculosis, the purpose of the examination is to identify people with active, infectious tuberculosis disease [5].

The overseas medical evaluation is performed by 1 of 400 panel physicians, appointed by US embassies. The content is provided by the CDC to these panel physicians via "Technical Instructions," updated in both 2007 and 2009 and available online [6]. Essentially, each evaluation of an applicant 15 years old or older should include documented medical history, focused on symptoms of active tuberculosis disease, including cough of greater than 3 weeks duration, dyspnea,

Table 5.1 Classification based on overseas TB evaluation

TB classification	TB status	Results of TB screening
Class A	Infectious TB	TB disease diagnosed (smear or culture+) and require treatment (either with full course overseas or with waiver described below)
Class B1: pulmonary	Active TB, not infectious	No treatment: history or CXR suggests TB but sputum/culture negative
		Completed treatment: diagnosed with pulmonary TB and finished treatment before immigration
Class B1: extrapulmonary	Active extrapulmonary TB, not infectious	Evidence of extrapulmonary TB
Class B2	TB, not clinically active	Abnormal CXR without symptoms. Needs LTBI evaluation
Class B3	TB, old or healed	Abnormal CXR but consistent with resolved disease. Needs contact evaluation
No TB class	No evidence of TB	Normal TB screening

fever, weight loss, or hemoptysis, as well as a physical examination and a chest X-ray [6]. If symptoms, physical examination, or chest X-ray is suggestive of active TB, three sputum smears are examined [6].

Evaluation of applicants ages 2–14 from countries with a WHO-estimated TB incidence rate of $\geq$20 cases per 100,000 population should have a screening test with tuberculin skin test (TST) or with interferon-gamma release assay (IGRA). (A list of those countries with incidence rates can be found in the WHO Global TB Report 2012, page 19.) If the TST is $\geq$10 mm or the IGRA is positive, or if the applicant has symptoms of tuberculosis, then a chest X-ray should be obtained. Again, if symptoms, physical examination, or chest X-ray is suggestive of active TB, three sputum smears are examined [6].

Evaluation of applicants less than age 2 from countries with a WHO-estimated TB incidence rate of $\geq$20 cases per 100,000 population or any child of age less than 15 from countries with a WHO-estimated TB incidence rate of <20 cases per 100,000 population should undergo a physical examination and have a history provided by a responsible adult. Those applicants with symptoms of TB should receive a TST or IGRA and a chest X-ray and have three sputum smears examined [6]. Children over age 15, for purposes of tuberculosis screening, are treated as adults.

Based on the results of these tests, each applicant is assigned a *class*. Each class and its requirements are documented in Table 5.1.

Anyone designated *Class A* cannot enter the United States until either (a) he/she has completed a course of therapy, his/her sputum smear converts to negative, and he/she is reclassified to a class permitted entry or (b) he/she initiates treatment overseas, demonstrates smear conversion to negative, and obtains a waiver to enter the United States, provided a US-based provider agrees to assume responsibility for the patient's completion of the full treatment course [6]. Anyone designated *Class B1*, *Class B2*, or *Class B3* is permitted entry.

Epidemiology of TB in Refugees

Although the WHO notes declining incidence of TB worldwide, many countries still have very poor control of TB. The 22 countries classified by the WHO as "high-burden countries" have an average TB incidence of 163 cases per 100,000 people, though there are several with TB incident rates on the order of 200–300 cases per 100,000 people. Most countries on the "high-burden countries" list are in Asia or Sub-Saharan Africa, the two regions from which most refugees come to the United States [1].

Concurrently, the current overseas medical screening identifies active tuberculosis disease and does not screen for latent tuberculosis infection (LTBI). It is estimated that among all immigrants to Canada, 30–50 % of them, or around 1.5 million people, have LTBI [7], while in the United States, the number of foreign-born persons with LTBI is likely closer to 7 million people [8]. While the probability of developing active TB disease from reactivation of LTBI in all immigrants is only 5–10 % annually [9], the risk of developing active TB disease from reactivation of LTBI in refugee populations is two times higher than that [10]. This doubling of risk is thought to be due to an overall higher prevalence of LTBI and increased rate of recent acquisition of exposure to tuberculosis [11].

Finally, though the overall incidence of TB reached its lowest level ever in the United States in 2011, it should be noted that 62.5 % of all incident cases were found in foreign-born persons [4]. Another retrospective review of the demographics of cases of active TB found that of the cases of foreign-born persons with active TB, fully 50 % had been in the United States for more than 5 years [12]. Such persistence of reactivation of LTBI speaks to the need for screening newly arrived refugees for LTBI, as well as the need to treat LTBI in this population.

Diagnosis

Because of the higher risk of reactivation of LTBI in the refugee population, domestic tuberculosis screening focuses on identification of LTBI cases among newly arrived refugees with the goal of prevention of reactivation of tuberculosis disease. It should also be noted that though the CDC TB technical instructions require a screening test for LTBI for certain populations, these are rarely done in practice overseas as part of the general medical evaluation. Once in the United States, LTBI diagnosis is made by screening for exposure to *Mycobacterium tuberculosis* antigens. To this end, diagnosis can be made using one of two screening tests: the tuberculin skin test (TST) or the interferon-gamma release assay, or IGRA [3].

The older of the two tests is the TST. The test requires that five units of purified protein derivative (PPD) of *M. tuberculosis* be injected subcutaneously, usually on the forearm, just beneath the skin to create a wheal [13]. This test is a universal screen, and it can be performed in children and pregnant women. The test is considered positive, and therefore represents the presence of *M. tuberculosis* antigen in the

Table 5.2 Interpretation of TB induration based on risk factors

5 or more millimeters	10 or more millimeters	15 or more millimeters
An induration of 5 or more millimeters is considered positive for: • HIV-infected persons • Recent contacts of persons with infectious TB • People who have fibrotic changes on a chest radiograph • Patients with organ transplants and other immunosuppressed patients (including patients taking a prolonged course of oral or intravenous corticosteroids or TNF-α antagonists)	An induration of 10 or more millimeters is considered positive for: • People who have come to the United States within the last 5 years from areas of the world where TB is common (e.g., Asia, Africa, Eastern Europe, Russia, or Latin America) • Injection drug users • Mycobacteriology lab workers • People who live or work in high-risk congregate settings • People with certain medical conditions that place them at high risk for TB (silicosis, diabetes mellitus, severe kidney disease, certain types of cancer, and certain intestinal conditions) • Children younger than 4 years • Infants, children, and adolescents exposed to adults in high-risk categories	An induration of 15 or more millimeters is considered positive for: • People with no known risk factors for TB

patient, if the radius of the indurated area at the injection site is larger than a predetermined size, which varies depending on a patient's medical risk factors (see Table 5.2 above) [14].

Though the TST has good sensitivity for LTBI, with a pooled estimate of 77 % in a recent meta-analysis [15], its specificity is rather poor, with false-positives possible if a patient has had exposure to other non-tuberculous mycobacteria or to vaccination with bacillus Calmette-Guerin (BCG), which is often administered to infants in countries with high burden of tuberculosis. It should be noted, however, that a cross-reaction between BCG vaccination and a positive TST rapidly wanes with time. It has been found that in those people vaccinated as infants, a TST done 10 years later will be positive in only 1–2 % of cases [10]. In addition, because those patients vaccinated with BCG come from high-burden countries, there is likely a high prevalence of LTBI among them. For these reasons, according to CDC screening policy, a positive TST in a patient immunized with BCG, regardless of the age at which the patient is screened, should still be treated as a case of true LTBI [5].

Due partially to concerns about the poor specificity of the TST, a blood test called the interferon-gamma release assay (IGRA) was developed, and two proprietary assays (the QuantiFERON Gold and T-SPOT.TB) have been approved by the FDA for use as an initial screening test for LTBI diagnosis. It should be noted that in the United States, though the IGRA test can be used in children 5 years old or older, its use is not recommended for children under 5, due in part to poorer sensitivity of the test in that age group [16]. Thus, in children under 5, the TST should be used [16]. These tests quantify amount of interferon-gamma formation or the number of T lymphocytes recruited in the patient's serum when combined with surface antigens found in *M. tuberculosis* and a small number of other rare mycobacteria, but, importantly, not found in BCG or in common environmental mycobacteria. Thus, the IGRA has improved specificity for LTBI [15]. It should be noted, however, that correct interpretation of the IGRA requires, just as that of the TST requires, active cellular immunity in the patient, so the sensitivities of the two tests are equivalent. Neither test is able to predict which 10 % of patients with LTBI will go on to develop active infection [3].

Currently, the CDC recommends the use of either the TST or the IGRA as a screening test for LTBI in adults [17]. In Canada, the latest guidelines recommend using the TST as the primary screening test and then to use the IGRA as the confirmatory test in those patients with a high likelihood of a false-positive TST result [10]. The Canadian approach is supported by a recent cost-effectiveness analysis [18]. But given that IGRA is unaffected by prior BCG vaccination, providers may choose to use it for initial testing in refugee populations. For children <5 years, CDC recommends TST as there is limited data on using IGRA in this age group.

Current CDC guidelines stipulate that every refugee should be screened for LTBI. It should be noted, however, that a given positive screen necessitates a willingness of the medical establishment to treat that patient. Since treatment is time-consuming (usually 6–9 months, detailed further in the following section) and costly, recent cost-effectiveness analyses have called that policy into question. Specifically, one study found that based on cost-effectiveness analysis, screening could be limited to those refugees coming from countries with a high burden of incident infectious tuberculosis cases (150 incident cases/100,000 population) [19], and one study found that cost-effectiveness analysis indicates that screening should focus on active tuberculosis cases and the intensive tracking and treatment of their close contacts [20].

Treatment

If a refugee has a positive screening TST or IGRA, he or she should be screened immediately for active tuberculosis disease. This screening should be similar to that done in the overseas medical evaluation and should again focus on symptoms of tuberculosis disease, such as cough of greater than 3 weeks duration, dyspnea, fever, weight loss, or hemoptysis. In children, symptoms may be more nonspecific and may include recurrent fevers or pneumonias or simply failure to thrive [5]. The screening should also include a physical examination, with a focus on forceful or productive cough or palpable lymph nodes, and a chest X-ray, with attention paid to cavitary or extensive lesions in the upper lobes [6]. Health providers should be aware that children are more likely than adults to have extrapulmonary tuberculosis

Table 5.3 Basic TB disease treatment regimens

Preferred regimen	Alternative regimen	Alternative regimen
Initial phase	Initial phase	Initial phase
Daily INH, RIF, PZA, and EMB[a] for 56 doses (8 weeks)	Daily INH, RIF, PZA, and EMB[a] for 14 doses (2 weeks), then twice weekly for 12 doses (6 weeks)	Thrice-weekly INH, RIF, PZA, and EMB[a] for 24 doses (8 weeks)
Continuation phase	Continuation phase	Continuation phase
Daily INH and RIF for 126 doses (18 weeks) or twice-weekly INH and RIF for 36 doses (18 weeks)	Twice-weekly INH and RIF for 36 doses (18 weeks)	Thrice-weekly INH and RIF for 54 doses (18 weeks)

[a]EMB can be discontinued if drug susceptibility studies demonstrate susceptibility to first-line drugs

disease, including meningitis, mastoiditis, or involvement of lymph nodes or bone [5]. If symptoms, physical examination, or chest X-ray is suggestive of active TB, three sputum smears should be obtained and examined.

It should be noted that provision of sputum can be difficult for very young children, so early morning gastric aspirate collection, which usually requires hospitalization, can substitute for sputum collection [6].

If, based on suggestive symptoms, chest X-ray, or at least one positive sputum smear, a refugee is thought to have active tuberculosis, he or she should be started on treatment immediately. Due to the slow growth of the mycobacteria, and its ability to develop resistance to drugs, treatment is for at least 6 months and requires an initial four-drug regimen (rifampin, RIF; isoniazid, INH; pyrazinamide, PZA; and ethambutol, EMB, the so-called RIPE regimen) for 2 months followed by modification of the drug regimen based on drug susceptibility from the patient's isolate [21]. See Table 5.3 above.

It should be noted that the treatment regimens above can also be used in infants, children, and adolescents, with the exception that EMB is not routinely used in children. The current first-line recommendation for children is 6 months of INH and RIF supplemented for the first 2 months with PZA [22]. Information on dosing in adults and children can be found online at http://www.cdc.gov/mmwr/preview/mmwrhtml/rr5211a1.htm.

If a refugee has a positive screening TST or IGRA but does not have symptoms or a chest X-ray concerning for active tuberculosis, CDC guidelines stipulate that he or she should be treated for latent tuberculosis infection (LTBI). As stated previously, refugees have a twofold higher incidence of reactivation of tuberculosis compared to other immigrant groups [10]. In addition, because reactivation of tuberculosis could then lead to transmission to others of active disease, treatment of LTBI in this population could serve as prevention of future cases of active tuberculosis.

Treatment of LTBI most commonly consists of 9 months of daily oral isoniazid (INH) for all ages. The efficacy of INH as compared to no treatment in reducing rate

Table 5.4 Latent TB infection treatment regimens

Drugs	Duration	Interval	Minimum doses
Isoniazid	9 months	Daily	270
		Twice weekly[a]	76
Isoniazid	6 months	Daily	180
		Twice weekly[a]	52
Isoniazid and rifapentine	3 months	Once weekly[a]	12
Rifampin	4 months	Daily	120

[a]Use directly observed therapy (DOT)

of incident active tuberculosis disease was established in a Cochrane review of 11 randomized controlled trials [23]. One known complication of isoniazid therapy is development of hepatitis, and while current guidelines do not require checking baseline liver function tests in all patients receiving treatment for LTBI, they suggest a check prior to treatment initiation in those with baseline liver disease, those who are pregnant, those with HIV, and those with daily alcohol use [17]. After initiation of treatment, liver function tests should be checked every 3 months, and treatment should be stopped if the test numbers rise to five times the upper limit of normal or if the patient develops signs and symptoms of overt hepatitis [17].

One of the difficulties in initiating treatment is its relatively long duration, and research has recently been done to devise equivalent, shorter treatment regimens. Rifampin, given for 4 months, is one acceptable alternative to 9 months of isoniazid [3]. In addition, a recent randomized controlled trial comparing directly observed administration of daily isoniazid and rifapentine for 3 months with standard self-administered isoniazid for 9 months found the shorter course non-inferior to the standard treatment [24]. The current CDC recommendations for treatment regimens for LTBI reflect these alternative regimens [25]. See Table 5.4 above.

Dosing is listed in Table 5.5 below, although the isoniazid/rifapentine dosing is not included in this figure [17]. It should be noted that the newer isoniazid/rifapentine regimen has not been assessed in a sufficient number of children younger than age 12, and in this population, the recommendation is still 9 months of daily INH [26].

In both cases of active tuberculosis disease and latent tuberculosis infection, case management is very important. In active tuberculosis disease cases, a contact investigation of close contacts to the index case should be initiated to screen and offer treatment for high-risk persons [27]. Guidelines for conducting a contact investigation are available online from the CDC at http://www.cdc.gov/mmwr/preview/mmwrhtml/rr5415a1.htm. Directly observed therapy for active and latent tuberculosis infection treatment is important for those patients with drug-resistant tuberculosis and for those treated for LTBI on a time-shortened regimen. Case management allows monitoring for adverse effects of medication [3]. Finally, thorough case management, including assuring adherence to a full course of treatment, greatly improves the chance of eradication of the infection, either active or latent, and lessens the chance of inducing secondary drug resistance. In this way, the burden of tuberculosis in this particularly vulnerable population can be reduced over time.

Table 5.5 Dosing regimens for LTBI

Drug/dose	Frequency/duration (doses)	Rating[a] (evidence)[b]	
		HIV negative	HIV positive
Preferred regimen			
Isoniazid			
Adult: 5 mg/kg	Daily × 9 months (270 doses)	A (II)	A (II)
Children: 10–20 mg/kg			
Maximum dose: 300 mg			
Alternate regimens			
Isoniazid			
Adult: 15 mg/kg	Twice weekly × 9 months[c]	B (II)	B (II)
Children: 20–40 mg/kg	(76 doses)		
Maximum dose: 900 mg			
Isoniazid			
Adults: 5 mg/kg	Daily × 6 months (180 doses)	B (I)	C (I)
Children: not recommended			
Maximum dose: 300 mg			
Isoniazid			
Adults: 15 mg/kg	Twice weekly × 6 months[c]	B (II)	C (I)
Children: not recommended	(52 doses)		
Maximum dose: 900 mg			
Rifampin			
Adults: 10 mg/kg	Daily × 4 months (120 doses)	B (II)	B (III)
Children: 10–20 mg/kg	Daily × 6 months (180 doses)		
Maximum dose: 600 mg			

Note: In situations in which rifampin cannot be used (e.g., HIV-infected persons receiving protease inhibitors), Rifabutin may be substituted

[a]Strength of the recommendation: A = preferred regimen; B = acceptable alternative; C = offer when A and B cannot be given

[b]Quality of the supporting evidence: I = randomized clinical trials data; II = data from clinical trials not randomized or from other population; III = expert opinion

[c]Intermittent regimen must be provided via directly observed therapy (DOT), i.e., health care worker observes the ingestion of medication

References

1. WHO. WHO global tuberculosis report 2012. Geneva: World Health Organization; 2012. http://www.who.int/tb/publications/global_report/gtbr12_main.pdf. Accessed Aug 2013.
2. Flynn JL, Chan J. Tuberculosis: latency and reactivation. Infect Immun. 2001;69:4195–201.
3. Bernardo J. Tuberculosis. In: Walker P, Barnett E, editors. Immigrant medicine. Philadelphia: Elsevier; 2007. p. 255–71.
4. CDC. Trends in tuberculosis—United States, 2011. MMWR Morb Mortal Wkly Rep. 2011;61(11):181–5.
5. CDC. Domestic tuberculosis guidelines. Atlanta: CDC; 2010. http://www.cdc.gov/immigrantrefugeehealth/guidelines/domestic/tuberculosis-guidelines.html. Accessed Aug 2013.
6. CDC. CDC immigration requirements: technical instructions for tuberculosis screening and treatment. Atlanta: CDC; 2009. www.cdc.gov/immigrantrefugeehealth/pdf/tuberculosis-ti-2009.pdf. 1-40. Accessed Aug 2013.

7. Public Health Agency of Canada. Canadian tuberculosis standards. 6th ed. Ottawa, ON: Tuberculosis Prevention and Control, Public Health Agency of Canada, Canadian Lung Association/Canadian Thoracic Society; 2007.

8. Barnett E. Infectious disease screening for refugees resettled in the United States. Clin Infect Dis. 2004;39:833–41.

9. Watkins RE, Brennan R, Plant AJ. Tuberculin reactivity and the risk of tuberculosis: a review. Int J Tuberc Lung Dis. 2000;4:895–903.

10. Greenaway C, Sandoe A, Vissandjee B, et al. Canadian Collaboration for Immigrant and Refugee Health. Tuberculosis: evidence review for newly arriving immigrants and refugees. CMAJ. 2011;183(12):E939–51.

11. Marras TK, Wilson J, Wang EEL, et al. Tuberculosis among Tibetan refugee claimants in Toronto: 1998 to 2000. Chest. 2003;124:915–21.

12. Cain KP, Haley CA, Armstrong LR, et al. Tuberculosis among foreign-born persons in the United States: achieving tuberculosis elimination. Am J Respir Crit Care Med. 2007; 175:75–9.

13. Lee E, Holzman RS. Evolution and current use of the tuberculin skin test. Clin Infect Dis. 2002;34:365–70.

14. CDC. Chapter 3: Testing for tuberculosis infection and disease. In: CDC, editor. Core curriculum on tuberculosis: what the clinician should know. Atlanta: CDC; 2011. p. 45–75.

15. Pai M, Zwerling A, Menzies D. Systematic review: T-cell–based assays for the diagnosis of latent tuberculosis infection: an update. Ann Intern Med. 2008;149:177–84.

16. Mazurek GH, Jereb J, Vernon A, et al. Updated guidelines for using the interferon gamma release assays to *Mycobacterium tuberculosis* infection—United States, 2010. Morb Mortal Wkly Rep. 2010;59(5):1–25.

17. CDC. Latent tuberculosis infection: a guide for primary health care providers. Atlanta: CDC; 2010. http://www.cdc.gov/tb/publications/ltbi/diagnosis.htm. Accessed Aug 2013.

18. Oxlade O, Schwartzman K, Menzies D. Interferon-gamma release assays and TB screening in high-income countries: a cost-effectiveness analysis. Int J Tuberc Lung Dis. 2007;11:16–26.

19. Pareek M, Bond M, Shorey J, et al. Community-based evaluation of immigrant tuberculosis screening using interferon gamma release assays and tuberculin skin testing: observational study and economic analysis. Thorax. 2013;68(3):230–9.

20. Dasgupta K, Menzies D. Cost-effectiveness of tuberculosis control strategies among immigrants and refugees. Eur Respir J. 2005;25(6):1107–16.

21. CDC. Treatment for TB disease. Atlanta: CDC; 2011. http://www.cdc.gov/tb/topic/treatment/tbdisease.htm. Accessed Aug 2013.

22. CDC. Treatment of tuberculosis: American Thoracic Society, CDC, and Infectious Disease Society of America. MMWR Morb Mortal Wkly Rep. 2003;52(RR11):1–77.

23. Smieja MJ, Marchetti CA, Cook DJ, et al. Isoniazid for preventing tuberculosis in non-HIV infected persons [review]. Cochrane Database Syst Rev. 2000(2):CD001363.

24. Sterling V, Borisov AS, et al. Three months of rifapentine and isoniazid for latent tuberculosis infection. N Engl J Med. 2011;365(23):2155–66.

25. CDC. Treatment of latent TB infection. Atlanta: CDC; 2012. http://www.cdc.gov/tb/topic/treatment/ltbi.htm. Accessed Aug 2013.

26. CDC. Recommendations for use of an isoniazid-rifapentine regimen with direct observation to treat latent *Mycobacterium tuberculosis* infection. MMWR Morb Mortal Wkly Rep. 2011;60:1650–3.

27. CDC. Guidelines for the investigation of contacts of persons with infectious tuberculosis: recommendations from the National Tuberculosis Controllers Association and CDC. MMWR Morb Mortal Wkly Rep. 2005;54(RR15):1–37.

Chapter 6
Intestinal Parasites

James Wallace, Anne E.P. Frosch, and William Stauffer

Intestinal Parasitic Infections in Refugees

On October 31, 2011, this planet welcomed its seven billionth inhabitant. Of that difficult to encompass number, roughly one-third harbor a parasitic infection, more than half of which are intestinal [1]. Although many of these intestinal parasitic infections are subclinical and patients who have them are asymptomatic, they can cause significant morbidity and may result in mortality. The United States welcomes immigrants from parts of the world where people are constantly and continuously exposed to intestinal parasites, many of which are diagnosed and treated upon arrival in the US. Methodological differences in studying the prevalence of a given parasite (e.g., stool ova and parasites versus serology) as well as differing characteristics of refugees such as country of origin, age, and education level render the task of determining exact numbers of immigrants affected by intestinal parasites difficult. What we do know is that they are among the most commonly seen infections in refugees, with estimates ranging from 8.4 to 84 % of refugees in North America being affected [1, 2]. See Fig. 6.1 for prevalence of intestinal parasites in a large sample of refugees in Minnesota. Starting in 1999, the CDC began implementing

J. Wallace, M.D., M.S.P.H. (✉)
Department of Medicine, University of Minnesota Medical Center,
420 Delaware St. S.E., MMC 284 PWB 14th floor Suite 100,
Minneapolis, MN 55455, USA
e-mail: walla474@umn.edu

A.E.P. Frosch, M.D., M.P.H. • W. Stauffer, M.D., M.S.P.H., CTropMed, F.A.S.T.M.H.
Division of Infectious Diseases and International Medicine,
Department of Medicine, University of Minnesota,
420 Delaware Street. S.E., Minneapolis, MN 55455, USA
e-mail: park0587@umn.edu; stauf005@umn.edu

A. Annamalai (ed.), *Refugee Health Care: An Essential Medical Guide*,
DOI 10.1007/978-1-4939-0271-2_6, © Springer Science+Business Media New York 2014

Parasite*	Total (N=26,956)	Somalia (N=11,602)	Ethiopia (N=3278)	Liberia (N=2723)	Other African Countries (N=1063)†	Laos (N=5959)	Vietnam (N=1215)	Burma (N=1116)
				number of refugees (percent)				
Any	4897 (18.2)	1775 (15.3)	423 (12.9)	565 (20.7)	242 (22.8)	1412 (23.7)	296 (24.4)	184 (16.5)
Multiple	436 (1.6)	138 (1.2)	41 (1.3)	85 (3.1)	34 (3.2)	75 (1.3)	55 (4.5)	8 (0.7)
Protozoans								
Any	2763 (10.3)	904 (7.8)	198 (6.0)	221 (8.1)	109 (10.3)	1119 (18.8)	57 (4.7)	155 (13.9)
Multiple	52 (0.2)	25 (0.2)	5 (0.2)	2 (0.1)	7 (0.7)	12 (0.2)	0	1 (0.1)
Giardia intestinalis	2368 (8.8)	629 (5.4)	179 (5.5)	204 (7.5)	80 (7.5)	1089 (18.3)	49 (4.0)	138 (12.4)
Entamoeba‡	447 (1.7)	300 (2.6)	24 (0.7)	19 (0.7)	36 (3.4)	42 (0.7)	8 (0.7)	18 (1.6)
Nematodes								
Any	1975 (7.3)	940 (8.1)	106 (3.2)	237 (8.7)	86 (8.1)	327 (5.5)	250 (20.6)	29 (2.6)
Multiple	172 (0.6)	27 (0.2)	12 (0.4)	37 (1.4)	10 (0.9)	34 (0.6)	45 (3.7)	7 (0.6)
Trichuris trichiura	1243 (4.6)	900 (7.8)	68 (2.1)	136 (5.0)	33 (3.1)	21 (0.4)	70 (5.8)	15 (1.3)
Hookworm	494 (1.8)	21 (0.2)	21 (0.6)	88 (3.2)	35 (3.3)	193 (3.2)	121 (10.0)	15 (1.3)
Ascaris lumbricoides	237 (0.9)	46 (0.4)	17 (0.5)	34 (1.2)	14 (1.3)	16 (0.3)	107 (8.8)	3 (0.3)
Strongyloides stercoralis	205 (0.8)	3 (<0.1)	13 (0.4)	23 (0.8)	15 (1.4)	132 (2.2)	13 (1.1)	6 (0.5)
Trematodes								
Schistosoma species	406 (1.5)	26 (0.2)	147 (4.5)	164 (6.0)	69 (6.5)	0	0	0

* A revised form for refugee screening data permitted reporting of additional infections to the Minnesota Department of Health beginning in 1998. The following intestinal parasites detected among newly arrived refugees were excluded from the analysis of the effect of albendazole treatment: *Blastocystis hominis* (1529 cases), *Hymenolepis nana* (360), *Dientamoeba fragilis* (100), *Clonorchis sinensis* (11), fasciola species (4), taenia species (17), *H. diminuta* (2), and diphyllobothrium species (1).
† Other countries included Benin, Burundi, Cameroon, Ivory Coast, Democratic Republic of Congo, Eritrea, Gambia, Ghana, Guinea, Guinea-Bissau, Kenya, Niger, Nigeria, Rwanda, Senegal, Sierra Leone, Sudan, Togo, and Uganda.
‡ This category includes pathogenic *Entamoeba histolytica* and nonpathogenic *E. moshkovskii* and *E. dispar*, which cannot be morphologically differentiated by means of standard light microscopy.

Fig. 6.1 Prevalence of intestinal parasites in a large refugee sample in Minnesota (Swanson SJ et al. N Engl J Med 2012;366:1498–1507)

recommendations for empiric antiparasitic treatment for refugees coming to the United States, both before departure and upon their arrival [3].

As one would expect, the prevalence of intestinal parasites in newly arriving refugees, especially the nematodes causing trichuriasis, ascariasis, and hookworm infection, has been significantly impacted by the implementation of pre-departure presumptive treatment in US-bound refugees [4]. Overall, there has been a decrease in intestinal parasitosis since starting empiric pre-departure therapy, as well as a shift in the most commonly found parasites when screened upon arrival to the United States [4] (see Fig. 6.2). Prior to implementation of pre-departure empiric therapy, the most commonly encountered organisms found during screening included hookworm infection and *Giardia* (a protozoan), whereas since 1999 the most commonly encountered helminth has become *Trichuris* [4]. Subsequent data has indicated that Strongyloides, which is not adequately treated with a single dose of albendazole, and schistosomiasis, which is not treated with albendazole, were highly prevalent infections in refugees [4]. These two parasites were of particular concern since not only are they common, they also cause chronic infection and can result in serious morbidity and even mortality. In 2007 ivermectin and praziquantel (for sub-Saharan African refugees) were recommended. Praziquantel was instituted in sub-Saharan Africans in 2010 but ivermectin has not been implemented to date [3].

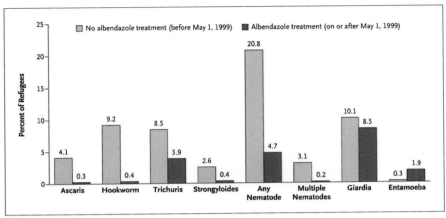

Swanson SJ et al. N Engl J Med 2012;366:1498-1507

Fig. 6.2 Change in intestinal parasitosis with empiric pre-departure therapy (Swanson SJ et al. N Engl J Med 2012;366:1498–1507)

Screening Recommendations

Optimally, refugees arriving to the United States from Africa, Asia, and Southeast Asia should receive some form of presumptive therapy for intestinal parasites. This is typically performed by the International Organization for Migration (IOM) in their home countries or in refugee camps. If they have undergone presumptive therapy, new arrivals may have documentation of their treatment course.

The term "presumptive therapy" encompasses treatment for intestinal parasites which refugees coming from certain parts of the world can be "presumed" to have based on prevalence data from a given area. The principal intestinal parasites that are targeted, as well as the medications used with presumptive therapy are:

1. Soil-transmitted helminths (STH) including the roundworms, hookworm, *Ascaris*, and *Trichuris* (albendazole)
2. *Strongyloides* (ivermectin)
3. Schistosomes (praziquantel)

It is recommended that all refugees from South and Southeast Asia, except those with contraindications, be treated with albendazole and ivermectin. It is also recommended that all refugees from Africa should be treated with albendazole and praziquantel and those from non-*Loa loa* endemic areas with ivermectin for *Strongyloides* [3]. Please see Table 6.1 for a summary of these recommendations. Of particular note when considering presumptive therapy for Africans is the importance of the parasite *Loa loa*. In areas of *Loa loa* endemicity (see Table 6.2), there have been reports of encephalitis resulting from ivermectin therapy (which targets *Strongyloides*) in patients who have a concomitant *Loa loa* infection and a high microfilarial parasite load. Because of this, any patient who comes from a *Loa loa*

Table 6.1 Recommended medication regimen for presumptive treatment of parasitic infections [3]

Refugee population	Regimens by pathogen		
	Soil-transmitted helminths: albendazole	Strongyloidiasis: ivermectin	Schistosomiasis: praziquantel
Adults			
Asia, Middle East, North Africa, Latin American, and Caribbean	400 mg orally for 1 day	Ivermectin, 200 μg/kg/day orally once a day for 2 days	Not recommended
Sub-Saharan Africa, non-*Loa loa* endemic area	400 mg orally for 1 day	Ivermectin, 200 μg/kg/day once a day for 2 days	Praziquantel, 40 mg/kg (may be divided and given in two doses for better tolerance)
Sub-Saharan Africa, *Loa loa* endemic area	400 mg orally for 1 day	If *Loa loa* cannot be excluded, treatment may be deferred until after arrival in the United States Or Albendazole 400 mg twice a day for 7 days	Praziquantel, 40 mg/kg (may be divided and given in two doses for better tolerance)
Pregnant women			
Asia, Middle East, North Africa, Latin America, and Caribbean	Not recommended	Not recommended	Not applicable
Sub-Saharan Africa	Not recommended	Not recommended	Praziquantel, 40 mg/kg (may be divided and given in two doses for better tolerance)
Children			
Asia, Middle East, North Africa, Latin America, and Caribbean	12–23 months of age: 200 mg orally for 1 day. Presumptive therapy is not recommended for any infant less than 12 months of age	Ivermectin, 200 μg/kg/day orally once a day for 2 days Should not be used presumptively if ≤15 kg	Not applicable
Sub-Saharan Africa	12–23 months of age: 200 mg orally for 1 day. Presumptive therapy is not recommended for any infant less than 12 months of age	Ivermectin, 200 μg/kg/day orally once a day for 2 days Should not be used presumptively if ≤15 kg or from *Loa loa* endemic country	Children under ≤4 years of age should not receive presumptive treatment with praziquantel. Only for children from sub-Saharan Africa

Adapted from the Centers for Disease Control and Prevention

Table 6.2 *Loa loa* endemic countries in Africa [3]

African countries *NOT* endemic for *Loa loa* (may use ivermectin for presumptive Strongyloides therapy)		African countries endemic for *Loa loa* (use albendazole for 7 days for presumptive Strongyloides therapy)
Algeria	Mauritania	Angola
Botswana	Mauritius	Burundi
Burkina Faso	Morocco	Cameroon
Côte d'Ivoire	Mozambique	Central Africa Republic
Egypt	Namibia	Chad
Eritrea	Rwanda	Congo
Gambia	Senegal	Democratic Republic of the Congo
Ghana	Somalia	Equatorial Guinea
Guinea	South Africa	Ethiopia
Kenya	Swaziland	Gabon
Liberia	Tanzania	Guinea-Bissau
Libya	Togo	Niger
Madagascar	Zambia	Nigeria
Malawi	Zimbabwe	Sierra Leone
Mali		Sudan
		Uganda

Table 6.3 Contraindications to presumptive therapy

Albendazole contraindications	Children <1 year of age, pregnancy, refugees with known neurocysticercosis, evidence of cysticercosis (e.g., subcutaneous nodules), or with a history of unexplained seizures
Praziquantel contraindications	Children <4 years of age, refugees with known neurocysticercosis, evidence of cysticercosis (e.g., subcutaneous nodules), or with a history of unexplained seizures
Ivermectin contraindications	Children <15 kg or measuring <90 cm, pregnant women in any trimester, or breastfeeding women within the first week after birth
	Refugee is departing or has lived in a *Loa loa* endemic area

endemic country should *not* be treated presumptively with ivermectin before coming to the United States. Rather, they should be tested for *Strongyloides* in the United States and if positive, treated with high-dose albendazole or screened for *Loa loa* with a daytime blood smear, and if negative, treated with ivermectin [3]. These recommendations are not uniformly implemented due to logistics and funding issues. An updated list of pre-departure therapy received by each major resettlement group may be found at http://www.cdc.gov/immigrantrefugeehealth/guidelines/overseas/interventions.html.

There are a number of important exceptions which limit receipt of presumptive therapy including pregnancy, breastfeeding, and restrictions on use of medications at young ages. Please see Table 6.3.

Once in the destination country, post-arrival screening recommendations are tailored to whether or not the refugee received pre-departure treatment [5]. Please see Table 6.4.

Table 6.4 Overview of post-arrival screening recommendations

No pre-departure treatment	Pre-departure treatment with albendazole	Pre-departure treatment with albendazole and praziquantel	Complete pre-departure treatment including ivermectin
• Eosinophil count (all refugees) • Stool O&Px2 or presumptive albendazole (all refugees) • Presumptive treatment or schistosome serology (refugees from sub-Saharan Africa) • Presumptive treatment or Strongyloides serology (all refugees except those from *Loa-loa* endemic areas of sub-Saharan Africa) • Strongyloides serology and treat only if no contraindications (refugees from *Loa loa* endemic areas of sub-Saharan Africa)	• Eosinophil count (all refugees) • Presumptive treatment or schistosome serology (refugees from sub-Saharan Africa) • Presumptive treatment or Strongyloides serology (all refugees except those from *Loa-loa* endemic areas of sub-Saharan Africa) • Strongyloides serology and treat only if no contraindications (refugees from *Loa loa* endemic areas of sub-Saharan Africa)	• Eosinophil count • Presumptive treatment or Strongyloides serology (all refugees except those from *Loa-loa* endemic areas of sub-Saharan Africa) • Strongyloides serology and treat only if no contraindications (refugees from *Loa loa* endemic areas of sub-Saharan Africa)	• Eosinophil count—if elevated recheck in 3–6 months

Adapted from CDC Guidelines on Domestic Intestinal Parasites

Parasites Commonly Encountered in Refugees

The most commonly found intestinal parasites seen in newly arrived refugees to the United States have changed somewhat since the introduction of albendazole pre-departure treatment in 1999. Based on data collected from Minnesota between 1993 and 2007, infection with *Giardia lamblia* and *Trichuris* are now the most prevalent intestinal parasites seen. Among the nematodes, *Strongyloides*, *Ascaris*, and hookworm are the most common behind *Trichuris* [4]. Of course, geographic origin will play a very important role in modifying the initial differential formed when seeing a refugee patient (see Table 6.5), especially with less common organisms such as the non-schistosome flukes (e.g., paragonimiasis) and the cestodes (e.g., *Taenia* spp. and *Hymenolepis*). A summary of common parasites encountered in refugees follows.

Table 6.5 Predominant geographic distribution of intestinal parasites found in refugee populations [5]

Global	Africa[a]	Asia[a]	Latin America[a]	Middle East[a]	Eastern Europe[a]
Ascaris lumbricoides	*Schistosoma mansoni*	*Fasciolopsis buski*	*Taenia solium*	*Echinococcus*	*Diphyllobothrium latum*
Trichuris trichiura	*Schistosoma haematobium*	Southeast Asia: *Opisthorchis viverrini*	*Schistosoma mansoni*	*Giardia*	*Opisthorchis felineus*
Hookworm	*Schistosoma intercalatum*	*Clonorchis sinensis*	*Opisthorchis guayaquilensis* (Ecuador)		
Strongyloides stercoralis	*Taenia saginata* (especially Ethiopia and Eritrea)	*Schistosoma japonicum*			
Enterobius vermicularis		*Schistosoma mekongi*			
Fasciola		South Asia: *Taenia solium*			
Hymenolepis					
Most protozoa, especially *Giardia intestinalis* (*lamblia*)					

[a]Organisms either unique to the location or particularly common or overrepresented

Protozoa

The protozoa are single-celled organisms which cause quite similar symptoms as a group, those being abdominal discomfort and diarrhea. They are also overall more likely *not* to cause disease than to cause disease in those who are affected.

Entamoeba histolytica. Although a causative agent of dysentery, *E. histolytica* more commonly causes mild gastrointestinal disease such as abdominal discomfort and loose stools. It can cause a more severe disease which involves bloody diarrhea (dysentery) and may become tissue invasive [6]. In this latter case, the most common site is the liver, where an abscess may form. It may also affect the lungs and brain, although these presentations are rare. In refugees *E. histolytica* causing clinical disease after arrival to the United States is rare. Although cysts are commonly reported in stool ova and parasite examination, these cysts are much more likely to be the indistinguishable, non-pathogenic, *E. dispar*. When reported in an asymptomatic person the diagnosis of *E. histolytica* should be confirmed with a stool antigen test prior to treating.

Giardia spp. This is the most commonly encountered parasite in refugee populations who receive ova and parasite stool screening. *Giardia* is the most common parasitic cause of diarrhea affecting people in both developed and developing countries, the latter far more than the former. Transmitted by fecal-oral contamination, it, like many others, preferentially affects those in poorer socioeconomic areas. Most infections are asymptomatic. There is lack of data regarding benefit versus cost and risk of adverse events in treating asymptomatic persons. Those with symptoms (e.g., bloating, burping, abdominal discomfort, diarrhea, or failure to thrive in small children) should be tested for this infection and treated accordingly. Routine screening in asymptomatic persons is not recommended; however, when encountered, most clinicians choose to treat. There is no consensus on this latter point.

Blastocystis hominis. Ubiquitous throughout the world, *Blastocystis* is the most commonly encountered organism in screening fecal cultures in new arrivals. In most individuals, this infection does not cause signs or symptoms and is not considered a pathogen. However, it has been associated with disease in certain individuals, particularly those with underlying immunodeficiency (e.g., HIV), and in travelers. If a person has gastrointestinal symptoms and no other etiology is found, it is reasonable to consider treatment.

Dientamoeba fragilis. A common parasite, D. fragilis, can cause abdominal pain, persistent diarrhea, and flatulence which may be chronic or acute, although many who are infected have no symptoms. It is transmitted via the fecal-oral route and when symptomatic should be treated.

Nematodes

Roundworms belong to the phylum Nematoda and are therefore commonly referred to as nematodes. Among the most abundant animals on earth, they are a common cause of infection and disease in the developing world, both acute and chronic, the latter having powerful effects on development.

Soil-transmitted helminths (STH) are a group which includes *Ascaris lumbricoides*, *Trichuris trichiura*, and the hookworms. They are commonly referred to together because of their very high prevalence, similarity in life cycle, and worldwide distribution. They also belong to the group of "neglected tropical diseases," along with several other infectious agents labeled so by the WHO because they affect a broad swath of humanity, often in developing countries, but do not garner the research and interest that other diseases often do [7, 8]. All soil-transmitted helminths need a soil cycle, and transmission in the United States is rare. They all have a limited life span, and within 5 years of leaving an endemic area, a refugee will be free of infection.

Ascaris lumbricoides (STH). The most common of the soil-transmitted helminths, nearly one in six people (roughly 1.2 billion humans) are infected [9]. The vast majority of infected individuals have no symptoms. However, with high numbers of worms, commonly referred to as a large worm burden, patients can suffer intestinal blockage. This is most common in children. In addition, the parasite may "wander" into areas where its presence may cause disease, such as blocking the gallbladder outlet (causing cholecystitis) or the appendix (causing appendicitis). Because of its life cycle, which involves passing through the lungs, patient may also present with respiratory symptoms such as cough, dyspnea, and wheezing.

Trichuris trichiura (STH). *Trichuris* is a parasite which inhabits the large intestine (most nematodes infect the small bowel) and is found in many areas where human feces are used as fertilizer (often referred to as "night soil"). One becomes infected by ingesting *Trichuris* eggs, and it can, like many other parasites, be asymptomatic or cause disease. More than 90 % of people infected are asymptomatic. Those who are symptomatic may experience watery, bloody, and painful bowel movements. In addition, it is associated with anemia. In children with heavy infections, growth retardation can occur. It has been associated with rectal prolapse.

Hookworm: *Ancylostoma duodenale*, *Necator americanus* (STH). Hookworm is found in areas where human feces are used as fertilizer or in areas where human wastes are deposited on the soil. Infection occurs via direct penetration of the skin, often of the lower extremities, and the first symptom is often an itchy rash at the site of infection. Once established in the small intestine, they can cause abdominal pain, as well as weakness and fatigue. They are most notable for the chronic anemia which may result from chronic infection, resulting in growth retardation in children. This is the most pathogenic of the soil-transmitted helminths.

Strongyloides stercoralis. Although a nematode that is very similar to hookworm, *Strongyloides* is generally not grouped with the other STHs. A roundworm roughly the size of a mustard seed, *Strongyloides* is a soil-transmitted helminth which, like *Trichuris* and hookworms, infects humans via skin penetration, often of the feet and legs. Found throughout the world, but predominantly in tropical areas, *Strongyloides* often manifests itself with dermatologic, pulmonary, and intestinal symptoms such as rash, dry cough, and abdominal discomfort.

NOTE: Unlike most other helminths, *Strongyloides* is capable of autoinfection, i.e., the host can continually reinfect himself/herself and thus have a persistent, even lifelong infection. Also, *Strongyloides* can become disseminated and result in "hyperinfection" which has a high mortality rate and is often misdiagnosed as Gram-negative sepsis; this is most often due to immunosuppression particularly following the administration of corticosteroids. Special attention must also be given when considering treatment of patients with *Strongyloides* who are from *Loa loa* endemic areas (please see Section "Screening Recommendations" above).

Loa loa. A nematode transmitted by the bite of deerflies of the genus *Chrysops*, loaiasis most often results in eye worm and red, itchy swellings of the skin referred to as Calabar swellings. It is found throughout west-central sub-Saharan Africa, in areas of high-canopied rain forest. One key factor making *Loa loa* infection of prime importance is that in patients treated with ivermectin for *Strongyloides* who were coinfected with Loa loa, there have been reports of encephalitis precipitated by the treatment; please see recommendations above.

Trematodes

Trematodes, also known as "flukes," are parasites which infect many different types of vertebrate hosts, including man. Their life cycle typically involves a freshwater snail as an intermediate before infection of the definitive vertebrate host.

Schistosoma spp. Widespread throughout the tropical world, Schistosome species are very important and at times overlooked parasites which can cause significant morbidity when chronic. Schistosomes have a complex life cycle which must involve certain freshwater snails, and humans are infected via the skin, usually by wading in areas populated by said snails. Initially, patients may have a dermatologic reaction at the site of skin penetration, including rash with vesicles and pruritus. Roughly 5–7 weeks after infection, patients may develop "Katayama fever," the syndrome of fever, headache, myalgias, abdominal pain (right upper quadrant often), and bloody diarrhea [10]. Serious neurologic complications can also occur at this time, including seizures and transverse myelitis. Untreated infections, which may last many years, lead to a chronic granulomatous disease which can cause liver disease and large intestinal symptoms with *S. mansoni*, *S. japonicum*, and *S. mekongi*, whereas chronic infection with *S. haematobium* can lead to renal disease and bladder cancer.

Opisthorchis spp., *Clonorchis sinensis*, *Fasciola hepatica* (liver flukes). Found in Asia, Southeast Asia, Eastern Europe, and countries of the former Soviet Union, liver flukes are contracted by eating undercooked freshwater fish. They inhabit the bile tree of humans, and when they cause disease it results in symptoms of abdominal discomfort, diarrhea, and constipation secondary to bile duct inflammation and biliary obstruction. Chronic infection results in inflammation and scarring of the biliary tree, which can lead to gallbladder and bile duct cancers. In fact, some species may be mistaken for gallstones and only be discovered upon surgery.

Of note, *Fasciola*, the common liver fluke, is found in a more broad geographical swath and is acquired not by uncooked or undercooked seafood, but by eating raw freshwater plants, such as watercress (as well as undercooked sheep or goat livers) [11]. Symptoms are similar to the other liver flukes, despite this parasite's actively burrowing through the liver parenchyma to arrive at the biliary tree. The most commonly encountered liver flukes in refugees are *Opisthorchis* and *Clonorchis* and are seen mainly in SEA refugees (e.g., Laotian).

Paragonimus westermani (lung fluke). Paragonimiasis is most common in South and Southeast Asia, where humans are infected by eating raw or undercooked crab or crayfish. Symptoms of infection first involve the abdominal tract, with nausea, vomiting, and diarrhea, and may then be followed by pulmonary symptoms including chest pain, fever, and cough which may be productive of bloody sputum [12]. Given the prominence of hemoptysis, tuberculosis is often considered along with paragonimiasis in the differential diagnosis [13]. This infection is seen primarily in SEA refugees, currently most common in Burmese refugees.

Cestodes

Inhabiting the intestines of humans, cestodes have long been regarded with revulsion by man, most probably second to passage in the feces of entire worms of great length (e.g., Diphyllobothrium which can be over 10 ft when excreted) or of gravid proglottids (large, egg-laden segments of the worms), seen primarily with *Taenia* spp.

Hymenolepis nana (dwarf tapeworm). Found throughout the world, and particularly where there is poor hygiene, this parasite is commonly called the "dwarf tapeworm." Humans are infected by fecal-contaminated food or water, and most patients are asymptomatic with infection because of the small size of this tapeworm compared to the members of genus Taenia. Symptoms if present are usually of abdominal discomfort and weakness, and children with heavy infections may have perineal pruritus and therefore be misdiagnosed with pinworm infection. This is particularly common in Ethiopian and Somali refugees.

Taenia saginata (beef tapeworm). Found throughout the world, *Taenia saginata* is the largest tapeworm to cause human disease, reaching lengths of up to 10 m. Humans are infected by eating raw or undercooked beef and when symptomatic will often have abdominal discomfort, weight loss, and anorexia.

Taenia solium (pork tapeworm). The pork tapeworm, like the beef tapeworm, is found throughout the world and causes a similar clinical presentation when it affects the gastrointestinal system. However, unlike the beef tapeworm, *Taenia solium* eggs can be directly infectious to humans (i.e., there is the possibility of human-to-human infection). When another human is directly infected by eating eggs, the parasite can migrate to any number of different tissues and develop into cysts; the most worrying location is the brain, which results clinically in neurocysticercosis, which is a significant cause of adult onset seizures in many parts of the developing world [14]. In an immigrant, particularly from Central or South America, who presents with new onset seizures, neurocysticercosis must be on the differential.

Diphyllobothrium latum (fish tapeworm). Obtained through eating raw or undercooked fish, diphyllobothriasis is found primarily throughout the northern hemispheres and is more common within the United States than in refugee populations entering the United States. Symptoms, when present, may be vomiting, diarrhea, and weight loss. Of note is the propensity for vitamin B12 deficiency and consequent anemia.

Table 6.6 outlines the therapeutic regimens for the above parasites for adults.

All medications are dosed for adults and orally taken unless otherwise noted [15].

More detailed descriptions of organisms discussed above, as well as therapeutic treatment regimens, can be found in these references [2, 11, 13, 15].

Eosinophilia

An elevated eosinophil count may be the result of any number of infectious and noninfectious processes (see Tables 6.7 and 6.8), but in certain groups it can help bring to the fore the possibility of a latent and perhaps asymptomatic, parasitic infection. Unfortunately things are not as straightforward as they may seem; eosinophilia, or an absolute eosinophil count greater than $400/mm^3$ in a peripheral blood sample, has both poor negative and poor positive predictive values as a marker of parasitosis in returning travelers [16]. However, as with all tests, a thorough history will reveal characteristics that render the above value more or less likely an indicator of parasitic disease. For example, in the case of patients who have had prolonged exposure to possible helminth infections, eosinophilia becomes much more useful as a possible indicator of underlying, chronic infection.

In the previous sections of this chapter, we have detailed the presumptive therapy which newly arrived immigrants should undergo upon arrival to the United States. It is important to recall that an elevated eosinophil count can take some time, from 3 to 6 months, to return to normal after treatment. Therefore, in patients who have been treated, a recheck of the peripheral eosinophil count should be performed 3–6 months afterward to ensure resolution. If the eosinophil count remains elevated, a more detailed work-up should be pursued, with particular emphasis on *Strongyloides*, soil-transmitted helminths, and *Schistosoma* species as these are the most common causes. During this work-up, it will as always be important to consider the

Table 6.6 Adult therapeutic regimens [15]

Intestinal pathogen	Treatment
Protozoa	
Entamoeba histolytica	Metronidazole 500–750 mg PO three times daily, duration 7–10 days; paromomycin 25–30 mg/kg per day/three doses per day for 7 days
Giardia intestinalis (aka *G. lamblia, G. duodenalis*)	Metronidazole 500 mg orally twice daily or 250 mg orally TID, duration 5–7 days
Blastocystis hominis	Metronidazole 750 mg TID, duration 5–10 days
Dientamoeba fragilis	Paromomycin 25–35 mg/kg per day in three divided doses, duration 7 days or metronidazole 500–750 mg TID, duration 10 days
Nematodes	
Ascaris lumbricoides	Albendazole 400 mg single dose
Trichuris trichiura	Albendazole 400 mg per day for 3 days
Ancylostoma duodenale, Necator americanus	Albendazole 400 mg single dose
Strongyloides stercoralis	Ivermectin 200 µg/kg for 1–2 days
Loa loa	Diethylcarbamazine 8–10 mg/kg orally in three divided doses daily for 21 days
Trematodes	
S. mansoni, S. haematobium	Praziquantel 40 mg/kg per day orally in two divided doses for 1 day, 6–8 h apart
S. japonicum, S. mekongi	Praziquantel 60 mg/kg per day orally in three divided doses for 1 day, 6–8 h apart
Opisthorchis viverrini, Clonorchis sinensis	Praziquantel 75 mg/kg/day orally, three doses per day for 2 days
Fasciola hepatica	Triclabendazole 10 mg/kg for 2 days
Paragonimus westermani	Praziquantel 25 mg/kg given orally three times per day for 2 consecutive days
Cestodes	
Hymenolepis nana	Praziquantel 25 mg/kg single dose
Taenia saginata, Taenia solium	Praziquantel 5–10 mg/kg single dose; <u>BEWARE</u> praziquantel with cysticercosis as it is cysticidal and may cause inflammation and provoke seizures
Diphyllobothrium latum	Praziquantel 5–10 mg/kg single-dose

geographic region from which the patient is coming, as this will be very important to help clarify the differential diagnosis and arrive at the most likely etiology. If 6 months after presumptive treatment the eosinophil count is still elevated, the differential must be broadened to include other infectious and noninfectious causes.

Finally, it should be noted that the duration of infection with parasites that result in an elevated eosinophil count can be very long, indeed with an organism such as *Strongyloides* it may last the entire life of the patient because of autoinfection. Other parasites with a long duration of infection are Schistosoma (32 years) and Loa loa

Table 6.7 Causes of eosinophilia (from CDC Domestic Intestinal Parasite Guidelines) [5]

Parasites causing eosinophilia commonly found on stool exam	Other parasitic infections associated with eosinophilia	Parasites commonly found in the stool NOT typically associated with eosinophilia	Nonparasitic causes of eosinophilia
Ascaris lumbricoides	Angiostrongylus	Entamoeba spp.	Asthma
Hookworm species	Anisakis	(*E. histolytica*,	Atopy
Trichuris trichiura	Capillaria spp.	*E. dispar*, others)	Drug allergy
Strongyloides	Cysticercosis	Cryptosporidium spp.	Eosinophilic leukemia
Tapeworms	Echinococcus spp.	*Giardia intestinalis*	Hodgkin's lymphoma
(*T. solium*	Filariasis	(a.k.a. *G. lamblia*	Hypereosinophilic
and *T. saginata*)		and *G. duodenalis*)	syndrome
Schistosoma			Pemphigoid
(*S. mansoni, S.*			Pemphigus
haematobium, S.			Polyarteritis nodosa
japonicum)			
Other flukes			
(Paragonimus,			
Opisthorchis,			
Fasciola)			

Table 6.8 Causes of eosinophilia in refugees, by region [5]

Region	Parasites causing eosinophilia
Africa	*Schistosoma mansoni, S. haematobium, S. intercalatum*
	Taenia saginata (esp. Ethiopia and Eritrea)
Asia	Overall: *Fasciolopsis buski*
	Southeast Asia: *Opisthorchis viverrini, Clonorchis sinensis, S. japonicum, Schistosoma mekongi*
	South Asia: *Taenia solium*
Latin America	*Taenia solium*
	Schistosoma mansoni
	Opisthorchis guayaquilensis (Ecuador)
Middle East	*Echinococcus*
Eastern Europe	*Diphyllobothrium latum*
	Opisthorchis felineus

(16–24 years). Hookworm and Ascaris are examples of parasites with relatively shorter life spans (3–5 years and 1–1.5 years, respectively) [17].

Treatment should be directed at the parasite identified during eosinophilia evaluation. However, despite a thorough investigation, it is quite possible that an etiologic cause may not be identified, in which case presumptive therapy may be reasonable. In this case, single-dose therapy with ivermectin and/or albendazole has been proposed [17].

Conclusion

Parasitic infections continue to be highly prevalent and an important cause of morbidity in newly arrived refugees. A complete history, including geographic risk factors and the screening recommendations outlined above, can help detect a majority of these intestinal parasitic infections. Recommendations on diagnosis and treatment of these infections are periodically updated by CDC and providers are encouraged to access this information for guidance on management.

References

1. Garg PK, Perry S, Dorn M, et al. Risk of intestinal helminth and protozoan infection in a refugee population. Am J Trop Med Hyg. 2005;73:386–91.
2. Mody R. Intestinal parasites. In: Walker PF, Barnett ED, editors. Immigrant medicine. China: Saunders Elsevier; 2007. p. 273.
3. CDC recommendations for overseas presumptive treatment of intestinal parasites for refugees destined for the United States. 2010 [last updated 2010 May 24]. http://www.cdc.gov/immigrantrefugeehealth/guidelines/overseas/intestinal-parasites-overseas.html. Accessed Aug 2013.
4. Swanson SJ, Phares CR, Mamo B, Smith KE, Cetron MS, Stauffer WM. Albendazole therapy and enteric parasites in United States-bound refugees. N Engl J Med. 2012;366(16): 1498–507.
5. CDC domestic intestinal parasites guidelines. 2013 [last updated 2013 Jun]. http://www.cdc.gov/immigrantrefugeehealth/guidelines/domestic/intestinal-parasites-domestic.html. Accessed Aug 2013.
6. Salles JM, Salles MJ, Moraes LA, et al. Invasive amebiasis: an update on diagnosis and management. Expert Rev Anti Infect Ther. 2007;5(5):893–901.
7. Knopp S, Steinmann P, Keiser J, et al. Tropical diseases: nematode infections. Infect Dis Clin North Am. 2012;26(2):341–58.
8. Savioli L, et al. Working to overcome the global impact of neglected tropical diseases—first WHO report on neglected tropical diseases. Geneva: WHO; 2010. ISBN 978 92 4 1564090.
9. Dold C, Holland CV. *Ascaris* and ascariasis. Microbes Infect. 2011;13(7):632–7.
10. Strickland GT, Ramirez BL. Schistosomiasis. In: Strickland GT, editor. Hunter's tropical medicine and emerging infectious diseases. 8th ed. Philadelphia, PA: WB Saunders Company; 2000. p. 804–32.
11. Roberts LS, Janovy J. Foundations of parasitology. New York: McGraw Hill; 2005. Chapter 17.
12. Lal C, Huggins JT, Sahn SA. Parasitic diseases of the pleura. Am J Med Sci. 2013;345(5):385–9.
13. Cook G, Zumla A. Manson's tropical diseases, Helminthic infections, vol. Section 11. 21st ed. London: WB Saunders; 2003.
14. Del Brutto OH. Neurocysticercosis: a review. ScientificWorldJournal. 2012;Article ID 159821.
15. Drugs for parasitic infections. The Medical Letter. 2004. http://www.mimg.ucla.edu/faculty/campbell/drugs_for_parasites.pdf
16. Seybolt LM, Christiansen D, Barnett ED. Diagnostic evaluation of newly arrived asymptomatic refugees with eosinophilia. Clin Infect Dis. 2006;42:363–7.
17. Kim Y, Nutman TB. Eosinophilia. In: Walker PF, Barnett ED, editors. Immigrant medicine. China: Saunders Elsevier; 2007. p. 309.

Chapter 7
Viral Hepatitis

Douglas J. Pryce and Asha M.J. Madhar

Viral Hepatitis A, B, C, D, and E in Refugees (Screening and Clinical Considerations)

Where you were born and where you have lived determines most of a refugee's viral hepatitis risk.

Introduction

Refugees, asylees, immigrants, and their families have been born in, or have lived in, regions highly endemic for the various viral hepatitides compared to the developed countries where they relocate. There are a variety of viruses that have an affinity for infecting the human liver, which are communicable and all can lead to acute hepatitis and hepatitis B, C, and D can develop into chronic liver infection. Chronic viral hepatitis B and C cause the majority of liver cancers in the world; it is the sixth most common cancer and third most deadly. The prevalence of each type of hepatitis varies by region and exposure due to poor public health infrastructure (water quality, medical practices, vaccine availability).

Acute hepatitis A and E are the most common types of viral hepatitis and present as a usually mild viral hepatitis. Refugees are infected abroad in the refugee's home country or region and in the refugee camps. It is possible that an asymptomatic young person or a symptomatic older individual with a very recent exposure could arrive as a new refugee. The short incubation and infection cycle, without a chronic phase, combined with the refugee's group immunity, decreases the chance of these becoming significant communicable diseases. Thus, new arrival screening of

D.J. Pryce, M.D. (✉) • A.M.J. Madhar, M.D.
General Internal Medicine, Hennepin Country Medical Center, University of Minnesota,
701 Park Avenue S, Minneapolis, MN 55415, USA
e-mail: douglas.pryre@hcmed.org

A. Annamalai (ed.), *Refugee Health Care: An Essential Medical Guide*,
DOI 10.1007/978-1-4939-0271-2_7, © Springer Science+Business Media New York 2014

refugees for infectious hepatitis A and E is not needed. Hepatitis B has infected about 2 billion worldwide and has a high prevalence estimated at 360 million in the chronically infected phase (hepatitis B surface antigen positive for more than 6 months). It is silent through the immunotolerant phase from birth into adulthood and can be spread sexually and by close contact, thus screening of refugees is indicated [1]. Chronic hepatitis C (CHC) is medically significant with morbidity and mortality similar to chronic hepatitis B (CHB), but is less prevalent than CHB and is mostly spread through percutaneous routes and less through communicable routes. Hepatitis C historically has not been recommended for routine screening. However, with improved and available curative treatment, there is cost benefit of screening refugees from high prevalence countries [2]. Current recommendation is to screen those born during 1945–1965 and those with risk factors, which is similar to guidelines for the general US population. Hepatitis D virus (HDV) infection is dependent on hepatitis B virus for replication and is of much lower prevalence, thus is not considered for screening. HDV is a progressive clinical entity which can be detected in regular clinical follow-up care recommended for all hepatitis B carriers.

Vaccinations for newly arrived refugees, to protect the susceptible, are available for hepatitis A and B. In general, the newly arrived refugees should receive the Advisory Committee on Immunization Practices (ACIP) recommended vaccinations hepatitis A and B for ages ≤18 or those that have risk factors, unless immunity is proven by serology. Most refugees, adults and children, are from hepatitis B endemic areas where the hepatitis B surface antigen (HBsAg) prevalence ≥2 % and those not immune should be vaccinated [3, 4].

In the US, refugee hepatitis B screening protocols and vaccination resources vary between the states, and refugees are free to move between states after arrival, thus clinicians caring for refugees need have awareness that individual refugees may have incomplete screening or need completion of their vaccination series for protection. National guidelines for medical screening and vaccination, including guidelines for viral hepatitis, in newly arrived refugees to the US are developed by the Center for Disease Control and Prevention's Division of Global Migration and Quarantine (CDC/DGMQ) and issued by the Office of Refugee Resettlement (ORR) Domestic Medical Screening Guidelines Checklist and promoted to each state's refugee health program by the Association of Refugee Health Coordinators (ARHC) [4–6].

A summary of the characteristics of viral hepatitides is presented in Table 7.1. The clinical presentation of the acute phase of all hepatitis is similar and shown in Table 7.2.

Summary: Viral Hepatitis Screening and Vaccination Recommendations for Refugees

Hepatitis B

Screen all refugees (adults and children) from hepatitis B endemic areas for HBsAg, anti-HBc, and anti-HBs. Vaccinate all unvaccinated children (ages 0–18 years old) for hepatitis B that are susceptible. Vaccinate all susceptible adults for increased

Table 7.1 Viral hepatitis characteristics

	A	B	C	D (requires Hep B Infection)	E
Chronic infection (worldwide prevalence)	No	360 million	170 million	10 million	No[a]
Acute hepatitis phase	Yes	Yes	Yes	Yes	Yes
Mild or asymptomatic	Children	Perinatal–young adult	Most	Coinfection with acute HBV	Children
Severe symptoms	In preexisting chronic liver disease (CLD)	Development of ESLD	Development of ESLD	Superinfection of CHB	In pregnancy
Vaccine preventable	Yes (age 1–18)	Yes (susceptible)	No	No	No
Treatment available	No	Yes	Yes, cure possible	Yes	No
Refugee screening test	No	HBsAg, anti-HBc, anti-HBs	anti-HCV[b]	No	No
Transmission	Fecal/oral Sexual contact Close contacts	Perinatal (up to 90 %) Sexual Contact Parenteral Close contacts	Parenteral Perinatal (6 %)	Close contacts Parenteral	Fecal/oral Perinatal
Referral[c]	No	Yes	Yes	Yes	No

[a]Hepatitis E can become chronic in persons on immunosuppressive treatments for solid-organ transplant and with HIV

[b]Test those high risk and born during 1945–1965. Positive anti-HCV results are confirmed with HCV RNA testing

[c]Chronic hepatitis B, C, and D should be assessed for disease severity and need for treatment consideration and monitored periodically for progression of liver disease and hepatocellular carcinoma

Table 7.2 Signs
and symptoms of acute
hepatitis infection from all
types of hepatitis

Fever
Fatigue
Decreased appetite
Nausea and emesis
Abdominal pain
Gray-colored stools
Dark-colored urine
Arthralgias
Jaundice
Abnormal lab tests (elevated liver transaminases and bilirubin)

risk for hepatitis B, which includes living in close contact with their community members from endemic hepatitis B areas.

Hepatitis A, D, and E

Routine testing for viral hepatitis A, C, D, or E infection in asymptomatic refugees is not recommended at any age. Refugees with signs or symptoms of disease should receive appropriate diagnostic testing.

Hepatitis C

Routine screening for hepatitis C is similar to guidelines for the general US population. Screen those born during 1945–1965 and those with risk factors. Risk factors include individuals with body art, those who have received blood transfusions or blood products in developing nations, history of intravenous drug use, HIV positive status and children born to hepatitis C-positive mothers [5].

Vaccination for Hepatitis A

ACIP recommends HAV vaccine for all children ages 1–18.

Chronic Hepatitis B

Chronic hepatitis B (CHB) infection is the most concerning hepatitis infection for newly arrived refugees due to high worldwide prevalence in the areas that refugees mostly come from (see Fig. 7.1) and the long-term health risk that 15–25 % will develop end-stage liver disease (ESLD) and/or hepatocellular carcinoma (HCC) [7].

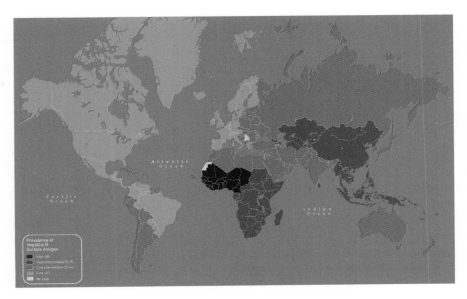

Fig. 7.1 Geographic distribution of chronic hepatitis B virus infection in adults; Reprinted from Vaccine. 30(12). Ott JJ, Stevens GA, Groeger J, Wiersma ST, Global epidemiology of hepatitis B virus infection: new estimates of age-specific seroprevalence and endemicity, pages 2212–9, Copyright (2012) with permission from Elsevier

The WHO estimated in year 2000 at least 600,000 people died due to acute and chronic HBV-associated liver disease [8]. CHB infection is the cause of 53 % hepatocellular carcinomas in the world [9].

US refugee health data on the prevalence of HBsAg in newly arrived refugees between 2006 and 2008 demonstrated 2.8 % overall prevalence, range 0.6–15.5 %, with 95 % confidence range 2.6–3.0 %. The highest prevalence was among refugees from Eritrea (15.5 %), Liberia (12.2 %), Myanmar (12.4 %), Ethiopia (9.1 %), Somalia (8.3 %), and Malaysia (8.8 %). Six other countries (Iran, Iraq, Laos, Russia, Thailand, and Vietnam) were noted to have substantially decreased rates when compared with 1991 prevalence data [10]. Thus, the prevalence is highly variable between countries and over time. Refugees themselves also vary greatly in their socioeconomic status, which correlates with previous risk of exposure, but overall, refugee groups are arriving in the US with disproportionately higher rates of CHB than the US population. The US population has about 1.3–2.2 million infected with CHB and the overall prevalence of CHB infection is less than 1 %, but foreign born account for about 47–70 % of those infected [11]. Antiviral treatment for hepatitis B is available and indicated for those with progressive chronic infection to reduce or postpone the development of end-stage liver disease. Further justification for referral and consideration of antiviral hepatitis B treatments is that the number on a list of liver transplant candidates was significantly reduced by 30 % due to clinical improvement with the institution of antiviral hepatitis B treatment [12]. Despite the need for clinical evaluation and monitoring for CHB, in 2010 the Institute of

Medicine report highlighted that 65 % of all persons with CHB in the US are undiagnosed and only half of those diagnosed receive appropriate care [13, 14].

Transmission of CHB worldwide is 90 % perinatal in the highly endemic areas. Good measures are available to prevent transmission of HBV at delivery that dramatically reduce the new CHB infection rate of infants to HBV-infected mothers, but still in the US, 1,000 babies are born yearly infected with HBV due to lack of pregnancy screening for mothers with CHB [13]. Treatment of newborns born to HBsAg-positive mothers with the hepatitis B immune globulin within 12 h of birth and the three-dose hepatitis B vaccination series is highly effective at breaking the chain of perinatal transmission.

It is important to realize that refugees in the US live their life and marry in their respective ethnic communities which have high prevalence rates of CHB. Testing for lack of protective immunity against hepatitis B while screening for hepatitis B infection in newly arrived refugees from increased prevalence areas will uncover about 30 % of the population that are susceptible and will benefit from the hepatitis B vaccination series [3, 4, 13].

Enhancing the prevention of new cases of hepatitis B in the US, many of which are now attributable to the foreign born, and reduction of morbidity and mortality from hepatitis B for newly arrived refugees can be achieved with initial screening, proper follow-up of those infected, and vaccination of those susceptible.

Refugee Hepatitis B Screening National Guidelines [4–6]

Administer a hepatitis B screening panel including hepatitis B surface antigen (HBsAg), hepatitis B surface antibody (anti-HBs), and hepatitis B core antibody (anti-HBc) to all adults and children (for interpretation see Table 7.3).

Vaccinate previously unvaccinated and susceptible children, 0–18 years of age.

Vaccinate susceptible adults who are at increased risk for HBV infection due to close interaction with their community members that are from endemic areas.

Refer all persons with chronic HBV infection for additional ongoing medical evaluation.

Table 7.3 Interpretation of positive hepatitis B serologic screening tests [16]

Test	Result	Interpretation
HBsAg	Positive	Infection, acute or chronic (CHB if positive for more than 6 months)
		False positive from recent (<1 month) hepatitis B vaccination
	Negative	Not infected, early acute infection, resolving infection or immune
Total anti-HBc	Positive	Becomes positive in acute infection and recovery, then remains positive for life (in recovery or with CHB)
IgM anti-HBc	Positive	Acute HBV infection
	Negative	CHB or never infected or recovered from infection or immune
Anti-HBs	Positive	Protective antibody: indicates immunity from either vaccination or natural infection

Other Hepatitis B Screening Considerations [4]

1. Test children born in the US, not vaccinated as infants, for HBsAg, if parents are from high HBV endemic regions ≥8 %.
2. Any refugee with potential exposure within the last 60 days of hepatitis B testing should have repeat testing in 3–6 months.
3. Testing for hepatitis B should be done regardless of prior hepatitis B vaccination. CHB infection is mostly silent and hepatitis B vaccination would not be protective if they are already infected prior to vaccination.
4. Testing for HBsAg should not be done within 1 month of vaccination; it may lead to a false-positive result.
5. Screen all pregnant women.

Prevention/Vaccination [4]

1. The first vaccination of the series may be done at the time of HBsAg testing; it will not be harmful in HBsAg-positive cases.
2. Some refugee camps in certain countries currently provide some hepatitis B vaccination.

   For example, in the year 2012 for ages 18 and under, hepatitis B vaccination is reported by the CDC as currently being administered in Thailand at the Burma border for Burmese refugees and in Nepal for the Bhutanese/Nepalese refugees [4].
3. Immunizations administered outside the US with written documentation (date, type of vaccination, and the location or name of clinic) and administration intervals at the appropriate age can be accepted as valid, if the schedule was similar to the standard US recommendations (inappropriate age at the time of the previous vaccine is unacceptable).
4. If one or two doses of the hepatitis B vaccine series were given abroad and properly documented, the series should be completed without restarting, continuing with an acceptable US schedule [3, 4]. The minimum intervals are 4 weeks between first and second doses and 8 weeks between second and third doses.

   A positive anti-HBs test after one documented dose of the hepatitis vaccine is not considered protective, and the three-dose series should be completed.
5. Severe malnutrition at the time of the vaccination could impair immune response to some vaccines; revaccination or checking serology for immunity could be considered.
6. Traveling - established refugees frequently will be returning to endemic areas to visiting friends and relatives (VFRs), thus their immune status should be reviewed and susceptible patients vaccinated [15].

Preventive Counseling: Identification of those infected with hepatitis B will lead to increased awareness and the opportunity for counseling to prevent spreading infection by careful hygiene, avoiding alcohol, and assessment of status of all household contacts and sex partners who may be infected or at risk and in need of protective vaccination.

Clinical/Referral: Confirm immunity to hepatitis A and rule out coinfection with HCV and HIV. Medical referral to gastroenterology or a liver specialist is indicated to assess for ESLD, periodic monitoring for HCC, and consideration of antiviral therapy for progressive liver disease.

Special Considerations for Serology Results

Total Anti-HBc Is the Only Detectable Serologic Marker (No HBsAg or Anti-HBs)

May be due to:

1. Resolving acute infection in the window period of acute hepatitis B (this can be confirmed by testing for IgM anti-HBc).
2. Resolved HBV infection, anti-HBs levels have waned over many years.
3. CHB with undetectable circulating HBsAg titer that has waned to below the cutoff level. This is most likely for populations with a high prevalence of HBV infection or CHB coinfection with HIV or HCV.
4. False positive seen mostly in low prevalence populations with no risk factors for HBV. These individuals are still considered susceptible to HBV.

Further evaluation for examples *2*, *3*, and *4*: Testing a HBV DNA viral load would identify those infected with hepatitis B that need to be followed.

HBsAg and Anti-HBs Are Both Positive

The antibodies are unable to neutralize the circulating virus. These individuals are HBV-infected carriers.

Hepatitis D Coinfection or Superinfection with Hepatitis B

Hepatitis D virus (HDV) requires HBV infection to replicate and infect humans. HDV infection prevalence is estimated to infect at least ten million people worldwide and is more common in some areas of the Middle East, Mediterranean basin, Central Asia, West Africa, the Amazon basin, and some Pacific Islands. Certain indigenous groups from South America appear more susceptible to severe, often fatal HDV acute and chronic infection [17, 18]. HDV infection is decreasing in areas of the world where CHB prevalence rates are decreasing, including the

Mediterranean basin [17]. Refugees with elevated prevalence rates of hepatitis B infection are susceptible to HDV, but specific refugee prevalence data is rare. Low prevalence has been reported in past surveys of HBV-infected Albanian refugees (1 case was detected from 91 HBsAg positive) and Southeast Asian refugees (no HDV detected) [19, 20].

Coinfection of HBV and HDV is an acute, simultaneous, hepatic infection of both viruses that is mild and 95 % of the time it clears. Superinfection of CHB infection with HDV presents as a severe acute hepatitis (Table 7.3) that leads to a chronic hepatitis D in up to 80 % of the cases. Transmission is associated with close personal contact, intravenous drug use, promiscuous sexual activity, and people exposed to unscreened blood and blood products.

HDV enhances the severity of acute and chronic hepatitis B. The mortality and fulminant hepatitis rates are tenfold higher than in CHB infection alone [17].

Screening: Routine testing is not recommended for HDV in newly arrived refugees.

Prevention: There is no HDV vaccine. HBV vaccination will protect those not infected with hepatitis B from HDV infection but cannot protect the estimated 360 million CHB carriers worldwide from HDV infection susceptibility [1].

Clinical: Referral to a liver specialist is indicated for a refugee if HDV is suspected (a concerning clinical presentation is a progressive appearing or severe hepatitis B infection). Serology testing antibody to HDV (total anti-HDV) is clinically available. Select antiviral treatments for hepatitis B may have an effect in HDV infection. Liver transplantation is an option for ESLD and fulminant hepatitis caused by HDV.

Hepatitis C

Hepatitis C virus (HCV) infection is a clinically mild chronic liver infection that over several decades of time causes cirrhosis and hepatocellular carcinoma. Most with HCV are asymptomatic and may be unaware of their infection until chronic liver disease complications develop. The world prevalence is 2.2–3 % or about 130–170 million people are chronically infected worldwide [21–23]. The highest country rates for HCV antibody seroprevalence (not confirmed infections) are found in Rwanda (17 %), Egypt (15 %), Cameroon (12.5 %), Bolivia (11.2 %), Burundi (11.1 %), Guinea (10.7 %), Mongolia (10.7 %), Libya (7.9 %), and Zimbabwe (7.7 %) [22]. HCV prevalence rates vary within countries, for example, Egypt has a confirmed active HCV infection prevalence rate of 10 % (7 % in urban and 12 % in rural areas) and Pakistan's average seroprevalence rate is 3.0 % with regions ranging on average from 1.8 to 4.3 % [24, 25]. The high rates in Egypt have been traced to use of contaminated needles during a rural campaign to eradicate schistosomiasis in the Nile River basin [24]. Historically refugee screening for asymptomatic HCV has not occurred, especially across all the diverse refugee groups. It has not been thought to be cost-effective in the past. Even though HCV infection has clear clinical significance as a major chronic disease at the individual level, it is not a major communicable disease threat to public health when compared with tuberculosis, hepatitis B, or syphilis. In the absence of screening data, newly arriving refugee groups can only be estimated to have similar HCV prevalence rates to the regions and countries that they originated from. HCV prevalence rates are below 2 % in North America, Europe, and Australia which accept many of the relocated refugees from around the world [22, 23].

HCV transmission in developing countries where most refugees originate is mainly through non-sterile and unsafe medical procedures from injections, equipment, and blood products. In developed countries, transmission is caused by intravenous drug users (IUD) sharing needles and previously by contamination of blood or serum products. Perinatal transmission of HCV occurs at a rate of 5–6 % and health care needle stick from an HCV infected patient has a 1.8 % infection rate. Although sexual contact (not monogamous) increases risk, it is a low rate compared to IUD. HCV is detected in breast milk, but breast-feeding is not associated with increased risk [26].

The clinical course of hepatitis C infection has an acute hepatitis phase that in most is asymptomatic. In the less than 30 % of those that symptoms occur, after an incubation period of 2 weeks to 6 months, it is indistinguishable from other acute hepatitis syndromes (Table 7.2) and lasts less than a month. Chronic HCV infection persists in about 75–85 % of those infected, and over two decades of chronic HCV infection, up to 20 % develop cirrhosis and about 1.5 % go on to develop hepatocellular carcinoma [23]. Chronic HCV infection is more progressive with moderate alcohol intake, infection at older age, coinfection with HIV, and in Egyptians with schistosomiasis [27–29].

Screening: Routine screening for HCV infection in refugees is similar to the general population.

Screening recommendations for hepatitis C virus chronic infection has evolved based on:

1. A more recent cost-benefit analysis by the Canadian Collaboration for Immigrant and Refugee Health—*Screening for hepatitis C infection: Evidence review for newly arriving immigrants and refugees*— recommended screening for hepatitis C antibody in all immigrants and refugees arriving in Canada originating from countries with an expected prevalence of ≥3 % and referral for all positive cases [2].
2. The Center for Disease Control (CDC) has issued national guidelines to screen all persons born during 1945–1965 as this age group has a hepatitis C prevalence rate of 3.25 % [30], which is higher than the overall prevalence rate of 1.0–1.5 %. Refugees designated to be relocated to the US have a path to US citizenship and are in the group recommended for screening based on their birthdate. Testing could be further considered for refugees when HCV infection prevalence rates in their country of origin are as high or higher than the US prevalence rates that are the basis for the CDC guidelines.
3. Treatments for chronic hepatitis C are improving with higher rates of cure >50 % and the potential for less of the side effects that currently limit treatment.

Prevention: There is no vaccination. Alcohol should be avoided. Illicit intravenous drug users should be offered treatment referrals or should use sterile injection equipment and not share needles. Physicians should discuss limiting and monitoring drugs that affect the liver. Safe sex practices should be endorsed. Although breast-feeding has not been associated with increased transmission, it should be avoided with cracked or bleeding nipples.

Clinical Testing and Referral: Clinical testing is indicated for those born during 1945–1965 and with risk factors for hepatitis C infection: former and present IUD, children born to HCV-positive mothers, refugees that have ever received blood products or clotting factor in a developing nation or those exposed to potentially unsafe medical injections and procedures in developing countries, HIV infection, history of tattooing or body piercing, history of multiple sex partners or sexually transmitted diseases, and in the work-up of abnormal liver function tests.

Test for antibody to HCV (anti-HCV) and if positive, HCV RNA detection is used to confirm the infection and rule out a false-positive result. Referral for those known to be infected by HCV is made to a gastroenterologist or liver specialist for evaluation of chronic liver disease for consideration of potentially curative treatment and hepatocellular carcinoma surveillance screening. Coinfection with HIV or hepatitis B should be ruled out and serology for hepatitis A immunity evaluated.

Hepatitis A

Hepatitis A virus (HAV) is the most highly prevalent acute viral hepatitis worldwide. HAV is shed through feces. The most common transmission is the fecal oral route from the contamination of water to the food supply. It can also be transmitted through sexual (oral/anal) contact. Most refugees are from areas in the underdeveloped world that are intermediate or highly endemic for HAV (see Fig. 7.2) and were exposed due to poor water sanitation. In HAV highly endemic areas, 90 % have been infected by the age of 10 years [31]. HAV infection is a self-limited infection in most children and usually lasts less than 2 months, but in about 10 % of cases, prolonged or relapsing symptoms can last 6–9 months. Symptoms and signs of acute hepatitis (Table 7.2) are more likely with increased age [32]. Most adult refugees were infected as children and have lifelong immunity. Unvaccinated children and young adults from areas with good water sanitation may be susceptible to HAV infection, including some urban middle class individuals from underdeveloped countries. In general, lower-income regions correlate with high hepatitis A endemicity and low susceptibility, and high-income regions and countries have low prevalence rates of hepatitis A virus infection and higher susceptibility. Intermediate-wealth regions correlate with intermediate HAV prevalence and susceptibility [33].

Screening: Routine testing for HAV infection in refugees is not recommended at any age.

Vaccination: ACIP recommends HAV vaccine for all children ages 1–18 [34].

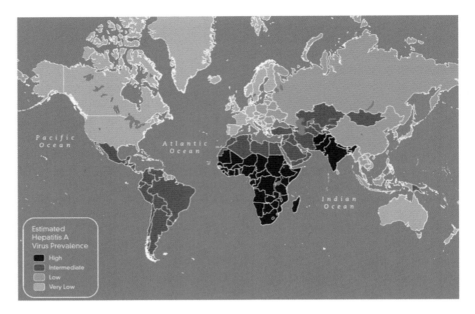

Fig. 7.2 Geographic distribution of hepatitis A endemicity. *Source*: CDC Travelers Health. Chapter 3. Infectious diseases related to travel. Hepatitis A. 2012

Hepatitis A serology (total anti-HAV IgG) to test for immunity is cost-effective, if the two-dose hepatitis A vaccination is being considered in adult refugees from regions of prevalence >33 % [34, 35].

Established refugee travelers are likely to be visiting friends and relatives (VFRs) in highly endemic areas. For unvaccinated VFRs <20 years old, serology testing or vaccination can be done. In VFRs age ≥20, it is cost-effective to check serology and vaccinate if susceptible [15].

In refugees with chronic liver disease, including CHB and CHC, hepatitis A immunity should be checked and susceptible individuals vaccinated.

Other Prevention: Access to sanitary water and avoidance of close contact or careful hygiene measures when in close contact with infected individuals.

Clinical: Supportive care and testing for IgM Anti-HAV serology for refugees with acute hepatitis signs and symptoms. HAV does not have a chronic phase.

Hepatitis E

Hepatitis E virus (HEV) liver infection is usually an acute mild self-limited infectious hepatitis. HEV infection is very common in developing countries due to fecally contaminated drinking water. Epidemics of HEV infection occur after natural disasters including flooding that causes water contamination, in overcrowded temporary housing, refugee camps, and across South and Central Asia, Southeast Asia, Africa, the Middle East, and Mexico [36]. High-risk groups according to the WHO include international travelers to regions of the world where HEV is endemic and refugees residing in overcrowded temporary camps following catastrophes, especially in Sudan, Somalia, Kenya, and Ethiopia [37].

Acute HEV infection incubation usually ranges from 15 to 60 days with acute hepatitis symptoms that more likely occur in older adolescents and young adults. It is usually asymptomatic in children. Most people recover completely. Pregnant women are most likely to experience severe hepatitis symptoms including fulminant hepatitis and death. HEV infection is different than HAV in that high mortality rates up to 30 % have been reported among pregnant women in some geographic areas [38]. Chronic infection may occur in HIV and in solid-organ transplant recipients on immunosuppression [39, 40]. In the US, returning travelers from endemic areas are most likely to be affected.

Screening: No screening for refugees is recommended for HEV infection.

Prevention: No vaccination is available. HEV infection is preventable by improving sanitation and water purity.

Clinical: HEV infectious hepatitis should be considered in a new arrival from an HEV endemic area (<3 months) with potential exposure and acute hepatitis symptoms (Table 7.2) and in whom other acute hepatitis syndromes (A, B, and C) have been ruled out. There is no FDA-approved test for HEV in the US. HEV testing (IgM and IgG antibodies to HEV and PCR assay for HEV RNA) can be requested from the CDC Division of Viral Hepatitis Laboratory for clinical evaluation [41]. Treatment is supportive, with hospitalization for fulminant hepatitis and severe illness in pregnancy.

References

1. World Health Organization position paper on hepatitis B vaccines. Weekly Epidemiological Record, No. 40, 2009;84:405–20.
2. Greenaway C, Wong DKH, Assayag D, et al. Screening for hepatitis C infection: evidence review for arriving immigrants and refugees. Appendix 7. Guidelines for immigrant health. CMAJ. 2011. doi:10.1503/cmaj.090313.
3. Weinbaum CM, Williams I, Mast EE, et al. Recommendations for identification and public health management of persons with chronic hepatitis B virus infection. MMWR Morb Mortal Wkly Rep. 2008;57(RR-8):1–20.
4. Center for Disease Control and Prevention. Evaluating and updating immunizations during the domestic medical examination for newly arrived refugees. Immigrant and refugee health domestic guidelines. 2012 [last updated 2012 Sep 27]. Available at: http://www.cdc.gov/immigrantrefugeehealth/guidelines/domestic/immunizations-guidelines.html. Accessed 3 May 2013.
5. Office of Refugee Resettlement. Medical screening protocol for newly arriving refugees. ORR's Domestic medical screening guidelines checklist attached to state letter 12-09

(07/24/12). Available at: http://www.acf.hhs.gov/programs/orr/resource/medical-screening-protocol-for-newly-arriving-refugees. Accessed 2 May 2013.

6. Association of Refugee Health Coordinators Medical Screening Committee Tools and Recommendations. Available at: http://www.astho.org/Programs/Infectious-Disease/Refugee-Health/ARHC-Medical-Screening-Recommendations/. Accessed 3 May 2013.

7. Beasley RP, Hwang LY. Overview of the epidemiology of hepatocellular carcinoma. In: Hollinger FB, Lemon SM, Margolis HS, editors. Viral hepatitis and liver disease. Proceedings of the 1990 International Symposium on Viral Hepatitis and Liver Disease: contemporary issues and future prospects. Baltimore, MD: Williams & Wilkins; 1991. p. 532–5.

8. Goldstein ST, Zhou F, Hadler SC, et al. A mathematical model to estimate global hepatitis B disease burden and vaccination impact. Int J Epidemiol. 2005;34:1329–39.

9. Perz JF, Armstrong GL, Farrington LA, et al. The contributions of hepatitis B virus and hepatitis C virus infections to cirrhosis and primary liver cancer worldwide. J Hepatol. 2006;45:529–38.

10. Rein DB, Lesesne SB, O'Fallon A, et al. Prevalence of hepatitis B surface antigen among refugees entering the United States between 2006 and 2008. Hepatology. 2009;51:431–4.

11. Kowdley KV, Wang CC, Welch S, et al. Prevalence of chronic hepatitis B among foreign-born persons living in the United States by country of origin. Hepatology. 2012;56:422–33. doi:10.1002/hep.24804.

12. Kim WR, Terrault NA, Pedersen RA, et al. Trends in waitlist registration for liver transplantation for viral hepatitis in the US. Gastroenterology. 2009;137:1680–6.

13. Institute of Medicine. Hepatitis and liver cancer: a national strategy for prevention and control of hepatitis B and C. Washington, DC: The National Academies Press; 2010.

14. Cohen C, Holmberg SD, McMahon BJ, et al. Is chronic hepatitis B being undertreated in the United States? J Viral Hepat. 2011;18:377–83.

15. Keystone JS. Chapter 58 Visiting friends and relatives. In: Walker PF, Barnett ED, editors. Immigrant medicine. Philadelphia, PA: Saunders Elsevier; 2007. p. 747.

16. Mast EE, Margolis HS, Fiore AE, Brink EW, Goldstein ST, Wang SA, Moyer LA, Bell BP, Alter MJ, Advisory Committee on Immunization Practices (ACIP). A comprehensive immunization strategy to eliminate transmission of hepatitis B virus infection in the United States: recommendations of the advisory committee on immunization practices. Part I: Immunization of infants, children, and adolescents. MMWR Morb Mortal Wkly Rep. 2005;54(RR-16):1–31.

17. World Health Organization. Hepatitis Delta. Geneva: World Health Organization; 2001. Available at: http://www.who.int/csr/disease/hepatitis/HepatitisD_whocdscsrncs2001_1.pdf. Accessed 3 May 2013.

18. Rizzeto M, Ponzetto A, Forzani I. Epidemiology of hepatitis delta virus: overview. Prog Clin Biol Res. 1991;364:1–20.

19. Chironna M, Germinario C, Lopalco PL, et al. HBV, HCV and HDV infections in Albanian refugees in Southern Italy (Apulia region). Epidemiol Infect. 2000;125(1):163–7.

20. Maynard JE, Hadler SC, Fields HA. Delta hepatitis in the Americas: an overview. Prog Clin Biol Res. 1987;234:493–505.

21. World Health Organization Hepatitis C fact sheet 2011. Available at: http://www.who.int/mediacentre/factsheets/fs164/en/. Accessed 2 May 2013.

22. World Health Organization. Hepatitis C—global prevalence (update). Wkly Epidemiol Rec. 1999;74:425–7.

23. Global Burden of Hepatitis C Working Group. Global burden of disease (GBD) for hepatitis C. J Clin Pharmacol. 2004;44(1):20–9.

24. CDC. Progress toward prevention and control of hepatitis C virus infection—Egypt, 2001–2012. MMWR Morb Mortal Wkly Rep. 2012;61(29):545–9.

25. Syed AA, Donahue RMJ, Qureshi H, et al. Hepatitis B and hepatitis C in Pakistan: prevalence and risk factors. Int J Infect Dis. 2009;13(1):9–19.

26. Centers for Disease Control and Prevention. Recommendations for prevention and control of hepatitis C virus (HCV) infection and HCV-related chronic disease. MMWR Morb Mortal Wkly Rep. 1998;47(RR-19):1–39.

27. Ghany MG, Strader DB, Thomas DL, et al. Diagnosis, management, and treatment of hepatitis C: an update. Hepatology. 2009;49:1335–74.
28. Kamal SM, Rasenack JW, Bianchi L, et al. Acute hepatitis C without and with schistosomiasis: correlation with hepatitis C-specific CD4+ T-cell and cytokine response. Gastroenterology. 2001;121(3):646–56.
29. Koshy A, al-Nakib B, al-Mufti S, et al. Anti-HCV-positive cirrhosis associated with schistosomiasis. Am J Gastroenterol. 1993;88(9):1428–31.
30. Centers for Disease Control and Prevention. Recommendations for the identification of chronic hepatitis C virus infection among persons born during 1945–1965. MMWR Morb Mortal Wkly Rep. 2012;61(RR-4):1–32.
31. WHO position paper on hepatitis A vaccines. Weekly epidemiological record No. 28–29, 2012;87:261–76.
32. Centers for Disease Control and Prevention. Chapter 8 Hepatitis A epidemiology and prevention of vaccine-preventable diseases. In: Atkinson W, Wolfe S, Hamborsky J, editors. The pink book—epidemiology & prevention of vaccine-preventable diseases. 12th ed. Washington, DC: Public Health Foundation; 2012. second printing.
33. Jacobsen KH, Wiersma ST. Hepatitis A virus seroprevalence by age and world region, 1990 and 2005. Vaccine. 2010;28(41):6653–7.
34. CDC. Prevention of hepatitis A through active or passive immunization. Recommendations of the Advisory Committee on Immunization Practices. MMWR Morb Mortal Wkly Rep. 2006;55(RR-7):1–23.
35. Bryan JP, Nelson M. Testing for antibody to hepatitis A to decrease the cost of hepatitis A prophylaxis with immune globulin or hepatitis A vaccines. Arch Intern Med. 1994;154: 663–8.
36. Center for Disease Control and Prevention Division of Viral Hepatitis. Hepatitis E information for health professionals. Overview and statistics. Available at: http://www.cdc.gov/hepatitis/HEV/HEVfaq.htm. Accessed 3 May 2013.
37. Previsani N, Lavanchy D. Hepatitis E. World Health Organization Department of Communicable Disease Surveillance and Response WHO/CDS/CSR/EDC/2001.12. http://www.who.int/csr/disease/hepatitis/HepatitisA_whocdscsredc2000_7.pdf
38. Navaneethan U, Al Mohajer M, Shata MT. Hepatitis E and pregnancy: understanding the pathogenesis. Liver Int. 2008;28:1190–9. doi:10.1111/j.1478-3231.2008.01840.x.
39. Dalton HR, Bendall RP, Keane FE, et al. Persistent carriage of Hepatitis E in patients with HIV infection. N Engl J Med. 2009;361:1025–7.
40. Kamar N, Selves J, Mansuy JM, et al. Hepatitis E virus and chronic hepatitis in organ-transplant recipients. N Engl J Med. 2008;358(8):811–7.
41. Center for Disease Control and Prevention Division of Viral Hepatitis. Hepatitis E Information for Health Professionals. 2012 [last updated 2012 Sep 14]. Available at: http://www.cdc.gov/hepatitis/HEV/LabTestingRequests.htm. Accessed 2 May 2013.

Chapter 8
Malaria

Kristina Krohn and William Stauffer

Introduction

The World Health Organization (WHO) estimated over 200 million cases of malaria and 660,000 deaths from malaria in 2010 [1]. Over 10,000 refugees entering the United States each year come from sub-Saharan Africa, where malaria is hyperendemic [2]. The WHO defines an area as hyperendemic when more than 50 % children aged 2–9 years old have malaria at any given time [3]. African children are at particular risk of contracting and dying from malaria; UNICEF estimates that malaria kills an African child every 30 seconds [4]. Most adults in hyperendemic areas have some immunity and therefore can be infected with malaria without showing signs of disease. In one study of Liberian refugees from refugee camps in four different countries, even 4 weeks after arriving in the United States, 60 % still had malaria parasites in their blood [5].

Malaria is believed to have been brought to the United States by European settlers and African slaves. Malaria was endemic until the 1950s when it was eradicated in the United States. Most of the United States continues to have the *Anopheles* mosquitoes, which can act as a good vector for malaria. Since the vector was not eradicated when malaria was eradicated in the United States, small outbreaks have been imported and spread within the United States [6, 7].

K. Krohn, M.D. (✉)
Department of Internal Medicine and Pediatrics, University of Minnesota,
14-100B Phillips Wangensteen Building MMC 913, 420 Delaware Street SE, Minneapolis,
MN 555455, USA
e-mail: kroh0040@umn.edu

W. Stauffer, M.D., M.S.P.H., C TropMed, F.A.S.T.M.H.
Division of Infectious Diseases and International Medicine, Department of Medicine,
University of Minnesota, 420 Delaware St. S.E., MMC 250, Minneapolis, MN 55042, USA
e-mail: stauf005@umn.edu

A. Annamalai (ed.), *Refugee Health Care: An Essential Medical Guide*,
DOI 10.1007/978-1-4939-0271-2_8, © Springer Science+Business Media New York 2014

The number of locally transmitted cases (156 since 1957) [6] pales in comparison to the more than 1,000 cases of malaria imported to the United States over a similar time frame; many of the imported cases occur in refugees [8–11].

Displaced populations have historically suffered more malaria than their stable countrymen, as they are exposed more to the elements during their flight and temporary housing in refugee camps [11, 12]. Even refugees who come from urban areas may have subclinical malaria infections. Once refugees arrive in the United States, they may be disenfranchised and have poor access to care due to language barriers, difficulty with transportation, stigma, or economic hardship. For all of these reasons, after being exposed to malaria, some refugees carry subclinical infection and may not present to a health-care provider with signs and symptoms for 3 months or more after they arrive in the United States [12–15]. Unfortunately, delayed diagnosis and inappropriate treatment of malaria infection by health-care professionals in the United States has led to fatal outcomes [16, 17].

There are four main species of malaria that infect humans: *Plasmodium falciparum*, *P. ovale*, *P. vivax,* and *P. malariae* [18]. *P. knowlesi* occasionally causes infection in humans, but its usual host is macaque monkeys [19].

P. falciparum causes most malaria deaths. It is highly endemic throughout sub-Saharan Africa and hyperendemic in many areas. In these areas most of the adults have partial immunity, and subclinical infection is common. Central Asia, South Asia, Southeast Asia, and parts of Latin America and the Caribbean have varying levels of all four species of malaria, but not to the same hyperendemic level seen in sub-Saharan Africa.

P. vivax, *P. ovale,* and *P. malariae* are also endemic in sub-Saharan Africa, but have a lower prevalence than *P. falciparum* and cause less severe disease. *P. vivax* and *P. ovale* cause relapsing human infection because they have an extended liver stage, where the sporozoites may live and reproduce without entering the blood stream. Most antimalarials do not treat the liver phase of infection, particularly hypnozoite infections of *P. vivax* and *P. ovale*. Therefore, these species can cause repeat infection if the liver stage is not treated [4]. Neither *P. falciparum* nor *P. malariae* have a dormant liver stage; therefore, they are not considered relapsing species. However, *P. malariae*-infected individuals may be asymptomatic for extended periods of time giving it the appearance of a recurrent or relapsed infection [14].

Refugees arriving from Southeast Asia, South Asia, Central Asia, and all areas in the Western Hemisphere generally come from areas with low or absent levels of malaria transmission. Because of the low level of malaria in these refugees, and higher rates of non-falciparum malaria, it is not currently feasible or cost-effective to do routine screening or to give presumptive treatment for refugees from areas other than sub-Saharan Africa according to the Centers for Disease Control and Prevention (CDC). For those refugees coming from or passing through areas with low level of malaria transmission, if signs and symptoms are present, physicians can do diagnostic testing for plasmodium and subsequent treatment for confirmed infections. The CDC malaria map (see Fig. 8.1) can be checked for information on malaria endemicity around the world.

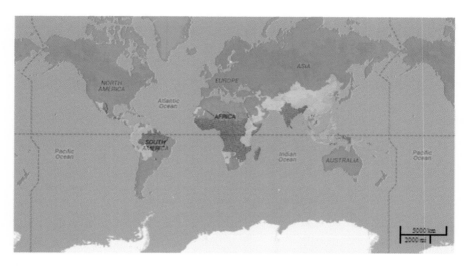

Fig. 8.1 CDC malaria map application http://www.cdc.gov/malaria/map/index.html

Predeparture Presumptive Treatment

Starting in 1999 the Centers for Disease Control and Prevention (CDC) recommend that all refugees departing for the United States from malaria endemic areas in sub-Saharan Africa receive presumptive therapy for malaria. Predeparture treatment is cost-effective in highly endemic areas in sub-Saharan Africa. Initially, a presumptive treatment course of sulfadoxine-pyrimethamine (SP, Fansidar™) was used, but as resistance emerged, the recommendation changed to artemisinin-based combination therapy (ACT) [14]. Malaria predeparture presumptive therapy must be administered and documented as directly observed therapy, and this documentation must be completed no sooner than 3 days prior to departure. Documentation is communicated to state health programs through the CDC's Electronic Data Network (EDN) and is in the paper copy carried by the refugee. Pregnant or lactating women and children <5 kg do not receive presumptive therapy prior to departure. After arrival, these refugees should either be presumptively treated if the contraindication no longer applies (e.g., postdelivery or weight of the infant is greater than 5 kg), or have testing and if positive should be treated [20, 21].

Post-arrival Presumptive Therapy

Once refugees arrive in the United States, if they have proper documentation of predeparture treatment, they require no further evaluation or treatment for malaria, unless they have clinical symptoms. If refugees are from sub-Saharan Africa and

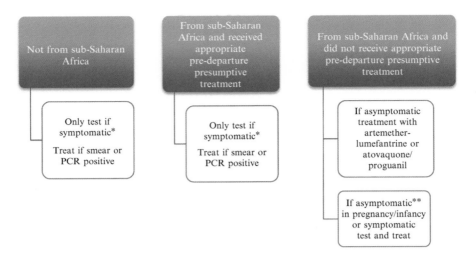

Fig. 8.2 When to screen or provide presumptive post-arrival treatment. *If symptomatic, test with blood smear or antigen PCR; rapid antigen test can be used if other tests not available or while waiting for other test results. **If asymptomatic, test with three blood smears every 12–24 h or antigen PCR

have not received appropriate predeparture therapy, they should receive presumptive treatment with atovaquone-proguanil or artemether-lumefantrine. The natural exceptions are for pregnant or lactating women, children less than 5 kg, and people with medication allergies who should not receive pre- or post-departure presumptive treatment [20, 21]. These special populations should receive post-arrival screening (see Fig. 8.2). However, universal post-arrival screening is not cost-effective.

Only refugees from highly endemic areas in sub-Saharan Africa who did not receive predeparture treatment should receive post-arrival treatment; all refugees from any area with endemic malaria should be monitored for malaria symptoms and for appropriate responses to treatment including watching for any side effects from treatment [21–23].

Life Cycle

When a female *Anopheles* mosquito bites a human, they can deposit malaria sporozoites into the person. First these sporozoites infect liver cells and mature into schizonts, which rupture and release merozoites. *P. vivax*'s and *P. ovale*'s dormant stage is known as hypnozoites and can hide out in the liver to invade the bloodstream weeks or even years later causing a relapsing infection. After the liver maturation, the merozoites infect red blood cells (RBCs). The merozoites then mature and rupture the

RBCs. Disease is caused by the maturation and replication in the bloodstream. Some of the malaria parasites differentiate into a sexual stage called gametocytes. Disease is passed on when another mosquito picks up the gametocytes while ingesting human blood. These gametocytes sexually reproduce in the mosquito with the offspring invading the mosquito's stomach wall and eventually moving to the mosquito's salivary glands to invade the next human the mosquito bites [24].

Symptoms and Signs

Physicians should suspect malaria in a newly arrived, or recently arrived, refugee with nausea, vomiting, fever, chills, sweats, headaches, muscle pains, hepatospleno-megaly, thrombocytopenia, or anemia. But, frequently newly arrived refugees from hyperendemic areas have subclinical infection or may have only incidentally noted abnormalities such as anemia, thrombocytopenia, hepatomegaly, or splenomegaly. The initial symptoms can be similar to common viral infections or the "flu." The classic cyclical fever pattern is helpful when it is present, but its absence does not rule out malarial infection. Later signs of severe malaria such as confusion, coma, neurologic focal signs, severe anemia, respiratory difficulties, and hepatospleno-megaly are more striking and may be specific to the type of malaria [25].

The most concerning malarial infection is *P. falciparum* malaria as it is common in refugees from hyperendemic areas and is the most life-threatening. Classic symptoms are the common symptoms listed above with cyclical fevers that spike around dusk and dawn. For *P. falciparum* the most common complications include neurologic changes indicating cerebral malaria, severe anemia due to hemolysis, hemoglobinuria, acute respiratory distress syndrome (ARDS), coagulation abnormalities, hypotension leading to cardiovascular failure, acute kidney failure, metabolic acidosis, and danger-ous hypoglycemia. Even if none of these are present, a parasite load with >5 % of infected red blood cells, called hyperparasitemia, is considered complicated malaria. Complicated malaria is life-threatening and requires aggressive treatment [23, 26].

P. ovale and *P. vivax* both may be called tertian malaria because their fever clas-sically spikes every 48 h. Otherwise symptoms are similar to *P. falciparum* malaria; complications are less likely but may still be seen. Both *P. ovale* and *P. vivax* may relapse, causing disease months to years after initial infection, due to sporozoites living in the liver without entering the bloodstream and causing symptoms.

P. malariae may cause a nephrotic syndrome where patients lose significant pro-teins in their urine and become edematous due the loss of blood proteins. This is different from the nephritic, blackwater fever, seen with *P. falciparum* where hemo-lysis causes dark urine from fragmented red blood cells in a patient's urine [27].

In general, physicians should have a low threshold to test for malaria in refugees who present with symptoms, especially fever, jaundice, and hepatosplenomegaly.

Diagnosis

As explained above, refugees coming from sub-Saharan Africa who have not received predeparture therapy with a recommended regimen should receive presumptive treatment on arrival in the United States; however, if there are contraindications to treatment (i.e., pregnancy or infancy), screening is appropriate. For newly arrived refugees without symptoms a single malaria thick and thin blood smear lacks sensitivity (<40 %) [20]. Three separate blood films taken at 12–24 h intervals is recommended as it has a greater sensitivity [20]. Rapid antigen testing also has poor sensitivity (<30 %) in asymptomatic individuals in small studies of refugees [14]. Another option for screening asymptomatic refugees is molecular testing (i.e., polymerase chain reaction (PCR)). In asymptomatic pregnant women and infants who cannot receive presumptive therapy, antigen PCR is preferred due to the poor predictive value of blood smears and rapid testing in people without symptoms [20, 23]. For asymptomatic individuals with a positive rapid antigen test, either blood smears or PCR confirmation should be done [20, 23].

Patients with symptoms should be tested for malaria utilizing a thick and thin blood smear, as it is highly specific for malaria infection. The specificity of blood smears depends on the practitioner's experience. Smears should involve thick smears to view more blood to increase sensitivity and thin smears to view individual parasites to improve specificity and allow identification of the specific species of malaria [25]. Initial blood smears may result in a false negative even in experienced hands. When malaria is suspected and the initial smear is negative, blood smears should be repeated at 12–24 h intervals [20]. The rapid antigen test approved by FDA has excellent sensitivity in symptomatic patients, and this may be used when experience with blood smears is limited or in conjunction with blood smears [20, 23].

Diagnosis and treatment for severe malaria infections or infection in specific populations (such as pregnant women and infants) is complicated. Providers can seek assistance from the *CDC Malaria Hotline* (770-488-7788 or 855-856-4713 toll-free) (M–F, 9 a.m. to 5 p.m., Eastern Time), especially in those cases where the treatment protocol may not be clear.

Treatment

Treatment of malaria depends on the disease severity, the species of malaria parasite causing the infection, and the resistance patterns in the part of the world where the infection originated [20]. A patient's age, weight, and pregnancy status may limit treatment options. Uncomplicated malaria may be treated with a single drug or a combination medication considering the resistance patterns where the malaria originated. Most areas have chloroquine resistance, with only a few areas of the Caribbean and Central America with malaria that remains sensitive to chloroquine [28]. Mefloquine resistance has emerged in Cambodia, Vietnam, Thailand, and Burma/Myanmar [28].

Complicated malaria requires two-drug treatment starting with intravenous quinine which can be combined with doxycycline, tetracycline, or clindamycin. Treatment for *P. vivax* and *P. ovale* also involves primaquine to eliminate the liver stage. Due to teratogenicity, pregnant women should not receive primaquine, but should receive chloroquine prophylaxis until the child is delivered and both can be tested for glucose-6-phosphate-dehydrogenase (G6PD) deficiency and safely given primaquine [29]. In patients with G6PD deficiency, primaquine can cause hemolytic anemia and should not be given [29].

For guidelines on treatment of malaria in the United States, please visit the CDC resource at http://www.cdc.gov/malaria/resources/pdf/treatmenttable.pdf.

Physicians may obtain consultation by calling the CDC's Malaria Hotline (770-488-7788) from 9:00 a.m. to 5:00 p.m. Eastern Time. After hours or on weekends and holidays, physicians may call the CDC Emergency Operation Center at 770-488-7100 and ask to page the person on call for the Malaria Branch.

Conclusions

Malaria can be imported into the country by refugees and transmitted locally. A complete history, including geographic risk factors, and the screening recommendations outlined above can help detect a majority of cases. Guidelines on screening for malaria in refugees and treatment recommendations are periodically updated by CDC, and providers are encouraged to access this information.

References

1. World Health Organization. World malaria report. 2012. http://who.int/malaria/publications/world_malaria_report_2012/wmr2012_full_report.pdf. Accessed Aug 2013.
2. US Department of State Bureau of Population, Refugees, and Migration Office of Admissions—Refugee Processing Center Summary of Refugee Admissions. http://www.wrapsnet.org/LinkClick.aspx?fileticket=qKPnYtpZDI4%3d&tabid=211&portalid=1&mid=630. Accessed Feb 2013.
3. World Health Organization. 2005. http://www.who.int/malaria/publications/atoz/incidence_estimations2.pdf. Accessed Aug 2013.
4. United Nations Children's Fund (UNICEF). 2003 [updated 2003 Jun]. http://www.unicef.org/media/media_7701.html. Accessed Aug 2013.
5. Maroushek SR, Aguilar EF, Stauffer W, Abd-Alla MD. Malaria among refugee children at arrival in the United States. Pediatr Infect Dis J. 2005;24(5):450–2.
6. Zucker JR. Changing patterns of autochthonous malaria transmission in the United States: a review of recent outbreaks. Emerg Infect Dis. 1996;2:37–43.
7. Filler SJ, MacArthur JR, Parise M, Centers for Disease Control and Prevention, et al. Locally acquired mosquito-transmitted malaria: a guide for investigations in the United States. MMWR Recomm Rep. 2006;55:1–9.
8. Kambili C, Murray HW, Golightly LM. Malaria: 30 years of experience at a New York City teaching hospital. Am J Trop Med Hyg. 2004;70(4):408–11.

9. Schlagenhauf P, Steffen R, Loutan L. Migrants as a major risk group for imported malaria in European countries. J Travel Med. 2003;10(2):106–7.
10. Taylor-Robinson A. Population migration and malaria: terms of reference. Trends Parasitol. 2001;17(7):315.
11. Mertans P, Hall L. Malaria on the move: human population movement and malaria transmission. Emerg Infect Dis. 2000;6(2):103–9.
12. Rowland M, Nosten F. Malaria epidemiology and control in refugee camps and complex emergencies. Ann Trop Med Parasitol. 2001;95(8):741–54.
13. Ndao M, Bandyayera E, Kokosin E, et al. Comparison of blood smear, antigen detection, and nested-PCR methods for screening from regions where malaria is endemic after a malaria outbreak in Quebec, Canada. J Clin Microbiol. 2004;42(6):2694–700.
14. Stauffer WM, Newberry AM, Cartwright CP, et al. Evaluation of malaria screening in newly arrived refugees to the United States by microscopy and rapid antigen capture enzyme assay. Pediatr Infect Dis J. 2006;25(10):948–50.
15. Collinet-Adler S, Stauffer WM, Boulware DR, et al. Financial implications of refugee malaria: the impact of pre-departure anti-malarial presumptive therapy. Am J Trop Med Hyg. 2007; 77(3):458–63.
16. Kain KC, Harrington MA, Tennyson S, et al. Imported malaria: prospective analysis of problems in diagnosis and management. Clin Infect Dis. 1998;27:142–9.
17. Newman RD, Parise ME, Barber AM, et al. Malaria-related deaths among U.S. travelers, 1963–2001. Ann Intern Med. 2004;141(7):547–55.
18. Centers for Disease Control and Prevention. Malaria parasites. 2010 [last updated 2010 Feb]. http://www.cdc.gov/malaria/about/biology/parasites.html. Accessed Aug 2013.
19. Jongwutiwes S, Buppan P, Kosuvin R, et al. Emerging infectious diseases. Centers for Disease Control and Prevention. 2011 [last updated 2011 Sep]. http://wwwnc.cdc.gov/eid/article/17/10/11-0349_article.htm. Accessed Aug 2013.
20. Centers for Disease Control. 2012 [last updated 2012 Oct]. http://www.cdc.gov/immigrantrefugeehealth/guidelines/domestic/malaria-guidelines-domestic.html. Accessed Aug 2013.
21. Phares CM, Kapella BK, Doney AC, et al. Presumptive treatment to reduce imported malaria among refugees from East Africa resettling in the United States. Am J Trop Med Hyg. 2011;85(4):612–5.
22. Division of Global Migration and Quarantine. Centers for Disease Control and Prevention. 2013 [last updated 2013 Aug]. http://www.cdc.gov/ncidod/dq/refugee/rh_guide/domestic.htm. Accessed Aug 2013.
23. Stauffer WM, Weinberg M, Newman RD, et al. Pre-departure and post-arrival management of P. falciparum malaria in refugees relocating from Sub-Saharan Africa to the United States. Am J Trop Med Hyg. 2008;79(2):141–6.
24. Malaria. DPDX CDC. 2009 [last updated 2009]. http://www.dpd.cdc.gov/dpdx/HTML/malaria.htm. Accessed Aug 2013.
25. Centers for Disease Control and Prevention. Malaria diagnosis (United States). 2012 [last updated 2012 Jun]. http://www.cdc.gov/malaria/diagnosis_treatment/diagnosis.html. Accessed Aug 2013.
26. Centers for Disease Control and Prevention. Malaria disease. 2010 [last updated 2010 Feb]. http://www.cdc.gov/malaria/about/disease.html. Accessed Aug 2013.
27. Eddleston M, Davidson R, Brent A, Wilkinson R, editors. Oxford handbook of tropical medicine. 3rd ed. New York: Oxford University Press; 2006. p. 31–65.
28. World Health Organization. Malaria. 2013 [last updated 2013 Mar]. http://www.who.int/mediacentre/factsheets/fs094/en/. Accessed Aug 2013.
29. Centers for Disease Control and Prevention. Treatment of malaria: guidelines for clinicians (United States). 2010 [last updated 2010 Feb]. http://www.cdc.gov/malaria/diagnosis_treatment/clinicians2.html. Accessed Aug 2013.

Chapter 9
HIV and Other Sexually Transmitted Infections: Testing and Treatment Considerations for Refugees

Sachin Jain and Jennifer Adelson-Mitty

This chapter will highlight key screening, testing, and management considerations relevant to refugee populations for human immunodeficiency virus (HIV) and other major sexually transmitted infections. We will begin with a discussion of HIV.

HIV

Global Burden of Disease

Per the United Nations Program on HIV/AIDS (UNAIDS) estimates, there were approximately 34 million people living with HIV at the end of 2011, which has been increasing over time. The overall global prevalence of HIV infection for people aged 15–49 is 0.8 % with the greatest burden of disease in sub-Saharan Africa (~5 % on average), followed by the Caribbean, Eastern Europe, and Central Asia (~1 % on average). The most common strain of HIV globally is HIV-1. HIV-2 is far more prevalent in West Africa but represents less than 1 % of global infections. While the prevalence of HIV has been on the rise due to people living longer with HIV, marked reductions in HIV incidence and deaths attributable to HIV/AIDS (acquired immunodeficiency syndrome) have been achieved over the past decade, primarily in sub-Saharan Africa and the Caribbean. That said, some regions are seeing increases in

S. Jain, M.D., M.P.H. (✉) • J. Adelson-Mitty, M.D. M.P.H.
Department of Infectious Diseases, Beth Israel Deaconess Medical Center,
Harvard Medical School, 110 Francis Street, LMOB Ground Floor, Boston 02118, MA, USA
e-mail: sjain4@bidmc.harvard.edu; jmitty@bidmc.harvard.edu

A. Annamalai (ed.), *Refugee Health Care: An Essential Medical Guide*, 103
DOI 10.1007/978-1-4939-0271-2_9, © Springer Science+Business Media New York 2014

new HIV infections, namely, central Asia, eastern Europe, Middle East, and North Africa, as well as men who have sex with men in urban areas across the world. Recent approaches to stemming the epidemic have focused on engaging more patients into care and treatment, risk reduction in injection drug use, biomedical prevention, vaccine development, accessibility to HIV testing, male circumcision, and reducing stigma and criminalization surrounding HIV, among others [1].

HIV in Refugees

HIV infection among refugees is not insignificant. As of 2006, there were an estimated 14.3 million refugees and 24.5 million internally displaced persons globally. Of those refugees and internally displaced persons affected by conflict, disaster, or displacement, 1.8 million were living with HIV. The precise burden of disease among refugees in the United States is unknown due to limited epidemiological data. Many refugees emigrate from settings that have a reported HIV prevalence from 2 to 28 %, with up to 14 % arriving from countries with a prevalence of >5 % based on earlier estimates. The countries that report high HIV prevalence and are also affected by conflict or humanitarian crisis include Nigeria, India, Mozambique, Democratic Republic of Congo, Tanzania, Kenya, Zambia, Uganda, China, Ethiopia, Malawi, and Russian Federation. Therefore, HIV prevalence may be largely influenced by the countries of origin and those through which refugees have transited. Concerns have been raised about incomplete data from underreporting, sampling challenges in conflict settings, or underdiagnosis [2].

In general, refugees may acquire several risk factors for HIV infection prior to resettlement, which are exacerbated by displacement. These risk factors include sexual violence, physical abuse requiring blood transfusions, drug use, exchange of sex for money or basic sustenance, and indirectly through depression or increased alcohol consumption. Disclosure of these exposures may not be forthcoming during initial post-resettlement intake assessments, especially when there is language and/or cultural discordance, even with the use of an interpreter. Refugees often do not have access to HIV treatment and prevention packages in many conflict-afflicted regions due to limited resources and regional priorities, so some have favored a human rights-based approach to understanding HIV in refugees [3]. There is unfortunately a greater degree of stigma, which may be perpetuated by preconceived notions that refugees have a higher prevalence of HIV disease than the host population. However, data suggest that the vast majority of refugee populations demonstrated a lower HIV prevalence than host populations where HIV prevalence data was available. Although refugees are integrated into communities within host countries in which they resettle, they may remain socially segregated and may not necessarily be targeted in broader regional public health campaigns, including but not limited to HIV. Therefore, refugee providers may need to elicit a thorough risk assessment over serial visits and offer appropriate prevention counseling [4].

HIV Entry Ban in the United States

It is essential to acknowledge the former HIV entry ban while discussing HIV in the refugee population. Historically, refugees had to be screened for HIV prior to departure from their originating country. However, this is no longer necessary. Dating back to 1952 prior to knowledge of HIV, there was a formal entry ban for any foreigners "who are afflicted with any dangerous contagious disease" that rendered them ineligible to receive a visa. Once HIV was identified, Congress added HIV infection to the list of dangerous contagious diseases on July 11, 1987. This was followed by the issuance of official regulations by the US Health and Human Services to enforce this on August 28, 1987, which enforced the above. Therefore, these laws required HIV testing to those wishing to enter the United States and prevented entry to any person who was found to be HIV positive [5]. The United States was not alone with such legislation. It was only 1 of 96 countries that imposed an entry ban on HIV-positive individuals per UNAIDS reports as of the year 2000.

In June of 2004, UNAIDS and the International Organization for Migration responded by issuing the "UNAIDS/IOM Statement on HIV/AIDS-related travel restrictions" that discounted the two most commonly cited reasons for travel restrictions by member States, which include public health threat of HIV being a communicable disease and the economic burden to treat HIV [6]. They additionally suggested that HIV-related travel restrictions may conflict with international human rights and humanitarian law and offered guidance regarding these issues. On June 2, 2009, the HHS and CDC published a Notice of Proposed Rule Making (NPRM), which proposed the removal of HIV infection from the definition of communicable disease of public health significance and removal of references to serologic testing for HIV from the scope of examinations. The final regulation was published on November 2, 2009 and ultimately went into effect on January 4, 2010. The new ruling removed the requirement for HIV testing for the immigrant medical exam and that HIV testing would be strictly voluntary and confidential [5, 7].

HIV Testing Considerations in Refugees

Given that there is no longer a requirement to test refugees prior to arrival, it is incumbent upon providers to offer routine HIV testing as part of general medical care in accordance with the 2006 CDC recommendations for all persons aged 13–64, although these age recommendations were based upon US epidemiology [8]. In addition, the Centers for Disease Control and Prevention (CDC) encourages screening refugees <13 and >64 years old. The current recommendation is to use whole blood or serum samples to perform enzyme-linked immunoabsorbent assay (ELISA), although rapid oral tests have also been utilized in health care settings with variable positive and negative predictive value [9, 10]. This should be done with oral or written consent as per the State law in the refugee's language, preferably with a medical interpreter, and being mindful of the refugee's cultural and societal norms. For example, in a retrospective case–control study of primarily Liberian refugees in Rhode Island, refugees were less likely to initiate antiretrovirals (ARVs) and also reported almost exclusive heterosexual contact as the primary risk factor for HIV transmission [11]. Therefore, queries about injected drug use or male-to-male sex may be perceived as offensive and should be framed in a culturally sensitive way.

Furthermore, counseling messages should be targeted to an individual's particular risk factors for future transmission. The refugee should have the option to opt out of testing and to ask questions before the test is performed. A thorough HIV risk assessment should be performed at the time of the initial medical evaluation to guide whether more or less frequent HIV testing is indicated. Review of prior potential HIV risk exposures should be revisited at subsequent visits since this information may not necessarily be volunteered at the intake evaluation shortly after arrival to a new country and enrollment into a foreign medical system. If someone reports a potential high-risk exposure and has a negative initial HIV test, the test should be repeated in 3–6 months to diagnose those who may have been in the "window period," or the time in which there is active infection but not yet detectable antibody to HIV. All positive HIV ELISA tests should be followed up with a confirmatory Western blot [4]. Once HIV infection is diagnosed, a viral load should be performed, which is a quantitative ribonucleic acid (RNA) test for HIV-1. There is currently no data to support routine HIV viral load testing, unless acute HIV infection is suspected.

Children born to HIV-infected mothers can be infected during childbirth and through breastfeeding. Since children have passively acquired maternal antibodies, infants should be screened with HIV viral load at day 14, at 1–2 months, and at 3–6 months of life. Diagnosis is confirmed with two positive DNA (deoxyribonucleic acid)/RNA tests and excluded with two negative DNA/RNA tests or antibody tests after 6 months of age per CDC guidelines. Negative disease should be confirmed with an antibody test at 18 months since maternal antibodies should have cleared by this time if the mother is HIV-infected [4].

Medical providers should determine whether an HIV-positive refugee has HIV-1 or HIV-2 since the treatment guidelines differ. The CDC recommends testing for HIV-2 infection for refugees that have traveled through or lived in the following countries: Angola, Benin, Burkina Faso, Cape Verde, Côte d'Ivoire (Ivory Coast), Gambia, Ghana, Guinea, Guinea-Bissau, Liberia, Mali, Mauritania, Mozambique, Niger, São Tomé, Senegal, Sierra Leone, and Togo. Some cases of HIV-2 have also been reported in India, Europe, Brazil, and the United States [12]. Most ELISA antibody assays can detect both HIV-1 and HIV-2 with high sensitivity. However, with one exception, this test itself does not distinguish between the two strains. The current Western blots done in the United States are only able to identify HIV-1. Dedicated HIV-2 antibody assays are available. However, unlike in HIV-1 where RNA viral load testing is widely used, this method is not widely available for HIV-2. In addition, HIV-2 viral load testing may be less reliable since it tends to cause a much lower-grade viremia as compared to HIV-1 [13]. Therefore, DNA testing can be used, but neither quantitative DNA nor RNA tests have been FDA-approved.

HIV Treatment Considerations in Refugees

Treatment is now recommended for HIV-infected individuals at all CD4 counts in the United States in light of emerging data that unchecked viral replication can cause chronic immune activation, leading to accelerated end-organ complications and even malignancy [14]. HIV treatment should be started early in the setting of opportunistic infections, including active tuberculosis. The major exception to starting early treatment is cryptococcal meningitis due to concern for cryptococcal immune reconstitution inflammatory syndrome (IRIS) [15]. The US Department of Health and Human Services offers extensive treatment guidance on their website: http://aidsinfo.nih.gov/guidelines. If the HIV viral load is found to be >1,000 copies/mL, a genotype analysis should be performed prior to initiating therapy to screen for transmitted drug resistance. HIV-2 is usually treated successfully with two nucleoside reverse transcriptase inhibitors (NRTIs) and a boosted protease inhibitor, even though natural polymorphisms of the reverse transcriptase and protease exist, which can theoretically impact the efficacy of either class of drug. Non-nucleoside reverse transcriptase inhibitors should not be used to treat HIV-2 due to intrinsic resistance to these agents and the fusion inhibitor enfuvirtide. Unfortunately, domestic guidelines are not currently available for HIV-2 viral load monitoring to assess response to therapy [16]. Once HIV infection is diagnosed, there should be a concerted effort to engage refugees in care, begin treatment, and address concerns related to cost, side effects, and prognosis. Additional data is needed to better understand how to optimize utilization of HIV care in different refugee populations within the United States.

To help providers determine an appropriate HIV regimen, patients should be screened for any comorbidities that may affect treatment choice such as depression, kidney disease, gastroesophageal reflux disease, anemia, hepatitis B/C coinfection, and nephrolithiasis, among others. Efavirenz-based regimens have been associated with neuropsychiatric manifestations, and as such, refugees started on efavirenz should be monitored closely given the high prevalence of depression and posttraumatic stress disorder at the time of arrival, both of which have been reported to flare with efavirenz use in case reports [17]. Many refugees are also of child-bearing age and may become pregnant after arrival, so treatment regimens should also take this into account for HIV-positive women. For example, efavirenz should be avoided in pregnancy and among those with child-bearing intentions due to risk of teratogenicity, especially in early pregnancy. In these cases, alternatives would include rilpivirine for patients with viral loads less than 100,000, or use of an alternative class of drug, such as a protease inhibitor or integrase inhibitor.

In addition to managing antiretroviral therapy, there are primary care issues that are unique to HIV-infected individuals, such as metabolic and cardiovascular disease. The Infectious Disease Society of America published HIV primary care guidelines, which include recommendations for lab monitoring, routine health maintenance, and immunizations, among many other primary care-related issues for HIV-positive patients [18]. Referral to an HIV specialist should be strongly considered for new diagnoses and particularly for patients with other comorbidities.

Other STDs

Mandatory predeparture testing overseas is required for the following sexually transmitted infections (STIs) that are supposed to be treated prior to arrival to the United States: syphilis, gonorrhea, chancroid, granuloma inguinale, and lymphogranuloma venereum. Laboratory diagnosis is only required for syphilis. Predeparture screening for the other above infections is based only on history and physical examination [4]. A retrospective study from a population of 25,779 refugees in Minnesota reported the following STI prevalence in their setting: 1.1 % were seropositive for syphilis, 0.6 % had Chlamydia, and 0.2 % had gonorrhea [19]. A survey of Iraqi refugees in San Diego, California, reported a prevalence of 2.5–2.6 % for syphilis among screened refugees [20]. Data for other STIs were not published in the San Diego cohort. This reflects that prevalence rates may vary across refugee populations across the United States depending on differential sexual practices and risk factors. Given that predeparture screening may not be very sensitive, proper evaluation should be performed upon arrival to the United States. As detailed previously, predeparture HIV testing is no longer required. Chlamydia, gonorrhea, and follow-up syphilis testing should be considered; however, the CDC acknowledges that aside from syphilis and chlamydia, currently "no data support the utility of routine testing for other non-HIV STIs in refugees." The Minnesota study authors suggested that perhaps chlamydia and gonorrhea screening for all newly arrived refugees may not be indicated given their extremely low prevalence, although additional data would aid future screening guidelines. As such, post-arrival screening for chancroid and granuloma inguinale is not recommended for refugees, and these will not be discussed here.

Syphilis

Syphilis is a sexually transmitted infection caused by *Treponema pallidum*. The major stages include primary, secondary, latent, and tertiary. The CDC recommends routine syphilis screening for the following groups: all persons 15 years old or above, individuals <15 years old that are sexually active, have been victims of sexual assault, or have lived in regions where nonsexually transmitted *Treponema pallidum* subspecies are endemic [4]. Primary syphilis is characterized by a painless ulcer that may be accompanied by regional lymphadenopathy. Secondary syphilis often presents with a diffuse, non-vesicular, reddish-brown, maculopapular rash classically involving the palms and soles. Tertiary or late syphilis is manifest by end-organ complications, including ascending thoracic aortic dilation, aortic regurgitation, tabes dorsalis, general paresis, meningitis, posterior uveitis, hearing loss, and gummas of the skin, bone, or visceral organs. Central nervous system symptoms warrant cerebrospinal fluid analysis, as this would impact dosing and duration of therapy. Most commonly used screening tests include the Venereal Disease Research Laboratory (VDRL) or rapid plasma reagin (RPR) assays.

Table 9.1 Syphilis treatment

Primary and secondary syphilis
Benzathine penicillin G 2.4 million units IM in a single dose
Penicillin allergy: Doxycycline 100 mg oral twice daily for 14 days
Early latent syphilis
Benzathine penicillin G 2.4 million units IM in a single dose
Penicillin allergy: Doxycycline 100 mg oral twice daily for 14 days
Late latent syphilis or latent syphilis of unknown duration
Benzathine penicillin G 7.2 million units IM administered as 3 doses of 2.4 million units IM each at 1-week intervals
Penicillin allergy: Doxycycline 100 mg oral twice daily for 4 weeks
Neurosyphilis
Aqueous crystalline penicillin G 18–24 million units per day, administered as 3–4 million units IV every 4 h or continuous infusion for 10–14 days
Penicillin allergy: Ceftriaxone 2 g either IM or IV once daily for 10–14 days

Positive screening tests should be confirmed with a fluorescent treponemal antibody absorption (FTA-ABS) or enzyme-linked immunosorbent assay (EIA). Treatment regimens are summarized in Table 9.1. Clinical response is reflected in a fourfold decrease in titers of either VDRL or RPR, so the same assay should be used on serial testing. Clearance of infection is indicated by a negative VDRL or RPR after 1 year for primary syphilis, 2 years for secondary syphilis, and 5 years for late syphilis. False-positive VDRL or RPR can occur in the setting of tuberculosis, hepatitis, other viral illnesses, malaria, rickettsial disease, HIV, systemic lupus erythematosus, rheumatoid arthritis, pregnancy, and after smallpox and MMR vaccinations. Patients should be counseled about the potential Jarisch–Herxheimer reaction, which may present with fevers, headache, myalgias, and malaise and can occur within 24 h after starting treatment for any stage of syphilis. Complicated infections should be referred to an infectious diseases specialist.

Endemic Treponematoses

For refugee populations it is important to keep in mind that nonsyphilitic treponemal subspecies that can produce a positive VDRL and RPR include *pertenue*, which causes yaws; *endemicum*, which causes bejel; and *carateum*, which causes pinta. These infections should be considered for positive syphilis tests without obvious risk factors or clinical manifestations of syphilis. Yaws, also known as frambesia and pian, is transmitted by direct skin-to-skin contact of ulcerative fluid leading to disfiguring bone and nose lesions in advanced disease, treated with either benzathine penicillin or azithromycin. Bejel, also known as endemic syphilis mostly found in the Sahel region of Africa and the Arabian Peninsula, is transmitted by mouth-to-mouth contact or sharing utensils that presents as an oral eruption or rash that can lead to skin gummas and bone inflammation. Pinta is a disease exclusive to Latin America that causes a papular rash characterized by "pintids" that can become disfiguring in later stages. Endemic treponematoses are most effectively treated with a single dose of IM benzathine penicillin G 600,000 units for children less than 10 years old and 1.2 million units for individuals 10 or more years old. Desensitization should be strongly considered for penicillin-allergic patients [21].

HIV and Syphilis Coinfection

Coinfection with HIV and syphilis presents unique diagnostic and treatment challenges. HIV infection has been reported to markedly decrease the sensitivity of RPR, presumably due to delayed antibody formation, making it more difficult to diagnose by serology [22]. Furthermore, primary syphilis lesions may be more numerous, larger, and deeper in HIV-infected patients. Similarly, secondary syphilis can occasionally manifest with more aggressive, ulcerative lesions than in HIV-uninfected patients. Primary and secondary syphilis can overlap in the HIV-uninfected population, but this is increased to as high as 75 % of patients with advanced HIV disease [23]. Several studies have reported an increased risk of ocular syphilis as well. Providers should maintain a low threshold for performing lumbar puncture to rule out neurosyphilis, even in those patients with primary or secondary syphilis. Studies, both prospective [24] and retrospective [25], have demonstrated that patients with HIV can have a delayed response to syphilis therapy as compared to HIV-uninfected patients, particularly in primary or early syphilis. In addition, there is a higher rate of treatment failure if initial RPR titers are high, so patients should be monitored closely for recurrent disease. While HIV has consequences for syphilis, syphilis can also impact management of HIV in that *T. pallidum* has been shown to causally decrease CD4 counts and increase HIV viral loads, but these changes have not yet been proven to be clinically significant [23, 26].

Chlamydia

The CDC recommends routine post-arrival screening for *Chlamydia trachomatis*, which is the most common STI reported in the United States, for all adults as well as those children that are sexually active or have been victims of sexual assault. The incidence has been increasing in the United States, which has been attributed to improved screening and sensitivity of available tests. Unfortunately, STI data among refugees settled in the United States is lacking. The Minnesota study cited above reported an overall prevalence of 0.6 % in refugees with a slightly higher predilection for those originating from the Middle East. Chlamydia can infect both the genitourinary tract and rectum. Most cases are asymptomatic, particularly in men. When chlamydia infection is symptomatic, it may result in urethritis, mucopurulent cervicitis, and pelvic inflammatory disease in women. Untreated chlamydia infection can be asymptomatic, but if left untreated has the greatest consequences for women, as it can lead to chronic pelvic pain, ectopic pregnancy, and infertility. This can have important implications since chlamydia can be transmitted vertically to neonates during childbirth, causing pneumonia and conjunctivitis, although the latter is routinely prophylaxed against in health care settings. Rarely, men can suffer epididymitis and infertility as long-term sequelae. Reactive arthritis can occur in men and women. However, the public health importance of testing men is prevention of infection in women. Rectal infection, which is mostly associated with anal intercourse, may cause proctitis or proctocolitis in rare instances. Lymphogranuloma venereum is a more aggressive form of *Chlamydia trachomatis* caused by L1, L2, and L3 strains endemic to tropical climates and can present with a painless ulcer with or without fever, followed by inguinal lymphadenopathy, and can lead to rectal strictures, rectovaginal fistulas, and perianal fistulas.

The preferred method of diagnosis is nucleic acid amplification testing of cervical swabs in women, urine for both men and women, and urethral swabs in men. Adults with chlamydia should be treated with a one-time oral dose of azithromycin 1 g or a 7-day course of doxycycline 100 mg twice a day [27]. It is also important to note that not only can chlamydia be co-transmitted with HIV through sexual contact but the presence of *Chlamydia trachomatis* can also biologically increase susceptibility and the infectivity of HIV [28]. Therefore, a positive test for chlamydia should prompt HIV testing as well. Additional data would help inform if more targeted testing is universally indicated.

Gonorrhea

The CDC recommends routine post-arrival screening for *Neisseria gonorrhoeae*, which causes gonorrhea, for all adults as well as those children that are sexually active or have been victims of sexual assault. Coinfection with *Chlamydia trachomatis* is common. Therefore, both should be screened for simultaneously with nucleic acid amplification testing from endocervical, male urethral, or urine specimens. As with chlamydia, there is equally limited prevalence data of gonorrhea among refugees upon arrival and over time. The Minnesota study cited above reported an overall prevalence of 0.6 % in their local refugee population, which is the same as that seen in chlamydia. In contrast to chlamydia, however, gonorrhea tends to be far more symptomatic. Men may present with dysuria, penile discharge, testicular swelling, and rectal pain. Women are less likely to have symptoms, but these can include dysuria, vaginal discharge, dysmenorrhea, and rectal pain. Whereas pharyngeal carriage can be seen with chlamydia, gonorrhea can actually cause a clinical pharyngitis, as well as arthritis and tenosynovitis. Reproductive complications in women are similar to those observed with untreated chlamydia infection. Vertical transmission to neonates can result in a more fulminant course than chlamydia, including complications such as sepsis, meningitis, and scalp abscesses.

Positive gonorrhea testing should also prompt HIV testing since gonorrhea can increase the risk of HIV transmission.

With regard to treatment, the standard of care is one-time ceftriaxone 250 mg intramuscular injection and azithromycin 1 g orally once or doxycycline 100 mg twice a day for 7 days, even if chlamydia nucleic acid amplification testing is negative. Cefixime had been used to treat GC, but the CDC revised this recommendation on August 10, 2012, to the above due to increasing resistance patterns based on surveillance data [29]. However, if ceftriaxone is not available, then cefixime can be used as long as a test of cure is performed 1 week after treatment. Fluoroquinolones are not recommended for treatment of gonococcal infections [30]. Patients with refractory disease should be referred to an infectious diseases specialist.

References

1. Global Report: UNAIDS Report on the Global AIDS Epidemic 2012. UNAIDS, Geneva. 2012. http://www.unaids.org/en/media/unaids/contentassets/documents/epidemiology/2012/gr2012/20121120_UNAIDS_Global_Report_2012_en.pdf. Accessed 21 Apr 2013.
2. Spiegel PB, Bennedsen AR, Claass J, et al. Prevalence of HIV infection in conflict-affected and displaced people in seven sub-Saharan African countries: a systematic review. Lancet. 2007;369:2187–95.
3. Holmes W. HIV and human rights in refugee settings. Lancet. 2001;358(9276):144–6.
4. U.S. Department of Health and Human Services (DHHS), Centers for Disease Control and Prevention (CDC), and National Center for Emerging and Zoonotic Infectious Diseases (NCEZID). Screening for HIV infection during the domestic medical examination for newly arrived refugees. 2012. http://www.cdc.gov/immigrantrefugeehealth/guidelines/domestic/sexually-transmitted-diseases.html. Accessed 9 Jul 2013.
5. Centers for Disease Control and Prevention (CDC), U.S. Department of Health and Human Services (HHS). Medical examination of aliens—removal of human immunodeficiency virus (HIV) infection from definition of communicable disease of public health significance. Fed Regist. 2009;74(210):56547–62. http://www.gpo.gov/fdsys/pkg/FR-2009-11-02/pdf/E9-26337.pdf. Accessed 21 Apr 2013.
6. Inter-Agency, UNAIDS/IOM Statement on HIV/AIDS-Related Travel Restrictions. June 2004. http://www.unhcr.org/refworld/docid/468249392.html. Accessed 21 Apr 2013.
7. Taylor K, Howard S. An end to the era of the US HIV entry ban. Clin Infect Dis. 2011;53(5):v. doi:10.1093/cid/cir548.
8. Branson BM, Handsfield HH, Lampe MA, et al. Revised recommendations for HIV testing of adults, adolescents, and pregnant women in health-care settings. MMWR Recomm Rep. 2006;55(RR-14):1–17.
9. Centers for Disease Control and Prevention (CDC). False-positive oral fluid rapid HIV tests—New York City, 2005–2008. MMWR Morb Mortal Wkly Rep. 2008;57:660–5.
10. Jain S, Lowman ES, Kessler A, et al. Seroprevalence study using oral rapid HIV testing in a large urban emergency department. J Emerg Med. 2012;43(5):e269–75.
11. Beckwith CG, DeLong AK, Desjardins SF, et al. HIV infection in refugees: a case-control analysis of refugees in Rhode Island. Int J Infect Dis. 2009;13(2):186–92.
12. Centers for Disease Control and Prevention (CDC). Human immunodeficiency virus type 2. HIV/AIDS fact sheets. Atlanta, GA: Centers for Disease Control and Prevention; 2007.
13. Popper SJ, Sarr AD, Travers KU, et al. Lower human immunodeficiency virus (HIV) type 2 viral load reflects the difference in pathogenicity of HIV-1 and HIV-2. J Infect Dis. 1999;180(4):1116–21.

14. Thompson MA, Aberg JA, Hoy JF, et al. Antiretroviral treatment of adult HIV infection: 2012 recommendations of the International Antiviral Society-USA panel. JAMA. 2012;308(4): 387–402.
15. Makadzange AT, Ndhlovu CE, Takarinda K, et al. Early versus delayed initiation of antiretroviral therapy for concurrent HIV infection and cryptococcal meningitis in sub-Saharan Africa. Clin Infect Dis. 2010;50(11):1532–8.
16. Campbell-Yesufu OT, Gandhi RT. Update on human immunodeficiency virus (HIV)-2 infection. Clin Infect Dis. 2011;52(6):780–7.
17. Moreno A, Labelle C, Samet JH. Recurrence of post-traumatic stress disorder symptoms after initiation of antiretrovirals including efavirenz: a report of two cases. HIV Med. 2003;4:302–4.
18. Aberg JA, Kaplan JE, Libman H, HIV Medicine Association of the Infectious Diseases Society of America, et al. Primary care guidelines for the management of persons infected with human immunodeficiency virus: 2009 update by the HIV medicine Association of the Infectious Diseases Society of America. Clin Infect Dis. 2009;49(5):651–81.
19. Stauffer WM, Painter J, Mamo B, et al. Sexually transmitted infections in newly arrived refugees: is routine screening for Neisseria gonorrhoeae and Chlamydia trachomatis infection indicated? Am J Trop Med Hyg. 2012;86(2):292–5.
20. Centers for Disease Control and Prevention (CDC). Health of resettled Iraqi refugees—San Diego County, California, October 2007–September 2009. MMWR Morb Mortal Wkly Rep. 2010;59(49):1614–8.
21. Hook EW. Endemic treponematoses. In: Mandell GL, Bennett JE, Dolin R, editors. Principles and practice of infectious diseases. 6th ed. Philadelphia, PA: Elsevier; 2005. p. 2785–8.
22. Ballard RC, Koornhof HJ, Chen CY, et al. The influence of concomitant HIV infection on the serological diagnosis of primary syphilis in southern Africa. S Afr Med J. 2007;97(11 Pt 3): 1151–4.
23. Rompalo AM, Joesoef MR, O'Donnell JA, Syphilis and HIV Study Group, et al. Clinical manifestations of early syphilis by HIV status and gender: results of the syphilis and HIV study. Sex Transm Dis. 2001;28(3):158–65.
24. Rolfs RT, Joesoef MR, Hendershot EF, et al. A randomized trial of enhanced therapy for early syphilis in patients with and without human immunodeficiency virus infection. The Syphilis and HIV Study Group. N Engl J Med. 1997;337:307–14.
25. Knaute DF, Graf N, Lautenschlager S, et al. Serological response to treatment of syphilis according to disease stage and HIV status. Clin Infect Dis. 2012;55(12):1615–22.
26. Zetola NM, Engelman J, Jensen TP, et al. Syphilis in the United States: an update for clinicians with an emphasis on HIV coinfection. Mayo Clin Proc. 2007;82(9):1091–102.
27. Workowski KA, Berman S, Centers for Disease Control and Prevention (CDC). Sexually transmitted diseases treatment guidelines, 2010. MMWR Recomm Rep. 2010;59(RR-12):1–110.
28. Fleming DT, Wasserheit JN. From epidemiological synergy to public health policy and practice: the contribution of other sexually transmitted diseases to sexual transmission of HIV infection. Sex Transm Infect. 1999;75:3–17.
29. Centers for Disease Control and Prevention (CDC). Update to CDC's Sexually transmitted diseases guidelines, 2010: oral cephalosporins no longer a recommended treatment for gonococcal infections. MMWR Morb Mortal Wkly Rep. 2012;61(31):590–4.
30. Del Rio C, Hall G, Homes K, et al. Update to CDC's sexually transmitted diseases treatment guidelines, 2010: oral cephalosporins no longer a recommended treatment for gonococcal infections. MMWR Morb Mortal Wkly Rep. 2012;61:590–4.

Chapter 10
Chronic Disease Management in Refugees

Peter Cronkright and Astha K. Ramaiya

Introduction

The medical literature regarding refugee populations in developed countries has predominantly focused on infectious communicable diseases and mental health [1, 2]; however, with changing lifestyles in developing countries and the process of acculturation within developed countries, refugees are facing an increased risk of non-communicable diseases by either having a preexisting condition or acquiring it once in a developed country [1–5]. Twenty-two industrialized countries admitted 79,800 refugees for resettlement during 2011, of which the United States of America (USA) received 51,500 [6]. The United States accounts for nearly 75 % of all permanently settled refugees worldwide [1]. Most recently, 65 % of refugees resettling in the United States originate from Iraq, Burma, and Bhutan. Of the refugees being tested within the first 8 months of arrival, 51.1 % had some chronic disease and 18.4 % had two or more [1]. Such prevalence rates support the need to address chronic conditions in refugees, but the literature provides little guidance for care of common non-communicable disorders in refugees. The objective of this chapter is to [1] synthesize the medical literature so as to offer clinicians an evidence-based approach for the care of common non-communicable disorders in adult refugees and [2] cite the systems challenges that caregivers face when providing chronic care to refugees.

P. Cronkright, M.D. (✉)
Department of Medicine, Upstate Medical University,
90 Presidential Plaza, Syracuse, NY 13202, USA
e-mail: cronkrip@upstate.edu

A.K. Ramaiya, M.Sc.
Department of Internal Medicine, SUNY Upstate Medical University,
750 East Adams Street, Syracuse, NY 13210, USA
e-mail: ramaiyaa@upstate.edu

A. Annamalai (ed.), *Refugee Health Care: An Essential Medical Guide*,
DOI 10.1007/978-1-4939-0271-2_10, © Springer Science+Business Media New York 2014

Common Symptomatic Diseases and Disorders

Chronic Pain

A common concern of newly resettled refugees is chronic pain, but very little is known about the long-term course. Clinicians currently assess and provide care based on the knowledge and management strategies of chronic pain for the general population. Among various populations, the frequency of chronic pain ranges from 7 to 40 % [7].

A Pain Framework

The conceptual models of pain vary both historically and culturally between being emotional and pathological. Today, in mainstream medicine, pain is often considered as "real" or "not real," which is a perception the author discourages. Rather, clinicians should approach pain as an expression of a complex and delicately balanced system. When functioning effectively, our pain system promotes life by avoiding harmful stimuli; however, an imbalance of its functions may result in chronic pain disorders and diminish life experiences [8].

Immigrant care providers should have a basic understanding of the healing traditions that are commonly practiced by patients from various geographic regions. Two popular practices of Asian medicine origin are *Qi* (pronounced chee) and *Gua Sha*. Proper circulation has long served as a metaphor for health and vitality. According to East Asian medicine, pain is related to the impedance in flow of life energy. Qi flows through channels within the body called meridians and exists in a state of balance between dark (Yin) and light (Yang) properties. An illness results when *Qi* is unbalanced and its flow is obstructed through the meridians. The meridians and *Qi* are in close proximity to the skin surface. By the placement of needles on specific points along these meridians, acupuncture attempts to right the balance of Yin and Yang, restoring Qi flow throughout the body [9]. *Gua Sha* is a traditional healing technique widely used by practitioners of traditional East Asian medicine worldwide. The term *Gua Sha* is Chinese: *gua* means to scrape or scratch and *sha* means sand or red, raised, millet-size rash. Different cultures have different terms for this practice, and refugees will not likely be familiar with the English terms of coining, scraping, and spooning. *Sha* is present when palpation results in superficial, slowly fading blanching of the skin. Unresolved *sha* may be associated with chronic pain and illness. *Sha* stasis can be liberated by sweating from fever or through treatments such as *Gua Sha* or cupping [10].

Clinicians of mainstream medicine typically gather patient information using a framework that classifies the pain according to its origin physiologically. The efficacy of this approach is often limited by the physiologic type, the limits of language and verbal skills required to verbalize pain, especially for the refugee, and the meaning of the pain, which draws in the patient's experiences, beliefs, culture, and coping mechanisms [8].

Pain is classified as either nociceptive or neuropathic. Nociceptive pain is divided into somatic or visceral. Neuropathic pain arises from abnormal neural activity secondary to disease, injury, or dysfunction of the nervous system [11]. The physiologic process of feeling pain (nociception) requires three conditions: an organ to receive an outside impression, a connecting passageway, and an organizational center to transform the sensation into a conscious perception [8].

Somatic pain is triggered by injury to a joint, muscle, tendon, bone, or skin. The injury activates the peripheral sensory neurons (nociceptors). Most experiences of acute pain are somatic, and the pain serves as an alarm that is localized in time and place. The most intense component has a fast onset after injury and typically dampens long before the injury leaves. The process of tissue disruption and inflammation causes the release of chemical mediators, triggering electrical signals in sensory nerves that carry the pain message to the brain. This response is often an intense, rapid, protective alarm that triggers a cascade of inflammatory mediators. The mediators excite nociceptors to carry the signal of pain to the spinal cord. The system is analogous to a fire alarm triggered by the first hint of smoke. The injured area is left with a persistent hypersensitivity that protects against trauma and promotes healing. Peripheral inflammation induces a sensitized state in which weak pain stimuli cause an exaggerated pain response (hyperalgesia). It also may trigger pain from a stimulus that is normally non-noxious (allodynia), such as light touch to a burned finger or movement of an inflamed joint. Recovery time limits the ability of nociceptors to fire repetitively, resulting in the intense but brief character of acute somatic pain [8].

The viscera do not have the same protective signals of tissue damage as connective tissues. Pain from the viscera is typically diffused and poorly localized. An acute myocardial infarct is at times missed by the patient and/or clinician because of its ill-defined pain character. While somatic fibers are precisely mapped in the spinal cord and brain, viscerosensory afferent fibers overlap each other and converge at several levels within the CNS. Visceral injury often results in a high degree of visceral-autonomic integration, and chronic visceral pain is often expressed as a functional disorder. Such disorders may feature extra-organ involvement, such as sexual dysfunction, sleep disruption, fatigue, and ill-defined pain. Irritable bowel syndrome is a common example of a functional visceral disorder [8].

Using the basic framework of nociceptive or neuropathic, neuropathic pain refers to a primary injury to the nervous system. A classic example of neuropathic pain is shingles. The nerve damage occurs along one or two dermatomes, does not cross the body's midline, and presents as an inflamed region of vesicles. Clinicians typically become skilled after seeing this clinical diagnosis once, as the condition typically follows the physiology familiar to clinicians of mainstream medicine. Less clear for clinicians is the physiology explaining why injury to the central nervous system, as in stroke or spinal cord injury, results in an inability to sense touch while having painful pressure ulcers or bladder infections. In these cases, the nervous system does not transmit touch signals, yet pain fiber regeneration can cause pain when the location is reinjured or inflamed [8].

Fig. 10.1 The total pain
concept

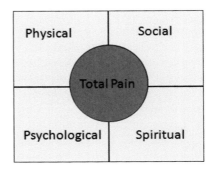

Under normal circumstances, we adapt to our pain rather than reliving it. If all
goes well, the responders put out the fire and the damage is repaired. The healing
process resets the pain alarms to standby and normalizes the stimuli response.
Chronic pain results when the balance is not reestablished. It is an illness, occurring
in many diseases. Chronic pain is pain that has lost its purpose [8].

Many physiologic factors contribute to the chronic pain state. The peripheral
nerve fibers become more responsive to a given stimulus, firing at lower thresholds
and generating more signals for a given stimulus. High-threshold nociceptors may
also reduce their threshold and become recruited into the generation of a more complex and intense pain signal. Peripheral concentrations of nerve growth factors are
increased, prolonging inflammation and pain. Prolonged pain firing of afferents
may also result in neurons carrying signals in both directions, a neurogenic inflammatory phenomenon called dorsal root reflex. The efferent signal heightens pain by
releasing more neurotransmitters and inflammatory agents. Finally, the central nervous system (CNS) undergoes physiochemical changes when pain signals are continuously transmitted from the spinal cord, resulting in hypersensitivity to pain,
increased pain with repeated stimuli (wind-up), and resistance to pain-relieving
inputs. The CNS response risks embedding a "painful memory" that no longer
requires a peripheral pain trigger [8].

Recognizing that chronic pain may occur without persistent peripheral stimuli,
all pain is "real." Historically, patients presenting with "unexplained" pain were
labeled as having a somatization disorder. In general, somatization refers to a tendency to experience and communicate psychological or social distress in the form
of somatic (i.e., physical) symptoms [12]. However, the term somatization has been
used in several different ways and does little to clarify the realities and meaning of
the symptoms [13].

The concept of Total Pain (Fig. 10.1) was first described by Cecily Saunders, the
founder of modern day Hospice, and offers clinicians a window to recognize the
refugees' pain and suffering [14]. Implementing the Total Pain concept requires
clinical skill. The clinician should strive to master the physical domain, be skilled in
the psychological, and work with a team of consultants to address the Social and
Spiritual domains. The author recommends a modification of LEARN (Fig. 10.2), a
model of multicultural communication, to effectively practice the skills of the physical and psychological domains [15].

Fig. 10.2 LEARN, a model
of multicultural
communication [15]

L = Learn
E = Examine (replaces Explain)
A = Acknowledge
R = Recommend
N = Negotiate

The Total Pain Concept in Practice

Practicing the behaviors of a modified LEARN model supports the assessment and management of chronic pain. The *Learn and Examine* portion of the mnemonic is performed during the clinician's history and physical. Primary care providers should be skilled in recognizing worrisome diseases that may present as various chronic pain syndromes, be it chronic arthralgias, headache, or fibromyalgia. Red flag physical concerns should be identified through performing an effective history, physical, and judicious use of tests. Identifying red flags differs from diagnosing by exclusion, which fosters "either-or," "real or not real" thinking. Avoiding the "psyche-soma" dichotomy allows the clinician and the patient to remain open to all factors that might influence the patient's pain symptoms.

Low back pain (LBP) is the most common pain complaint presenting to primary care providers in the United States. The following approach to LBP is derived from the literature, and the author recommends it serve as a framework for assessing the various chronic pain syndromes. It is intended to offer clinicians and refugee patients a plan of care that detects worrisome conditions, probes for emotional distress, and identifies ways to effectively manage pain and improve function [16, 17].

Clinicians assessing LBP need to be skilled at identifying red flag concerns for spine-related malignancy, inflammatory/infectious diseases, or fractures. The red flags to consider in the history and physical exam are onset after age 50 years, current or past diagnosis of cancer, unexplained weight loss, or no improvement of acute LBP after one month, and symptoms of cauda equina syndrome consisting of acute fecal incontinence or bladder dysfunction, saddle anesthesia, or motor deficits at more than one level. The historical absence of acute urinary retention has a very strong negative predictive value. Lumbar-sacral spine X-ray is appropriate if there is a history of trauma or osteoporosis. CT scan or MRI is considered appropriate if red flag concerns are present. No imaging is typically needed for patients with non-specific LBP and/or sciatica without red flag concerns, as MRI abnormalities do not correlate with symptoms [18, 19].

The best predictor of acute LBP becoming a chronic pain syndrome (>3 months) is the presence of emotional distress [18], and emotional issues are common in refugees [17]. Patients with PTSD, depression, and chronic anxiety disorders often present to the primary care office with somatic complaints [12]. As a result, clinicians need to be skilled in the psychological domain of the Total Pain concept, and all patients with chronic pain should be assessed for emotional distress.

The author recommends the following approach for assessing emotional distress. Of the current tools available, the Refugee Health Screener-15 has been validated for use in refugees of many languages and cultures [20] (see also Chap. 12). The PRISM tool has yet to be tested in refugee populations but does not require patient literacy and has been validated for assessing noncancerous pain and PTSD [21]. The 2-question depression screen is efficient and effective when used for the general population [12]. The PHQ-9 is a screening and diagnostic tool for depression which has been translated to several languages [22]. Finally, following the modified LEARN model, clinicians should listen for emotional metaphors or expressions as the refugee tells his/her illness story. The following are examples of expressions that led to the recognition of suffering: For a Sudanese single mother, "every corner of my body I have pain." Pain for a Somali father of nine children was verbalized as "burning pain from head to toe." The headache of an Iraqi male with TBI was characterized as "lost in myself since the explosion." Emotional expressions of pain open the door for clinicians to acknowledge and address the patient's suffering.

Acknowledge

Opportunities arise to acknowledge pain and suffering as a clinician assesses the refugee patient in pain. The following are examples of acknowledgement statements that can be used to build a trusting rapport: "it is clear that you have been suffering" or "it is clear that the pain has been running your life." Once acknowledged, the clinician can direct the discussion toward identifying the patient's worries, assessing coping skills, and recommending a care plan. This approach can be applied in a compassionate manner for various chronic pain complaints, be it headache, back pain, pelvic pain, or total body pain [16].

Recommend

Refugee care clinicians currently recommend a care plan based on the knowledge and management strategies of chronic pain for the general population. Historically, allopathic providers and patients have often been dissatisfied with the management of chronic pain syndromes. Over the past three decades, the use of opioids therapy for noncancerous chronic pain was supported by many medical societies. Chronic pain visits in which opioids were prescribed have doubled from 1980 to 2000 (8–16 %) [23]. Yet, disabling chronic LBP increased from a prevalence of 3.9 % in 1996 to 10.2 % in 2006. The most prescribed medication in the United States from 2006 through 2011 was hydrocodone. Non steroidal anti-inflammatory drugs (NSAIDs) and narcotics are modestly superior to placebo for acute LBP, but the benefit of narcotics for treatment of chronic LBP is unclear and may result in harm [19, 24]. In populations at risk, opioid dependence and misuse behaviors have been noted to be 24–31 % and 20–40 %, respectively. Fatal overdoses in the United States increased sharply, resulting in more deaths yearly from prescription opioids than cocaine and heroin combined [24]. Such concerns are a cause for clinicians to pause and consider alternative treatment options for the refugee patient with chronic pain.

Besides opioids, the clinician may consider prescribing the following medications chronically. NSAIDS are effective for acute pain but risk considerable multiorgan damage when used long term. Refugees are often receptive to a trial of acetaminophen, which is relatively safe when taken appropriately. Tricyclic antidepressants, serotonin–norepinephrine uptake inhibitors, and gabapentin act centrally to relieve pain. All have been studied and found to be beneficial for improving chronic pain and/or function. However, as a general rule, the prescribing of any one analgesic effectively decreases pain by about 50 % in a third of patients. Clinicians often prescribe a combination of analgesic medications with differing modes of action; however, a 2012 Cochrane Database Review of combination pharmacotherapy for neuropathic pain noted only 21 eligible studies, and the pain condition for 18 of the 21 studies was either diabetic peripheral neuropathy [11] or postherpetic neuralgia [7]. Chronic sciatica was the pain condition in only one study. No studies assessed the safety or efficacy of combination analgesics for greater than 6-week duration [25].

Allopathic providers often consider non-pharmacologic treatments. Continuing to use LBP as the pain syndrome, physical therapy-directed exercise and advice for patients with subacute LBP (6–12-week duration) are slightly more effective than placebo [26]. Despite the common use, repeated studies have shown no benefit from epidural injections for chronic LBP [27]. Surgery should be considered for subacute severe sciatica, but there are no studies showing benefit for chronic LBP. Treatment with transcutaneous electrical nerve stimulation (TENS) is no more effective than placebo and adds no benefit to that of exercise alone [19].

Complementary and alternative medicine (CAM) practices are available in most communities and may better align with the refugee's cultural and healing beliefs than pharmacologic solutions. CAM can be organized into the broad categories of mind–body medicine, manipulative and body-based practices, and natural products. CAM is practiced in various forms around the world and has potential benefit for chronic pain syndromes. There are a number of limitations in designing studies to evaluate complementary and alternative medicine practices. Even if well designed, it is not clear that the findings can be generalized to the refugee population and the spectrum of pain syndromes. However, there is usually little risk of adverse events, especially with mind–body medicine. The multiple natural product options will not be reviewed, and the following synopsis stems from a PubMed search for recent review articles of common CAM practices for LBP [9].

Mind–Body Medicine

Evidence-based literature on the effectiveness of non-pharmacologic therapies for LBP is increasing and requires periodic updates by clinicians. To date, superficial heat is the only non-pharmacologic therapy effective for acute LBP [28]. Cognitive behavioral therapy, exercise, spinal manipulation, and interdisciplinary rehabilitation are therapies with moderate efficacy for either subacute or chronic LBP.

In 2012, the Ottawa Panel reviewed the literature and determined that massage therapy for adults suffering from acute, subacute, and chronic LBP provides short-term improvement of subacute and chronic LBP symptoms. Massage interventions decrease short-term disability when combined with therapeutic exercise and education [28]. There is moderate evidence that physical therapy and rehabilitation interventions for chronic LBP reduce pain intensity and disability in the short term compared with nontreatment/waiting list controls. Exercise therapy compared to usual care improved posttreatment pain intensity and disability, and long-term functioning. Behavioral treatment offered short-term effectiveness in reducing pain intensity compared with nontreatment/waiting list controls. There is no evidence that the Pilates method improves pain or functionality of adults with nonspecific chronic LBP [29].

Behavioral therapies attempt to alter the experience of the sick role in patients with LBP. Operant therapies strive to reduce pain through increased social engagement and physical activity. Cognitive therapy addresses the patterns of thoughts, feelings, and beliefs that have a negative impact on the adjustment of a patient. Biofeedback and progressive muscle relaxation are respondent therapies that allow patients to interrupt the pain–tension cycle by applying relaxation techniques. Many types of biofeedback exist, but electromyogram (EMG) feedback is the primary type used for patients with muscular tension. This technique involves the placement of EMG sensors on the body in areas that experience significant tension during the pain–tension cycle. During the cycle, the sensors visually register this tension on a computer screen, and patients can then attempt to modulate their response [9].

Given the life adjustments required of the refugee, behavioral therapies should be considered in refugees with chronic LBP. For the general population, operant therapy or respondent therapy alone (not CBT) or in combination was more effective than wait list for reduction of pain in the short term. Functional status improved using progressive muscle relaxation but not other behavioral therapies [9].

Yoga attempts to create physical and emotional balance through the use of body postures and breathing techniques. A systematic review found five randomized control trials (RCT) noting that yoga leads to a significantly greater reduction in LBP than usual care or education or conventional therapeutic exercises. Two RCTs showed no between-group differences. It is concluded that yoga has the potential to alleviate LBP [30].

Tai Chi is an aerobic exercise that provides muscle strengthening and improves balance and coordination. Tai Chi exercise teaches "stillness in movement" and constant transfer of body weight, reflecting the simultaneous separation and merging of yin and yang energy in the form of Qi. It involves gentle, flowing circular movement of the upper limbs, constant weight shifting of lower limbs, meditation, breathing, moving of Qi, and various techniques to train mind–body control. There are many styles, but a simplified form of the traditional Yang family style Tai Chi is commonly practiced as 24 postures. There is evidence to suggest that Tai Chi is beneficial for pain relief, physical function, and psychological well-being among patients with LBP, osteoarthritis of the knees, and fibromyalgia [31].

Manipulative and Body-Based Practices

Spinal manipulative therapy (SMT) provides a high-impact-velocity thrust at the synovial joint. The mode of action remains unclear, but the intent of SMT is to create fluid-free areas or bubbles by reducing pressure within the synovial fluid. The dynamics of the bubbles accounts for the audible popping sound that is characteristic of SMT and indicates proper application of the technique. A systematic review of SMT studies notes no significant pain reduction at 3 and 6 months compared to sham SMT; however, compared with all other interventions for LBP, SMT produced statistically significant greater pain reduction at 1 and 6 months, but not at 12 months. In terms of functional status, SMT produced greater statistically significant improvement at 1 month, but no difference compared with other interventions at 3, 6, or 12 months [9].

Failure of conservative management often leads to the more invasive alternative of injection therapy. Prolotherapy involves the injection of various irritant solutions to facilitate a local inflammatory response. Studies of prolotherapy alone have not shown statistically significant reductions in pain or disability scores [9]. Epidural corticosteroid injections have become increasingly popular worldwide but lack evidence of long-term benefit for pain control or disability [32].

Negotiation

The Total Pain concept and modified LEARN model offer a framework for clinicians to establish a positive rapport with refugee patients [15]. Patients are more receptive to recommendations and willing to negotiate a care plan from a trusted clinician. The goal of pain management is to support the patient in managing the pain rather than have the pain manage them. Improvement of function and quality of life are important measures for success that likely require skilled negotiation.

Disability assessment is a common occurrence in the care of a refugee, and clinicians should consider the appropriateness of the patient's "sick role" [12, 16]. Sociologist Talcott Parsons described the "sick role" as allowing persons to be exempted from normal social obligations and responsibilities without blame. In a normal response to illness, taking on the sick role is adaptive and not pathological. At the other end of the spectrum, patients readily embrace the sick role or are resistant to giving it up [12]. The experience of the "sick role" is affected by a patient's culture, socialization, family, and personal experience and traits. A cohort of Sudanese refugee patients with "somatization" shared their illness stories and revealed narrative styles that highlight the interconnection of bodily illness and refugee-related trauma. They articulated the cause of the illness as threatening assaults on their sense of self and as part of their community and culture. As described earlier, the use of embodied metaphors to understand and cope with their current and past traumatic experiences was common, such as "traveling pains," "the heart," "blood," and "body constriction." In their narratives, an illness was perceived as a process and continued threat rather than a prior event [13]. Such embodied expressions are often accompanied by a normal neuromuscular examination.

The examination lacks the objective evidence of tissue damage or organ dysfunction that is typically required for disability. Recovery does not follow a predictable course [8]. As such, disability determination for chronic pain syndromes is a challenge.

There is a paucity of literature to guide the clinician in management of disability, and none target the resettled refugee. For cases of work-related injury, half of the patients with disability beyond 120-day duration continue to have a protracted disability. There is no proven formulary to assess the likelihood of protracted disability [8]. Recovery from the sick role does not follow a predictable course. Recommendation and negotiation of a care plan are challenging and may alter the clinician–patient relationship. The focus of care should be to empower the patient in moving from the sick role to behaviors that improve function. Cognitive behavioral therapy that is provided by a psychologist has reduced work-related disability [8]. Encouraging refugees to manage chronic pain through participation in mind–body therapies is reasonable; however, the impact on disability has not been defined.

Other Chronic Pain Syndromes

The previously described approach to LBP can be utilized for the evaluation and management of other chronic pain syndromes, such as chronic pelvic pain, headache, or fibromyalgia. The clinician's history and examination should identify red flag concerns, such as infectious signs in a female with chronic pelvic pain or early morning stiffness in a patient with arthralgia complaints. The history should probe for signs of emotional distress and sleep disturbance. It is important to recognize that coping with chronic pain from various diseases can be difficult and be associated with depression or other psychiatric diagnoses. Women with chronic pelvic pain are likely to report depression, anxiety, and sleep disturbances, in addition to limitations in sexual activity and mobility [33]. Depression and/or anxiety is present in 30–50 % of patients at the time of being diagnosed with fibromyalgia, and 30–70 % of fibromyalgia patients meet the criteria for irritable bowel syndrome and chronic fatigue syndrome, two common functional somatic syndromes. Clinicians should avoid, if possible, being a diagnostic "splitter" of such patients into multiple subspecialty diagnosis [34]. As with chronic back pain, the clinician's role is to perform a skilled clinical exam and consider appropriate diagnostic tests to objectively assess red flag symptoms and signs. Acknowledgement of the patient's suffering while providing compassionate reassurance and continued availability is often the best approach.

Deficiencies

Anemia

Globally, anemia affects 24.8 % of the population, and refugees emigrate from countries where anemia is of moderate to severe public health significance.

The prevalence is highest in preschool age children (47 %) and lowest in men (12.7 %), but the population group with the greatest number of individuals affected is nonpregnant women [35]. Regionally, the highest proportion of affected children and women is in Africa (47.5–67.6 %), while the greatest number affected is in Southeast Asia [35]. Studies report prevalence rates of 12–19 % for anemia in refugees resettling in developed countries, but the rate varies with the gender and age of resettled refugees [36]. Surveyed Canadian clinicians noted that iron deficiency anemia (IDA) was one of the top 20 conditions in need of guidelines for resettled immigrants and refugees [37]. Anemia has often been excluded from chronic disease studies on refugees because it is typically due to nutritional deficiencies and thought to resolve within a year of immigration [1].

Etiology of Anemia

Iron deficiency is the most common nutritional deficiency [35]. The WHO estimates that 50 % of the cases of anemia are due to iron deficiency, but the proportion may vary among population groups and regions. The main risk factors for iron deficiency anemia (IDA) are a low intake of iron, poor absorption of iron from diets high in phytate or phenolic compounds, and periods of life when iron requirements are especially high (i.e., growth and pregnancy). Heavy blood loss as a result of menstruation or parasite infections such as hookworms, ascaris, and schistosomiasis can result in IDA [35].

IDA often coexists with other acquired or inherited causes. Malaria infects the RBC and is endemic to most of the equatorial areas of the world. The prevalence of malaria in immigrants has been reported to be as high as 15 % [38]. Hemolytic anemia is the most common manifestation of an acute malaria infection. Acute and chronic infections can result in anemia of chronic disease (ACD), which typically is a normochromic–normocytic anemia but can progress to a microcytic anemia. ACD is the most common manifestation of HIV infection. Refugees are at risk for other micronutrient deficiencies that cause anemia, including vitamins A and B12, folate, riboflavin, and copper [35].

Endemic malaria regions are also geographic regions of high prevalence for genetic red blood cell (RBC) disorders and should be considered as a cause of anemia in such patients. Genetic defects of the RBC result in disorders of hemoglobin quantity (thalassemias) or quality (hemoglobinopathies), RBC enzyme dysfunction (G6PD deficiency), or membrane defects. The thalassemic syndromes are autosomal recessively inherited disorders that cause a decrease in β- or α-hemoglobin chain production. Thalassemias often present as mild microcytic anemia (thalassemia trait) but may cause profound anemia and growth retardation (thalassemia major). Thalassemias are common in Africa, the Mediterranean, India, and Southeast Asia. Isolated β-thalassemia traits should not be prescribed iron, and patients of reproductive age should consider genetic counseling. It is advisable to check a hemoglobin (Hgb) and mean corpuscular volume (MCV) on partners of prenatal patients with α-thalassemia. Glucose-6-phosphate dehydrogenase (G6PD) is important for the production of glutathione, which prevents oxidative damage to the RBC. Clinical hemolytic anemia can be induced in G6PD deficient patients by neonatal jaundice, infection, certain foods, or drugs. G6PD deficiency has the same geographic distribution as the thalassemias plus Central and South America. The diagnosis is made by measuring G6PD levels in red blood cells [38].

Hemoglobinopathies to consider in refugees are sickle-cell disease and hemoglobin E. A diagnosis is confirmed by hemoglobin electrophoresis. Heterozygous and homozygous HbE exist primarily in Southeast Asia. HgbE produces a mild microcytic anemia and should be identified to avoid unnecessary iron treatment. Sickle-cell anemia is characterized by moderate to severe chronic hemolytic anemia with recurrent painful vaso-occlusive crisis. Sickle-cell trait presents as mild anemia and urinary concentration defects but does not cause vaso-occlusive crisis unless severe hypoxia occurs [38].

Hereditary elliptocytosis is a RBC membrane defect seen in Northern Africa, and hereditary ovalocytosis occurs in Southeast Asians. Elliptocytosis and ovalocytosis are thought to confer resistance to malaria. Both produce a mild normochromic–normocytic anemia with elliptical- or oval-shaped RBCs on peripheral blood smear [38].

The RBC indices provide clues to the cause of the anemia. The MCV is used to classify an anemia as microcytic (MCV < 80 fL), normochromic–normocytic (MCV 80–100 fL), or macrocytic (MCV > 100 fL). A microcytic anemia is noted in IDA, thalassemia and HgbE, and severe ACD [38]. A normochromic–normocytic anemia is typical due to ACD. Less common causes are acute blood loss, early nutritional deficiencies, bone marrow disorders, and dimorphic-coexisting anemias (vitamin B12 and iron deficiency). Macrocytic anemia in the refugee raises concern of vitamin B12 deficiency, hypothyroidism, or liver disease [38].

The RBC number is often normal or increased in HbE and thalassemia, whereas the RBC number is reduced in IDA. Additional tests include serum ferritin and a hemoglobin electrophoresis. Ferritin is an acute phase reactant, elevated in ACD and diminished in IDA. A cutoff ferritin value of <100 ng/mL identifies 98 % of IDA. Serum iron and total iron-binding capacity are insensitive at distinguishing IDA from severe ACD. A hemoglobin electrophoresis identifies β-thalassemic syndromes and hemoglobinopathies but is normal in microcytic α-thalassemias and severe ACD [38].

Vitamin D Deficiency

Vitamin D deficiency is highly prevalent in refugees resettling from various regions of the world, due to nutritional deficiencies and or reduced skin absorption of the sun's ultraviolet radiation (UVR). Risk factors for reduced UVR light exposure are age <5 years, female gender from cultures/religions that cover extensively in clothing, and decreased daylight exposure [36, 39]. Considering geographic origin, immigrants from the Middle East and Eastern Africa have the highest prevalence of vitamin D insufficiency (25–50 nmol/L) or deficiency (<25 nmol/L). Karen refugee females also had a high prevalence of vitamin D deficiency and hypocalcemia [36]. Insufficiency or deficiency was less prevalent (33 %) among immigrants/refugees from Eastern Europe in comparison to other immigrant/refugee populations; this rate was comparable to the US-born population prevalence of 35 %. Such findings suggest that vitamin D deficiency should be considered a chronic deficiency in resettled refugees and warrants testing 25-OH vitamin D levels in all resettled refugees [40–42]. Some experts recommend vitamin D replacement in all newly resettled refugees.

Vitamin D deficiency results in osteomalacia, a disorder of bone characterized by decreased mineralization of newly formed osteoid at sites of bone turnover. Osteomalacia may be asymptomatic and present radiographically as osteoporosis. Symptoms of osteomalacia include bone pain of the lower spine, pelvis, and lower extremities, where fractures have taken place. The pain is described as dull and aching and is aggravated by activity and weight bearing. The muscle weakness is typically proximal and produces a waddling gait. Other abnormalities commonly present in vitamin D deficiency besides a low 25-hydroxyvitamin D (calcidiol) level are an elevated serum alkaline phosphatase, a reduced serum calcium and phosphorus, and an elevated serum parathyroid hormone (PTH) [42].

Vitamin D supplementation in deficient patients may improve muscle strength and bone tenderness within weeks, and bone density may improve within 3–6 months. In most cases, serum calcium and phosphate normalize after a few weeks of treatment, but alkaline phosphatase remains elevated for several months. Serum 25-hydroxyvitamin D should be measured approximately 3–4 months after initiating therapy. The dose should be adjusted to prevent hypercalciuria or hypercalcemia [42].

Multiple preparations of vitamin D and its metabolites are available, but vitamin D2 or D3 is least costly. Vitamin D metabolites are only necessary for disorders of vitamin D metabolism, as in liver or kidney disease. There is no standard dosing regimen for treating vitamin D deficiency. One common approach is to treat with 50,000 IU of vitamin D2 or D3 orally once per week for 6–8 weeks and then either 800 IU of vitamin D3 daily or 50,000 IU monthly thereafter. In addition to vitamin D supplementation, all patients should maintain a calcium intake of at least 1,000 mg per day, since inadequate calcium intake may contribute to the development of osteomalacia [42].

Vitamin B12 Deficiency

The Center for Disease Control (CDC) recommends that all Bhutanese refugees be given nutrition advice and receive supplemental vitamin B12 upon arrival in the United States. Vitamin B12 deficiency, defined as serum concentration <203 pg/mL, was found in 64 % (63 of 99) of overseas specimens collected during medical examinations in Nepal and a prevalence of about 30 % in resettled Bhutanese refugees to the United States [43]. Hematologic manifestations are a late clinical sign of vitamin B12 deficiency, and thus a complete blood count is not a sufficient screening test. Approximately 5–10 years are required for body stores of vitamin B12 to become depleted. The most likely cause of deficiency in this population is thought to be inadequate dietary intake. A possible secondary cause is chronic gastritis, and a small study has linked *H. pylori* infection to a greater prevalence of vitamin B12 deficiency [43, 44].

The 2005 Cochrane Database Systematic Review concluded that oral vitamin B12 was as effective as intramuscular treatment. Two RCTs compared oral with intramuscular administration of cyanocobalamin (vitamin B12). Kuzminski et al. in 1998 concluded that 2,000 µg oral daily was as effective as 1,000 µg administered intramuscularly every month. Bolaman et al. in 2003 concluded that 1,000 µg of oral or intramuscular vitamin B12 daily for 10 days followed by once weekly for 4 weeks and once monthly for life was equally effective for treatment of patients with megaloblastic anemia [45].

Based on a Morbidity and Mortality Weekly Report, the author recommends treatment for at least 30 days after arrival. As of yet, no studies have determined the necessary duration of treatment [43]. Due to the systems need of scheduling the refugee for regular injection visits, it is reasonable to opt for oral treatment of indefinite duration.

Iodine Deficiency

Iodine deficiency is a modifiable global health problem causing clinical disorders that include thyroid goiter, hypothyroidism, and cognitive impairment. Severe deficiency during pregnancy is associated with cretinism and increased neonatal and infant mortality. Mild deficiency during childhood is associated with goiter formation and learning disabilities. The goiter in children and adolescents is usually diffuse but becomes nodular in adults due to varied foci of thyroid follicle proliferation. Thyroid follicular cell replication also increases the chance of mutations. Large goiters mask coexisting foci of thyroid cancer and may compress on the trachea or esophagus [46].

The inland mountainous soil of the Andes, Alps, and Himalayas are iodine deficient. Coastal regions are typically rich in iodine food sources like fish, kelp, and vegetables grown in iodine-sufficient soil. However, sea salt naturally contains only a small amount of iodine, and iodine deficiency also occurs in coastal populations lacking dietary sources of iodine. Repletion from iodization of salt or in prenatal supplements has few adverse effects. However, goiter patients from regions of endemic iodine deficiency are at risk for iodine-induced hyperthyroidism following salt iodization. Increased incidences of both hypothyroidism and hyperthyroidism have also been observed after the introduction of iodized salt in various countries [47]. Clinicians should be aware that refugees with thyroid nodules may develop hyperthyroidism when iodine intake is supplemented. The actual prevalence of iodine deficiency in refugees is unknown.

The evaluation of a thyroid goiter includes assessing function with serum TSH and consideration of an ultrasound. In refugees from iodine-deficient regions, clinicians may elect to reserve sonography for patients with thyroid asymmetry or palpable nodules. However, the physical examination of goiter is highly inaccurate. Glands that are diffuse on physical exam are often nodular by ultrasound, and most enlarged thyroids with a single palpable nodule on physical exam will have multiple nodules by ultrasound [48]. Thus, there should be a low threshold for performing sonography on thyroid goiters. Nodules with indeterminate or suspicious ultrasound features should be considered for biopsy [48].

Skin Problems

Skin Findings Due to Traditional Healing/Rituals

Clinicians providing care for refugees will likely encounter skin findings of scarification, coining, and cupping. The practice of traditional healing occurs worldwide, and traditional healers in Africa provide the first line of care for 70 % of the population [49].

Scarification is a common skin finding in refugees from sub-Saharan Africa and is a result of small incisions into the skin. According to traditional healers, the illness leaves the body through bleeding (see Fig. 10.3). Sometimes the incision is used as a depot for herbal medicines. Scarification can also result from participation in cultural ceremonies and be unrelated to illness [49].

Coining is practiced in Southeast Asian communities and is used for a wide variety of illnesses. Coins are rubbed on the skin of the chest and back in symmetrical bands, creating linear petechiae and ecchymosis that may last several days [50] (see Fig. 10.4).

Cupping is a traditional Chinese practice used primarily to treat respiratory conditions, pain disorders, and gastrointestinal complaints. Traditionally, "dry"

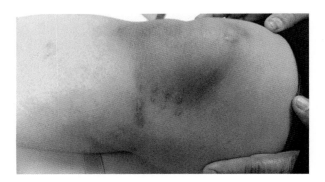

Fig. 10.3 Scarification

Fig. 10.4 Coining. Image
appears with permission
from VisualDx © Logical
Images, Inc.

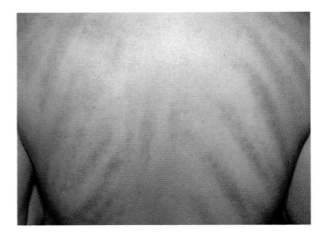

Fig. 10.5 Cupping

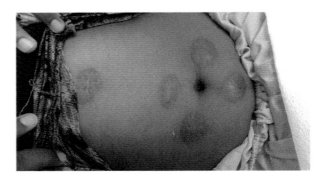

cupping involves burning a flammable substance inside a cup, which removes
oxygen and creates a vacuum. The cup is turned upside down on the skin as the
substance burns, typically on the back or abdomen. The vacuum draws the skin
upward, the skin vasodilates, creating a circular bruise. In "wet" cupping, a suction
pump is used rather than a flammable substance, and the skin is punctured to
stimulate surface blood flow [10, 50] (see Fig. 10.5).

Melasma

Melasma is a common condition in darker-skinned members of the refugee population [51]. Chloasma faciei or "the mask of pregnancy" is a form of melasma associated with pregnancy that presents as patchy facial hyperpigmentation thought to be
due to stimulation of melanocytes by estrogen and progesterone in sun-exposed
skin [51]. Melasma is a common condition, occurring in up to 75 % of Asian and
Hispanic women [51]. Predisposing factors are genetics, oral contraceptives, sun
exposure, and thyroid disorders [51–54].

Absolute recognition of its features is necessary, since treatment of melasma can involve teratogenic agents, as with retinoic acid and hydroquinone [51]. Expensive treatment, such as light therapy, may also be an unnecessary financial burden. Pregnancy should immediately be ruled out prior to any treatment of melasma, given its association with chloasma [51]. Typically, the condition resolves spontaneously within months after delivery, although in some women, hyperpigmented skin changes persist.

Pruritus

Itching is a common complaint in primary care [55]. Dry skin (xerosis) is one of the most common causes of itch in adult patients. Changes of the environment and daily routine often expose the refugees to conditions that promote xerosis, such as lower humidity, frequent bathing, and excessive use of defatting soaps. The approach to pruritus includes determining if the itch is caused by a primary skin condition or due to secondary skin changes of itching and subsequent scratching. Treatment of a primary skin condition usually relieves the itch. Atopic and allergic contact dermatitises are common causes of itching. Other, noninfectious causes include medication reactions and primary dermatoses, such as psoriasis and lichen planus [55]. In the refugee patient with itch, the following infectious conditions should also be considered as possible causes.

Cutaneous Infectious Disorders Causing Pruritus

Infestations should be one of the first diagnoses considered in a refugee with generalized pruritus.

Scabies is a mite that is transmitted mainly by direct personal or sexual contact. The diagnosis should be considered when household members itch; however, the absence of such history does not exclude scabies. Primary scabies lesions are burrows, typically a white or gray linear papule with a small vesicle at one end, but their absence should not delay the diagnosis. The lesions are found in the web spaces of fingers and flexor surfaces of the wrists and elbows; on the genitals, umbilicus, and beltline; and on the areola of women's breasts. It is uncommon for scabies to involve the head and neck areas of adults. The immune response to the infection and scratching may cause prominent secondary lesions and result in persistent itching for weeks after treatment [50].

The major symptom of *pediculosis* (lice) is itching and presents as three clinical conditions: head, body, and pubic lice. Head lice are transmitted by direct contact or commonly from shared combs, hats, or bedding [50, 55].

Bedbug bites are usually painless, located on the neck or extremities that are not covered by blankets or sheets, and are linearly distributed (or a "breakfast, lunch, supper" pattern). The bedbug hides in cracks of beds, furniture, baggage, and clothing. A clue to the infection is blood spots on the sheets, corresponding to the nocturnal feeding bite sites on the patient [50, 55].

Various parasitic diseases should be considered as possible causes of pruritus in a refugee.

Loiasis is a filarial disease occurring only in Central and West Africa. Its most distinctive clinical manifestation is the "eye worm," but loiasis infection often presents as pruritus with urticaria and transient migratory non-pitting edema (Calabar swellings) [56]. The transient edema is most commonly located on the extremities and is thought due to hypersensitivity reaction and lasts a few days to several weeks. Eosinophilia and elevated serum IgE are characteristic. Symptoms may continue for years after leaving an endemic region [56].

Onchocerciasis, or African river blindness, is a filarial infection of the subcutaneous tissue that causes intense pruritus. The infection is rarely seen outside its endemic regions of tropical Africa, Yemen, and Saudi Arabia and pockets of Central and South America [57, 58]. Many infected individuals are asymptomatic. Cutaneous lesions are the most common clinical presentation and are due to the inflammatory response of the host to dying microfilariae. The dermatitis often does not appear for at least 2 years after infection. The dermatologic manifestations are classified as acute papular dermatitis, larger chronic papular dermatitis, a lichenified dermatitis (Sowda) with hyperpigmented papules and plaques usually confined to one extremity, atrophic aged skin with little subcutaneous tissue, and depigmentation areas of the shins interspaced with normal pigment skin (leopard skin) [57]. The diagnosis is usually made by noting microfilariae in skin snips taken from the iliac crest (Africa) or scapula (Americas). Subcutaneous, mobile, painless nodules can occur as a result of tissue reaction to the adult worms, and ultrasound can distinguish these onchocercomata from lymph nodes or other masses. Microfilariae access the cornea via the skin and conjunctiva [57, 58].

Dracunculiasis, or Guinea worm, is a tropical disease primarily of Africa and India that may present as a raised tortuous track of the subcutaneous worm; an urticarial reaction lasting a few hours; and a pruritic, burning vesicular lesion most commonly over the lateral malleolus. The vesicle is often the initial sign of the disease [58].

Strongyloidiasis is endemic in many regions of the world and may persist in patients for decades after leaving endemic areas. The majority of patients are asymptomatic. The skin is the port of entry for acute infections, producing a pruritic urticarial reaction within 24 hours of infection. Chronically, cutaneous lesions are present in 90 % of patients, with 2/3 having intermittent maculopapular or urticarial eruptions. Larva currens, an intensely pruritic or serpiginous urticarial lesion produced by migrating filariform larvae, are transient and usually located on the buttocks or thighs [58].

Schistosomiasis skin lesions have been classified as the invasive cercarial dermatitis, or swimmer's itch, which produces pruritic erythematous papular eruptions acutely, and the nonspecific erythematous macules or papules of Katayama fever. Grouped papules may progress to form verrucous plaques [58].

Diffuse itching in the absence of an underlying skin condition requires evaluation for a systemic cause. Clinicians should consider and examine the patient for possible hematologic malignancy, cholestatic liver disease, renal disease, iron deficiency, thyroid disease, medications, and human immunodeficiency virus (HIV) infection. The following tests are recommended: complete blood count and differential, ferritin level and iron studies, thyroid-stimulating hormone (TSH) and free T4, blood urea nitrogen (BUN) and creatinine, liver panel, chest X-ray, and age- and sex-appropriate malignancy screening [55].

Treatment of pruritus is most successful when an underlying cause is identified. Skin care includes regular use of emollients. Histamine-mediated itching often responds to antihistamines, avoidance of hot water bathing, and use of cool compresses. Topical corticosteroids are the standard treatment for eczematous dermatitis. Refugees who struggle with both itch and insomnia or anxiety/depression may benefit from doxepin or mirtazapine nightly [55].

Other Cutaneous Infectious Disorders

Dermatophytes are fungi that cause superficial fungal infections and are named according to the body site involved [55]. Tinea pedis typically causes dry scales on the soles and sides of the feet in a moccasin distribution and may itch. Tinea corporis presents as annular, scaly plaques. The typical "ringworm" has central clearing and a surrounding ring of vesicles. Tinea capitis infects the scalp and is most common in children. Symmetrical scaling of the inguinal folds, typically sparing the scrotum in men, suggests tinea cruris. Tinea versicolor (pityriasis versicolor) thrives in warm humid weather and is common in refugees from tropical regions. Clinically, it presents as scaled oval patches that can be hyper- or hypopigmented. The fungal infection may penetrate the hair follicles in high sebaceous gland areas and cause a persistent folliculitis of the upper back and abdomen. Cutaneous candidiasis occurs most commonly on opposed surfaces of skin and causes bright red patches [55].

Leishmaniasis may occur in immigrants from Central and South Asia, North and East Africa, the Middle East and Mediterranean, and Latin America. Transmitted by the sand fly, the primary hosts include dogs and rodents. Humans are usually incidental victims. The incubation period between bite and lesion may be weeks to several months [59].

Acute cutaneous Leishmaniasis has been classified into either wet-rural type, which heals within 3–12 months, or the dry-urban type that typically resolves after a couple of years. The initial erythematous papule(s) occur(s) at the site of the sand fly bite and steadily enlarge over weeks to nodule(s) measuring about 2.5 cm in diameter. The lesions are often located on exposed areas, are only slightly pruritic, and commonly have satellite lesions. The lesions may progress to a volcano-shaped ulceration with raised margins and often are secondarily infected. Healed lesions leave a depressed, white or pink, cribriform scar. Punch biopsy from the ulcer margin confirms the diagnosis [59].

Leishmaniasis manifests in other ways than the acute cutaneous form. Chronic lesions persist in 3–10 % of cases and are commonly located on the face or ear (*Chiclero ulcer*). Mucocutaneous leishmaniasis, usually called espundia, presents in Latin America as ulcerative mucus membranes of the nose, mouth, and pharynx.

A visceral leishmaniasis (VL) patient is typically from India or Bangladesh and in Hindi is known as kala-azar (black fever). VL manifests clinically as fever, spleno-megaly, lymphadenopathy, cachexia, and pancytopenia. Diagnosis historically required tissue biopsy of the involved organ, but serologic diagnosis is increasingly an option [59].

Leishmaniasis recidivans (*lupoid leishmaniasis*) may occur months to years after the primary lesions heal or develop at the periphery of partially healed primary lesions. Soft erythematous plaques with whitish scales resemble lupus vulgaris. Disseminated anergic cutaneous leishmaniasis occurs in immune compromised individuals, usually starting as a single, non-ulcerated nodule of the face. Eventually the entire skin becomes nodular [59].

Leprosy primarily infects skin and peripheral nerves and may have a prolonged incubation period of many years before presenting clinically. It is a rare diagnosis in a refugee, and further details of clinical manifestations are beyond the scope of this chapter; however, it is recommended that the diagnosis be considered when clini-cians are uncertain of a dermatologic diagnosis. Skin biopsy and skin smears are needed for all clinical forms of leprosy [60].

Dyspepsia

Dyspepsia is defined as a chronic or recurrent pain or discomfort centered in the upper abdomen and is a common complaint in the care of adults. The discomfort is a subjective negative feeling that does not translate well verbally, especially for refugees, and often results in a broad differential diagnosis and risks excessive test-ing. The discomfort can include symptoms of early satiety, upper abdominal full-ness, bloating, or nausea [61]. However, bloating, nausea, or belching alone is insufficient for identifying dyspepsia. The predominance of epigastric discomfort helps to distinguish dyspepsia from gastroesophageal reflux (GERD), which is managed differently. The predominant complaints in GERD are typically heartburn and acid regurgitation. Heartburn is typically a burning sensation in the retrosternal area, often experienced postprandial. Regurgitation is the perception of flow of refluxed gastric content into the mouth or hypopharynx. Patients with predominant or frequent (more than once a week) heartburn or acid regurgitation should be considered to have GERD [62].

Dyspeptic patients over 55 years of age or those with alarm features should undergo prompt esophagogastroduodenoscopy (EGD). Upper GI malignancy is rare in younger patients without alarm features—unintended weight loss, persistent vomiting, progressive dysphagia, odynophagia, unexplained anemia or iron defi-ciency, hematemesis, palpable abdominal mass or lymphadenopathy, family history of upper gastrointestinal cancer, previous gastric surgery, or jaundice [61]. One exception is the consideration of prompt endoscopy in a refugee from regions where gastric or esophageal cancer is common. Over 70 % of gastric cancers occur in developing countries, and the incidence is greatest in Eastern Asia, Eastern Europe, and South America [63]. Strongyloidiasis should be considered in dyspeptic refugees whose symptoms do not respond to proton-pump inhibitor (PPI) treatment (see Sect. "Variations on Common Conditions").

For dyspeptic patients without alarm concerns, the care plan depends on their likelihood of *H. pylori* infection. *H. pylori* prevalence varies by ethnicity, geographic region, socioeconomic class, and age. Transmission typically occurs during childhood through an oral–oral or a fecal–oral route, and *H. pylori* is most common in impoverished areas with overcrowding and poor sanitation. A moderate to high prevalence of *H. pylori* infection is considered to be ≥10 % of the population [61].

Few studies target resettled pediatric refugees, but the geographic origin and prior living conditions for refugees place them in a high prevalence group for *H. pylori* [64, 65]. Four studies from Africa recorded *H. pylori* prevalence rates ranging from 41.3 to 91.3 %. Several studies on children and adolescents in Asia showed prevalence rates ranging from 20 to 84 %. The *H. pylori* prevalence rates from the Asia-Pacific region were high except among the white population of Australia and New Zealand [66] Serology was the most common method of diagnosis used in these studies [66]. Approximately 30 % of new refugee arrivals to Australia were positive for *H. pylori* stool antigen [67].

Current guidelines recommend a test-and-treat approach for patient populations of high prevalence for *H. pylori* infection (Grade A evidence), and the appropriate test varies according to the individual patient. Urea breath testing is not readily available, and the choice for clinicians is typically serologic testing of IgG antibodies using ELISA technology or a stool antigen assay. Both are inexpensive. The serologic test can be obtained at the time of the visit and while a patient is taking a proton-pump inhibitor (PPI). Large studies have found the serologic test to have a high sensitivity (90–100 %) but variable specificity (76–96 %), depending on the cohort's background prevalence of *H. pylori* infection. The sensitivity and specificity of the *H. pylori* stool antigen test are 94 % and 86–92 %, respectively. Concomitant PPI or Bismuth therapy results in false-negative stool antigen rates of 25 % and 15 %, respectively. However, ranitidine use does not alter the test sensitivity. Given the relative ease of testing and the pretest probability for infection in refugees, it is reasonable to perform serologic testing of *H. pylori*. A positive serology does not typically require a second confirmatory test. A negative result in the presence of symptoms may require secondary testing with either stool antigen assay or urea breath test to confirm negativity. The stool antigen assay and urea breath test are effective tests to determine eradication when performed at least 4 weeks after completion of treatment. The American College of Gastroenterology provides guidelines for determining who needs confirmation of eradication [68].

If *H. pylori* is present, the current treatment of choice for *H. pylori*-infected patients is a combination of PPI (standard dose twice daily) with amoxicillin (1 g twice daily) and clarithromycin (500 mg twice daily) administered for 7–10 days (7-day therapy is approved with rabeprazole; 10-day therapy is approved with lansoprazole, omeprazole, pantoprazole, and esomeprazole). Metronidazole (400 mg twice daily) may be substituted for amoxicillin in penicillin allergic patients. An alternative strategy is the combination of bismuth (Pepto-Bismol) 525 mg QID, metronidazole 250 mg QID, and tetracycline 500 mg QID combined with a PPI for 14 days [61].

Dental Disorders

Dental disorders in refugees arise due to limited accessibility to dental services in the native and host country [69]. Within refugee camps, individuals may be subject to violent physical trauma resulting in complications of oral health [69, 70]. Changes in diet after resettlement and poor nutrition within refugee camps increase the chance of developing cavities [70]. Cost of services, lack of coverage by insurance, communication barriers, and traditional beliefs about oral health contribute toward poor oral health in refugees [69–71].

The prevalence of dental disorders among refugees ranges from 22 to 51 %. This rate is variable between settings when compared to national rates [70, 72, 73]. Prevalence of tooth decay is significantly higher among refugees [72, 73]. Frequently observed dental disorders include dental caries, periodontal diseases, malocclusion, orofacial trauma, missing and fractured teeth, and oral cancer [70].

Dental disorders differ by geographic regions and ethnicities. Africans show lower oral disorders due to traditional diets low in sugar, dental practices using miswak stick brushes, and genetic protection [70–74]. The use of betel nut is common among Asians from the Indian subcontinent, Far East, and Pacific Rim. The betel nut has a hard texture and may cause tooth breakage. The habit causes oral submucous fibrosis, leading to diseases of the oral cavity, pharynx, and upper digestive tract. Betel nut in the Indian subcontinent is typically combined with sugar, tobacco, and betel leaf leading to tooth staining, hypersensitivity reaction, oral submucous fibrosis, and oral cancer [75].

Among refugees entering host countries, the prevalence of visiting dental services at least once since resettlement ranged from 23 to 85 % over a period of 5–10 years [69, 71, 73]. This range is varied among different settings based on dental insurance coverage. In the United States, there is limited coverage of dental services under Medicaid [71, 73].

With acculturation after resettlement, demand for dental services increases due to limited access, low education, and socioeconomic status. Dental care should target refugees because of low health literacy, low prior exposure to dental care, and the increased influence of American food habits after resettlement [73].

Various care models have been implemented to curb dental disorders, including biannual fluoride varnish among high-risk populations, school-based dental services, and early screening. Biannual dental visits have been shown to ensure tooth retention and decrease complications. Fluoride varnishing at the visits is recommended [76]. Children of refugees can undergo a school-based oral care program which incorporates education, screening, and counseling [77]. Refugees who use betel nut should be encouraged to stop and be screened for oral cancers. Treatments to prevent progression of oral submucous fibrosis include submucosal injection of triamcinolone acetonide and intralesional injections of collagenase or interferon gamma. In severe cases, surgery such as release of intraoral fibrous bands, coronoidectomy, masticatory muscle myotomy, and soft-tissue reconstruction is needed in combination with physical therapy [75].

Variations on Common Conditions

Obesity, Hypertension, and Diabetes

Given the high rates of micronutrient deficiencies in refugees, it seems counter intuitive that obesity, hypertension, and diabetes should be commonly encountered. Yet, despite a cohort of mostly young adults, over half of adult refugees received at an academic US clinic were overweight (31.3 %) or obese (23.3 %, BMI > 29), 13 % were noted to be hypertensive, and 4.4 % had diabetes [4]. Refugees emigrating from Europe and Central Asia are at significant risk of obesity, hypertension, coronary artery disease, and anemia [4]. Few newly arrived refugee adults resettling in the United States are underweight, and the proportion decreases from the time of US arrival to 8 months after arrival [1]. In part, recent data reflects the fact that many refugees resettling in the United States are originally from Iraq (24.6 %), where the prevalence of adult obesity nearly equals that in the United States [3]. Systems of care delivery for these common conditions should be adapted to meet the needs of the refugee (see sections below).

Chronic Lung Disease

Tobacco use and its related illnesses are common in refugees, especially among men [1]; however, refugees are also at risk of COPD and lung cancer from exposure to biomass smoke. Labeled "hut lung," the COPD is attributed to inhalation of biomass fuel smoke and fine sand dust from grinding maize or wheat on soft stone. The risk of COPD from exposure to biomass smoke is similar to that seen in smokers and greater than the risk of COPD due to passive smoking [78]. Biomass fuels, such as crop residues, animal dung, and wood, are used for cooking and heat in much of the world, especially Southeast Asia and Africa. Women who cook are at greatest risk, but children and elderly who remain indoors are also at risk from exposure. The clinical presentation is typically middle-aged or elderly women with complaints of breathlessness rather than cough. Having recurrent exacerbations of respiratory infections but without a smoking history, such patients are often diagnosed as having asthma. The findings on pulmonary function tests are similar to tobacco-related COPD. High-resolution computed tomography of biomass smoke-related COPD patients usually shows diffuse emphysema, bronchial wall thickening, thickening of interlobular septae, increased bronchovascular arborization, nodular opacities, ground-glass appearance, and pleural thickening [40]. Several studies have shown that exposure to biomass smoke is a risk factor for the development of lung cancer, most commonly adenocarcinoma [40].

Refugees with previously treated pulmonary tuberculosis are at risk for chronic lung disease from residual damage, which is often symptomatic with chronic productive cough. Pulmonary function testing up to 16 years after treatment has noted obstructive as well as restrictive disease in the majority of patients, and the degree of abnormality correlates with the extent of disease on the original chest radiograph [79].

Strongyloides

Like tuberculosis, clinicians should always consider the possibility of strongyloides in ill refugees. Strongyloides is endemic in many regions of the world, may remain lifelong in the host after leaving endemic areas, and can be transmitted to household or family members. Most infected carriers are asymptomatic or may present with diffuse gastrointestinal, dermatologic (see Sect. "Skin Problems"), or respiratory symptoms [80]. Strongyloides should be considered in refugees with dyspepsia that does not respond to proton-pump inhibitors. Asthma-like illness occurs in as much as 10 % of strongyloides-infected patients. Misdiagnosed as asthma, treatment with systemic steroids risks acute hyperinfection with strongyloides and septic shock [80].

Rheumatic Heart Disease

Rheumatic heart disease (RHD) is a disease of poverty and remains a major cause of cardiovascular disease in the regions of refugee emigration. For adults less than age 40 in endemic countries, RHD is the leading cause of heart disease and often results in heart failure [81]. Chronic, progressive valvular disease typically develops years after one or more episodes of acute rheumatic fever. A prospective study of children with acute rheumatic fever in Brazil found that 72 % developed chronic valvular disease and 16 % progressed to severe disease. Echocardiogram screening has been recommended in areas endemic for rheumatic fever [82]. Clinicians should assess all refugees for heart murmur and have a low threshold for performing an echocardiogram [83].

The mitral valve is involved in almost all cases of RHD, and the aortic valve is involved in 20–30 % [81]. Mitral stenosis is a diastolic murmur. When symptomatic, the primary complaint is dyspnea, often triggered by exercise, emotional distress, fever, or pregnancy. Fatigue and effort intolerance curtails activities as the stenosis progresses. Patients with mitral stenosis are at risk for atrial fibrillation due to atrial dilatation and the fibrotic changes from the prior carditis. Among acquired valvular heart disease, mitral stenosis has the highest risk for systemic thromboembolism, and the risk increases markedly following the onset of atrial fibrillation. All patients with mitral stenosis should be assessed for warfarin anticoagulation prophylaxis. Chronic mitral regurgitation (MR) can be well tolerated for years, and surgery is influenced by the patient's age, the severity of symptoms, coexistent coronary artery disease, preoperative left ventricular function, the type of surgery (repair vs. replacement), and the presence of atrial fibrillation [83].

Chronic, severe aortic regurgitation often remains asymptomatic as it leads to volume and pressure overload, and the rate of progression to systolic dysfunction is <6 % per year. Most patients can be safely monitored with regular exams and periodic echocardiograms. Clinicians should consider treating asymptomatic patients with vasodilator medications, such as hydralazine, nifedipine, or ACE inhibitors [83]. Mixed aortic valve disease is challenging and should be managed by a cardiologist if available.

Rheumatic heart disease should be assessed periodically (at least once per year) with echocardiography. There are defined echocardiographic criteria for surgical assessment that are independent of the patient's symptoms [83].

Individual and System Level Challenges and Recommendations

Refugees arriving in developed countries face individual and system level challenges [1]. Monitoring chronic disorders requires identification of factors that influence their health-care utilization [2]. Their experience with the health-care system is often shaped by their region of origin, duration of resettlement, language, expectations, functional status, and beliefs [1, 4, 84–86]. Language competency has been documented as a barrier to seeking health care. Many refugees are not able to communicate their symptoms and conditions to physicians and only seek health care when they get the symptoms, delaying a diagnosis and treatment [1, 87–90]. Cultural beliefs support their use of traditional medicine to overcome their condition. A study among Hmong Shaman noted that 90 % of individuals reported using traditional Shamanic treatment for their illness, and most only took the allopathic prescribed medicine when they felt sick [84].

Once refugees have entered a developed country, they face the risk of poor health outcomes [85]. In many instances, the country of origin plays a big factor in the utilization of the health-care system. As stated earlier, refugees from Europe and Central Asia are at significant risk of obesity, hypertension, coronary artery disease, and anemia [4]. Resettled Iraqis had the same prevalence of obesity as California residents (24.6 % vs. 24.8 %) and a higher prevalence of non-communicable diseases (56.8 % vs. 44.6 %) [1, 3]. Many refugees live in low-income, marginalized communities which affects nutritional intake [4]. Resettled refugees tend to maintain their food traditions, but their children acculturate nutritionally, resulting in an increased risk of childhood obesity [5]. Refugees from Africa had a higher risk of anemia in comparison to other regions [4]. A nutritional assessment is therefore recommended for resettled refugees. Furthermore, there should be a linkage to chronic disease management programs and clinics with culturally sensitive counseling to reduce burden of disease [3, 4].

Refugees are typically provided with health insurance when they enter the country. However, if resettled in the United States, Medicaid insurance is only assured for

9 months, and employment places the refugee at risk for loss of health insurance [2]. Lack of health insurance in individuals with chronic disorders is associated with increased health complications and decreased likelihood of seeking health services [2].

Refugees with behavioral and psychological consequences of trauma often do not seek or are not offered appropriate care. According to a study in California, prevalence of mental and emotional problems was higher for older resettled Vietnamese refugees in comparison to older non-Hispanic white adults [88]. However, acknowledgement and discussion of the trauma with a primary care provider was lower [88]. War-wounded refugees with and without chronic pain were assessed 8 years post-resettlement in Sweden. Although 91 % of the patients with chronic pain sought health care, only 9 % sought a psychiatrist [89].

The healthy migrant effect postulates "first-generation immigrants to the United States are healthier than people of similar ethnic backgrounds who were born in this country" [91]. In the Netherlands, refugees were more likely to be educated and have better health in comparison to their Dutch counterparts. Within this study, ethnic differences were vast, especially in terms of health outcomes and employment status [86].

Health-care delivery systems should consider the refugee patient's cultural differences, beliefs, and expectations of care. A study on female Somali Bantus demonstrated that women expected to be seen by a female physician to effectively communicate their health status [85]. Refugees have differing perceptions to treatment of the condition based on their financial situation and cultural beliefs. This belief may contradict physician recommendations [5, 90]. Language communication barriers lead to discontinuation of treatment and/or use of traditional medicine [84, 85].

Management of chronic disorders is often lifelong, yet many refugees stop taking medicines when the prescription is completed unless they are reminded by their physician or pharmacist [85]. Detrimental outcomes have been linked to refugee's belief that illnesses are short term and curable. Such beliefs are associated with random frequency of medication use, limited knowledge about associated complications, and use of traditional medicine [5, 84].

Providing care delivery to refugees is challenging, and the unique barriers to care are well defined [1, 2]. Screening agencies should link refugees to primary care in order to ensure continuum of care in the management of chronic conditions. Linking to primary care will aid in monitoring the health of this population and ease the integration process into the health-care system [4].

The chronic care model has been tested as an intervention within the general population for chronic disease management [92], and the author recommends it as a best practice model for refugee care. The model outlines that a multifaceted approach is warranted between patients, providers, and organization. Patients require physical, psychological, and social support which can be achieved through patient-centered education to facilitate self-management of the illness [92]. Providers require continuing medical education and feedback from practice through expert-based teams for clinical and behavioral management [92]. Organizational changes include changing personnel role, facilitating accurate and timely information systems, linkage with the community, multidisciplinary teams, innovative scheduling, and organization of visits [92]. This model has shown moderate evidence of being beneficial in terms of health-care utilization, health-care costs, health behavior of patients, perceived quality of care, and satisfaction of patients and caregivers [93]. Although there is no documented data on the chronic care model within refugees, it is applicable within this population. In order to monitor trends within countries, there is a dire need to collect timely data and collaborate to understand which programs are working and are cost effective [3].

Currently, there is very little collaboration between countries that provide care for refugee populations. In order to understand best practices and develop evidence-based programs, data needs to be accurate, reliable, and time bound to help in understanding refugee health and communicating results to both patients and national agencies [3]. Timely collection of data would increase early detection and increase referral to primary care providers [3]. In the long run, understanding conditions which are origin and culture specific would aid in developing high-impact cost-effective programs which benefit the health indicators of a country [3].

References

1. Yun K, Hebrank K, Graber LK, Sullivan M-C, Chen I, Gupta J. High prevalence of chronic non-communicable conditions among adult refugees: implications for practice and policy. J Community Health. 2012;37(5):1110–8.
2. Dicker S, Stauffer WM, Mamo B, Nelson C. Initial refugee health assessments: new recommendations for Minnesota. Minn Med. 2010;93(4):45–8.
3. Ramos M, et al. Health of resettled Iraqi refugees—San Diego County, California, October 2007–September 2009. MMWR Morb Mortal Wkly Rep. 2010;59(49):1614–8.
4. Geltman PL, Dookeran NM, Battaglia T, Cochran J. Chronic disease and its risk factors among refugees and asylees in Massachusetts, 2001–2005. Prev Chronic Dis. 2010;7(3):A51.
5. Palinkas LA, Pickwell SM. Acculturation as a risk factor for chronic disease among Cambodian refugees in the United States. Soc Sci Med. 1995;40(12):1643–53.
6. UNHCR. Asylum levels and trends in industrialized countries. Geneva: UNHCR; 2011.
7. Stanos SP, Mahajan G. Appropriate use of opioids in chronic pain: caring for patients and reducing risks. Englewood, CO: Postgraduate Institute for Medicine; 2012.
8. McCarberg B, Passik SD. Expert guide to pain management. 1st ed. Philadelphia, PA: American College of Physicians; 2005. p. 357.
9. Marlowe D. Complementary and alternative medicine treatments for low back pain. Prim Care. 2012;39(3):533–46.
10. Nielsen A, Knoblauch NTM, Dobos GJ, Michalsen A, Kaptchuk TJ. The effect of Gua Sha treatment on the microcirculation of surface tissue: a pilot study in healthy subjects. Explore. 2007;3(5):456–66.
11. Smith H. Definition and pathogenesis of chronic pain. In: Aronson M, Douchette K, editors. UpToDate; 2013.
12. Schneider RK, Levenson JL. Psychiatry essentials for primary care. Philadelphia, PA: ACP; 2008.
13. Coker EM. "Traveling pains": embodied metaphors of suffering among Southern Sudanese refugees in Cairo. Cult Med Psychiatry. 2004;28(1):15–39.
14. Mehta A, Chan LS, Saunders C. Understanding of the concept of "total pain". J Hosp Pallat Nurs. 2008;10(1):26–32.

15. Culhane-Pera KA, Borkan JM. Multicultural medicine. In: Walker PF, Barnett ED, editors. Immigrant medicine. China: Saunders Elsevier; 2007. p. 69–81.
16. Barsky A, Borus JF. Functional somatic syndromes. Ann Intern Med. 1999;130(11):910–21.
17. Cronkright P. Suffering with low back pain: you, me, and the refugee. Rochester, NY: North American Refugee Healthcare Conference; 2012.
18. Chou R, et al. Clinical guidelines diagnosis and treatment of low back pain: a joint clinical practice guideline from the American college of physicians and the American. Ann Intern Med. 2007;147:478–91.
19. Laine C, Goldman D, Wilson J. In the clinic: low back pain. Ann Intern Med. 2008;144(9): 1–16.
20. Hollifield M, Verbillis-Kolp S, Farmer B, et al. The Refugee Health Screener-15 (RHS-15): development and validation of an instrument for anxiety, depression, and PTSD in refugees. Gen Hosp Psychiatry. 2013;35(2):202–9.
21. Kassardjian CD, Gardner-Nix J, Dupak K, Barbati J, Lam-McCullock J. Validating PRISM (pictorial representation of illness and self measure) as a measure of suffering in chronic non-cancer pain patients. J Pain. 2008;9(12):1135–43.
22. Kroenke K, Spitzer RL, Williams JB. The PHQ-9: validity of a brief depression severity measure. J Gen Intern Med. 2001;16(9):606–13.
23. Manchikanti L, Vallejo R, Manchikanti KN, Benyamin RM, Datta S, Christo PJ. Effectiveness of long-term opioid therapy for chronic non-cancer pain. Pain Physician. 2011;14(2):E133–56.
24. Martell B, et al. Annals of internal medicine review systematic review: opioid treatment for chronic back pain: prevalence, efficacy, and association with addiction. Ann Intern Med. 2007;146(2):116–47.
25. Chaparro L, Wiffen P, Moore R, Gilron I. Combination pharmacotherapy for the treatment of neuropathic pain in adults. Cochrane Database Syst Rev. 2012;7:CD008943.
26. Pengel LHM, Refshauge KM, Maher CG, Nicholas MK, Herbert RD, McNair P. Physiotherapist-directed exercise, advice, or both for subacute low back pain: a randomized trial. Ann Intern Med. 2007;146(11):787–96.
27. Iversen T, Solberg TK, Romner B, et al. Effect of caudal epidural steroid or saline injection in chronic lumbar radiculopathy: multicentre, blinded, randomised controlled trial. BMJ. 2011; 343:d5278.
28. Brosseau L, Wells GA, Poitras S, et al. Ottawa Panel evidence-based clinical practice guidelines on therapeutic massage for low back pain. J Bodyw Mov Ther. 2012;16(4):424–55.
29. Pereira LM, Obara K, Dias JM, et al. Comparing the Pilates method with no exercise or lumbar stabilization for pain and functionality in patients with chronic low back pain: systematic review and meta-analysis. Clin Rehabil. 2012;26(1):10–20.
30. Posadzki P, Ernst E. Yoga for low back pain: a systematic review of randomized clinical trials. Clin Rheumatol. 2011;30(9):1257–62.
31. Peng PWH. Tai chi and chronic pain. Reg Anesth Pain Med. 2012;37(4):372–82.
32. Pinto RZ, Maher CG, Ferreira ML, et al. Epidural corticosteroid injections in the management of sciatica: a systematic review and meta-analysis. Ann Intern Med. 2012;157(12):865–77.
33. Alappattu MJ, Bishop MD. Psychological factors in chronic pelvic pain in women: relevance and application of the fear-avoidance model of pain. Phys Ther. 2011;91(10):1542–50.
34. Goldenberg D. Clinical manifestations and diagnosis of fibromyalgia in adults. In: Schur P, Romain P, editors. UpToDate; 2012.
35. Benoist B, et al. Worldwide prevalence of anaemia. Geneva, Switzerland: WHO; 2005.
36. Johnston V, Smith L, Roydhouse H. The health of newly arrived refugees to the Top End of Australia: results of a clinical audit at the Darwin Refugee Health Service. Aust J Prim Health. 2012;18(3):242–7.
37. Swinkels H, Pottie K, Tugwell P, Rashid M, Narasiah L. Development of guidelines for recently arrived immigrants and refugees to Canada: Delphi consensus on selecting preventable and treatable conditions. CMAJ. 2011;183(12):E928–32.
38. Hurley R. Anemia and red blood cell disorders. In: Walker P, Barnett E, editors. Immigrant medicine. Philadelphia, PA: Saunders Elsevier; 2007. p. 611–22.

39. McGillivray G, Skull SA, Davie G, et al. High prevalence of asymptomatic vitamin D and iron deficiency in East African immigrant children and adolescents living in a temperate climate. Arch Dis Child. 2007;92(12):1088–93.
40. Campagna AM, Settgast AM, Walker PF, DeFor TA, Campagna EJ, Plotnikoff GA. Effect of country of origin, age, and body mass index on prevalence of vitamin D deficiency in a US immigrant and refugee population. Mayo Clin Proc. 2013;88(1):31–7.
41. Benson J, Skull S. Hiding from the sun—vitamin D deficiency in refugees. Aust Fam Physician. 2007;36(5):355–7.
42. Menkes C. Clinical manifestations, diagnosis, and treatment of osteomalacia. In: Drszner M, Mulder J, editors. UpToDate; 2012.
43. MW Report. Vitamin B12 deficiency in resettled Bhutanese refugees—United States, 2008–2011. MMWR Morb Mortal Wkly Rep. 2011;60(11):343–6.
44. Benson J, Maldari T, Turnbull T. Vitamin B12 deficiency. Aust Fam Physician. 2010;39(4):215–7.
45. Butler C, Goringe A, Hood K, Mccaddon A, Mcdowell I. Oral vitamin B12 versus intramuscular vitamin B12 for vitamin B12 deficiency. Cochrane Database Syst Rev. 2005;20(3):CD004655. 2009.
46. Vitti P. Iodine deficiency disorders. In: Ross D, Mulder J, editors. UpToDate; 2012.
47. Leung AM, Braverman LE. Iodine-induced thyroid dysfunction. Curr Opin Endocrinol Diabetes Obes. 2012;19(5):414–9.
48. Ross D. Diagnostic approach to and treatment of goiter in adults. In: Cooper D, Mulder J, editors. UpToDate; 2012.
49. Winkler A, Mayer M, Ombay M, Mathias B, Schmutzhard E, Jilek-Aall L. Attitudes towards African traditional medicine and Christian spiritual healing regarding treatment of epilepsy in a rural community of northern Tanzania. Afr J Tradit Complement Altern Med. 2010;7(2):162–70.
50. Keystone JS. Skin problems. In: Walker PF, Barnett ED, editors. Immigrant medicine. Philadelphia, PA: Saunders Elsevier; 2007. p. 375–91.
51. Montemarano AD. Melasma. Medscape. 2012. http://emedicine.medscape.com/article/1068640-overview.
52. Hughes BR. Melasma occurring in twin sisters. J Am Acad Dermatol. 1987;17(5 Pt 1):841.
53. Foldes EG. Pharmaceutical effect of contraceptive pills on the skin. Int J Clin Pharmacol Ther Toxicol. 1988;26(7):356–9.
54. Lutfi RJ, Fridmanis M, Misiunas AL, et al. Association of melasma with thyroid autoimmunity and other thyroidal abnormalities and their relationship to the origin of the melasma. J Clin Endocrinol Metab. 1985;61(1):28–31.
55. Collier VU, et al. MKSAP 16 dermatology. Philadelphia, PA: MKSAP 16 American College of Physician; 2012.
56. Barnett ED. Loiasis. In: Walker PF, Barnett ED, editors. Immigrant medicine. Philadelphia, PA: Saunders Elsevier; 2007. p. 467–71.
57. Barnett ED. Onchocerciasis. In: Walker PF, Barnett ED, editors. Immigrant medicine. Philadelphia, PA: Saunders Elsevier; 2007.
58. Mackey S, Wagner K. Dermatologic manifestations of parasitic diseases. Infect Dis Clin North Am. 1994;8:713–43.
59. Juckett G. Leishmaniasis. In: Walker PF, Barnett ED, editors. Immigrant medicine. Philadelphia, PA: Saunders Elsevier; 2007. p. 447–54.
60. Joyce M. Leprosy. In: Walker PF, Barnett ED, editors. Immigrant medicine. Philadelphia, PA: Saunders Elsevier; 2007. p. 455–65.
61. Talley NJ, Vakil N. Guidelines for the management of dyspepsia. Am J Gastroenterol. 2005;100(10):2324–37.
62. Kahrilas PJ, Talley NJ, Grover S. Clinical manifestations and diagnosis of gastroesophageal reflux in adults. UpToDate; 2012.
63. Chen A, et al. Epidemiology of gastric cancer. UpToDate; 2013.
64. Mutch RC, Cherian S, Nemba K, et al. Tertiary paediatric refugee health clinic in Western Australia: analysis of the first 1026 children. J Paediatr Child Health. 2012;48(7):582–7.

65. Cherian S, Forbes D, Sanfilippo F, Cook A, Burgner D. The epidemiology of Helicobacter pylori infection in African refugee children resettled in Australia. Med J Aust. 2008;189(8): 438–41.
66. Goh K-L, Chan W-K, Shiota S, Yamaoka Y. Epidemiology of Helicobacter pylori infection and public health implications. Helicobacter. 2011;16 Suppl 1:1–9.
67. Benson J, et al. The prevalence of Helicobacter pylori infection in recently arrived refugees to South Australia. Toronto, ON: North American Refugee Healthcare Conference; 2013.
68. Chey WD, Wong BCY. American College of Gastroenterology guideline on the management of Helicobacter pylori infection. Am J Gastroenterol. 2007;102(8):1808–25.
69. Singh HK, Scott TE, Henshaw MM, Cote SE, Grodin MA, Piwowarczyk LA. Oral health status of refugee torture survivors seeking care in the United States. Am J Public Health. 2008;98(12):2181–2.
70. Davidson N, Skull S, Calache H, Murray SS, Chalmers J. Holes a plenty: oral health status a major issue for newly arrived refugees in Australia. Aust Dent J. 2006;51(4):306–11.
71. Willis MS, Bothun RM. Oral hygiene knowledge and practice among Dinka and Nuer from Sudan to the U.S. J Dent Hyg. 2011;85(4):306–15.
72. Cote S, Geltman P, Nunn M, Lituri K, Henshaw M, Garcia RI. Dental caries of refugee children compared with US children. Pediatrics. 2004;114(6):e733–40.
73. Geltman P. The impact of health literacy on the oral health status and other health outcomes of Somali refugees. Rochester, NY: Refugee Health Care Conference; 2012.
74. Angelillo IF, Nobile CG, Pavia M. Oral health status and treatment needs in immigrants and refugees in Italy. Eur J Epidemiol. 1996;12(4):359–65.
75. Aziz SR. Coming to America: betel nut and oral submucous fibrosis. J Am Dent Assoc. 2010;141(4):423–8.
76. Azarpazhooh A, Main PA. Fluoride varnish in the prevention of dental caries in children and adolescents: a systematic review. Hawaii Dent J. 2009;40(1):6–7. 10–3; quiz 17.
77. Melvin CS. A collaborative community-based oral care program for school-age children. Clin Nurse Spec. 2006;20(1):18–22.
78. Kodgule R, Salvi S. Exposure to biomass smoke as a cause for airway disease in women and children. Curr Opin Allergy Clin Immunol. 2012;12(1):82–90.
79. Wilkox P. Chronic obstructive airway disease following treatment of pulmonary tuberculosis. Respir Med. 1989;83(3):195–8.
80. Boulware D. Strongyloides. In: Walker PF, Barnett ED, editors. Immigrant medicine. Philadelphia, PA: Saunders Elsevier; 2007. p. 509–13.
81. Bongani M. Natural history, screening, and management of rheumatic heart disease. In: Gaasch W, Yeon S, editors. UpToDate; 2010.
82. Mayosi B. Natural history, screening, and management of rheumatic heart disease. In: Gaasch W, Yeon S, editors. UpToDate; 2010.
83. November O. Rheumatic fever and rheumatic heart disease. Report of a WHO Expert Consultation; Nov 2001. 2004.
84. Helsel D, Mochel M, Bauer R. Chronic illness and Hmong shamans. J Transcult Nurs. 2005;16(2):150–4.
85. Parve J, Kaul T. Clinical issues in refugee healthcare: the Somali Bantu population. Nurse Pract. 2011;36(7):48–53.
86. Schuring M, Burdorf A, Kunst A, Voorham T, Mackenbach J. Ethnic differences in unemployment and ill health. Int Arch Occup Environ Health. 2009;82(8):1023–30.
87. Harris M, Zwar N. Refugee health. Aust Fam Physician. 2005;34(10):825–9.
88. Sorkin D, Tan AL, Hays RD, Mangione CM, Ngo-Metzger Q. Self-reported health status of Vietnamese and non-Hispanic white older adults in California. J Am Geriatr Soc. 2008;56(8):1543–8.
89. Hermansson AC, Thyberg M, Timpka T, Gerdle B. Survival with pain: an eight-year follow-up of war-wounded refugees. Med Confl Surviv. 2007;17(2):102–11.
90. Muller J, Karl A, Denke C, et al. Biofeedback for pain management in traumatised refugees. Cogn Behav Ther. 2009;38(3):184–90.

91. Fennelly K. The "healthy migrant" effect. Healthy Gener. 2005;5(3):1–3.
92. Wagner EH, Austin BT, Davis C, Hindmarsh M, Schaefer J, Bonomi A. Improving chronic illness care: translating evidence into action. Health Aff. 2001;20(6):64–78.
93. De Bruin SR, Versnel N, Lemmens LC, et al. Comprehensive care programs for patients with multiple chronic conditions: a systematic literature review. Health Policy. 2012;107(2–3): 108–45.

Part III
Mental Health

Chapter 11
Risk Factors and Prevalence of Mental Illness in Refugees

Paula Zimbrean

Introduction

Identifying mental illness in refugees poses multiple challenges to providers and organizations worldwide. These challenges range, from technical aspects of language barriers and accessibility, to phenomenological questions such as the definition of mental illness across cultures.

Nevertheless, most Western societies now consider refugees as a population with high prevalence of mental illness and multiple efforts are ongoing toward standardizing screening methods and identifying risk factors early in the process of resettlement.

Screening

Overseas Screening

The Secretary of Health and Human Services promulgates, under the authority of the Immigration and Nationality Act (INA) and the Public Health Service Act, regulations outlining the requirements for the medical examination of aliens seeking admission into the US [1]. The Division of Global Migration and Quarantine provides the Department of State (DOS) and the US Citizenship and Immigration Services (USCIS) with medical screening guidelines for all examining physicians. The purpose of this overseas medical examination, for the DOS and USCIS, is to

P. Zimbrean, M.D. (✉)
Department of Psychiatry, Yale University, 20 York St Rm F611,
New Haven, CT 06504, USA
e-mail: paula.zimbrean@yale.edu

A. Annamalai (ed.), *Refugee Health Care: An Essential Medical Guide*,
DOI 10.1007/978-1-4939-0271-2_11, © Springer Science+Business Media New York 2014

identify applicants with inadmissible health-related conditions: any physical or mental disorder with associated harmful behavior, any drug abuse or dependence.

Any person applying for refugee status must undergo this medical examination aimed at detecting these inadmissible health related conditions. The requirements for this evaluation are included in the technical instructions for medical examination of aliens (TIs), last revised in 2010. Following this evaluation, refugees with a history of mental disorder with associated harmful behavior that may pose a threat to property or welfare of the alien or others, may be classified as follows:

- *Class A refugees* need the approved waiver for travel. An approved US health care provider is identified for the refugee. When the class A refugee arrives in the US, he or she must report promptly to the identified US health care provider.
- *Class B refugees* are diagnosed with a mental disorder with no current associated harm or behavior, or there is a history of harmful behavior judged not likely to recur. Refugees with a class B mental disorder do not require a waiver but it is recommended that they are evaluated by a mental health specialist soon after arrival.

Domestic Screening

The center for disease control (CDC) recommends that mental health screening be performed at the first medical evaluation that refugees undergo in the US. This screening consists of the following steps:

1. Review of records from overseas.
2. History and physical examination related to mental health.
3. Mental status examination.
4. Screening for depression and posttraumatic stress disorder (PTSD).
5. Referral for refugees considered at significant risk.

The importance of records from overseas is described above. The screening should give particular attention to history of head trauma with loss of consciousness, known psychiatric conditions, history of treatment, substance use, and exposure to traumatic events. The physical examination should look for signs of maltreatment (such as torture) and unexplained somatic symptoms that may be related to psychological distress [1].

CDC recommends that all refugees over 16 years old should be screened for major depression and PTSD. It is important however to prepare the patient before asking specific questions related to trauma. Attempts should be made at normalizing the emotional stress associated with the experience of trauma and with immigration. Structured instruments are also available for screening: for depression, PHQ—9 or the depression section of the Hopkins symptoms checklist; for PTSD, questions 1–16 of the PTSD portion of the Harvard trauma questionnaire as well as Primary Care PTSD screen (PC-PTSD). Some of these instruments are available for public use, while some must be purchased [2]. Many of these instruments have been translated in multiple languages. It is important however to keep in mind that psychiatric diagnosis should not be made based on psychological instruments alone. Anyone meeting the threshold scores for depression or PTSD on the screening questionnaire should be referred for a full evaluation with a mental health professional. A more detailed discussion on screening follows in Chap. 12.

Other countries have also issued guidelines regarding refugee mental health screening. For instance the Canadian Collaboration for Immigrant and Refugee Health (CCIRH) recommends screening for four mental health conditions: abuse and domestic violence, anxiety and adjustment disorder, depression, and torture and PTSD [3]. In Sweden, use of the health screening interview by social workers has been shown to be reliable in identifying PTSD in refugees [4].

Screening for mental health problems can be challenging due to many factors, patient or provider related. Refugees often arrive from places where stigma surrounding mental health issues is significant. Some of them cannot cope with recollection of traumatic events. In addition, the clinician may feel uncomfortable asking about psychiatric problems for fear that "it may open a can of worms" with strong emotional content that may delay the delivery of medical care. It is helpful to normalize the refugee's experience as much as possible (not only the trauma: "many refugees in your situation have been through traumatic experiences such as…" but also the mental health screening itself: "every refugee that we see here in this clinic is asked these questions"). Another helpful approach is to emphasize the importance of addressing these problems, if needed, for their overall adjustment and success in their new life. Refugees are usually quite open to talking about their stories, often with little prompting. Sometimes refugees decline mental health intervention, even if it is indicated. In these cases, psycho-education about the impact of symptoms upon their quality of life and available treatments prompts some refugees to return later for treatment. Also, personal contact established at screening is important since the refugees tend to ask for the clinician they spoke with when they were initially offered mental health care.

Risk Factors for Psychiatric Problems in Refugees

Risk factors can be broadly considered under three phases of migration: pre-migration, post-migration, and during migration.

Pre-migration Factors

Age

Studies looking at age of refugees and prevalence of mental illness have produced variable results. Some studies showed that refugees of younger ages experience more depression [5] while other studies showed that adolescents do better than older adults, especially in the Ethiopian population [6].

Gender

In most studies, women have a higher prevalence of PTSD and depression than men in Middle Eastern, Central African, Southern Asian, and Southeastern European refugees [7]. Other psychiatric conditions such as anxiety and pain disorder are also more common in women: tortured Bhutanese women reported higher prevalence of generalized anxiety disorder, pain disorder, and dissociative disorders than men. Several studies, however, found depression more common in male refugees than in female refugees [5]; oftentimes this is a reverse of the ratio seen in the country of origin. One study found an abnormal (80 %) prevalence of psychosis in men in a Somali refugee clinic population [8].

Education

Overall, more educated refugees scored lower on the mental health indices [6], which is thought to be related to loss of status that these refugees experience during the resettlement. At the same time, patients with limited education have more difficulties with integration and are more likely to have depression [5].

Rural Versus Urban Area of Origin

Refugees from rural areas had poorer outcomes [6].

Region of Origin

Refugees from Europe had worse mental health outcomes than those from Asia or the Middle East [6]. In addition, Southeastern European subjects had more somatic complaints than Central African refugees [9].

Trauma/Torture

There are multiple studies showing that a history of torture increases the risk of mental health problems [10]. The concept of "cumulative trauma" summarizes the fact that more episodes of trauma were related with more intensive symptoms of PTSD in refugees (with the exception of avoidance, which did not correlate with number of traumatic events experiences) [11]. In addition, there is evidence that in victims of torture, mental health problems may persist long after the resettlement [12, 13].

Death of a Relative

Having lost a relative or a close friend in the home country or during the resettlement has been associated with increased likelihood of psychiatric problems [14].

Migration Factors

The following factors characterizing the migration process have been associated with poorer mental health status:

Being detained after leaving country [15]
Time spent in refugee camp
Long time to be granted refugee status/asylum status
Incidence of torture [10]
One positive impact on mental health is being granted the refugee status [16]

Post-migration Factors

Although emphasis is often placed on the refugees' experience of trauma in their country of origin, there is a growing body of evidence that factors related to their post-settlement period can contribute more to mental health problems than experiences prior to fleeing their country [17].

Communication Problems

Lack of knowledge of the language of the adoptive country can affect the prevalence of mental health problems in two ways: on the one hand, it can seriously impact the quality of adjustment to the new environment and therefore increase the prevalence of depression or anxiety. At the same time, communication barriers can cause underdiagnosis and poor access to care leading to underreporting of psychiatric problems.

Housing Accommodations

Permanent private accommodations were related to better mental health than institutional or temporary accommodations [6]. In addition, residential mobility (frequent changes in residence) was seen as stressful and worsened mental health [18]. Living in unsafe neighborhoods and being concerned for own physical safety can also contribute to psychiatric problems [14].

Restricted Economic Opportunity

Lack of employment or loss of economic status has been associated with worse mental health [6].

Other post-migration factors associated with worse mental health outcomes:
Repatriation to a country they had previously fled [6]
Initiating conflict not resolved [6]
Worry about family not in the host country [19, 20]

Prevalence of Common Mental Illnesses

Determining the prevalence of various psychiatric disorders in the refugee populations presents multiple levels of challenges. Most of the prevalence studies have been done in clinical populations, typically refugees who were seen either in mental health clinics or in general health programs, which already introduces a selection bias. Epidemiologic studies attempt to overcome this bias, but face communications difficulties, fear of stigma and local beliefs about mental illness, and how it is integrated in everyday life. These factors lead to low rates of participation and minimizing of symptoms on questionnaires. In addition, the measures used to identify mental health problems have to meet the demands of being at the same time, culture specific, standardized, and practical for the provider. A study looking at how refugee trauma and health status were measured in English language publications identified over 125 different screening or diagnostic instruments used [21]. This illustrates the complexity of studying the prevalence of mental illness in the refugee population.

Communication can be particularly difficult when working with refugees due to multiple factors: language and cultural differences, the effect of culture on symptoms and illness behavior, differences in family structure, acculturation, and intergenerational conflict. Aspects of acceptance by the receiving country as reflected in employment and social status can also interfere with the process of evaluation and mental health treatment. These difficulties can be addressed through specific inquiry, use of trained interpreters, culture brokers, meetings with families, and community organizations [22].

Working with interpreters, when available, must be done with a culturally informed approach. The first step in working with an interpreter is selecting the language in which the interview will be conducted. Refugees, like many migrants, oftentimes speak more than one language. Although it may be convenient to conduct the interview in a language that is known to both patient and clinician, effort must be made in order to identify the language in which the patient can be most accurate. This will help avoid abbreviated statements and allow the expression of emotional content. In certain situations it may be possible to dispense with interpreter services: patients speak some English and insist on conducting the interview in English or later in treatment when patients' mastery of English improves. Interpreters or translators should be familiar with the psychiatric assessment, and they need to be able to translate (to find the corresponding words from one language to another while retaining the same meaning) but also to interpret which implies the transmission of denotative meaning, in addition to the connotative meaning [23]. It is important to train the interpreter to be able to translate in such a way that the clinician can assess the more important parts of the mental status exam such as the process, association, affect.

A frequent model uses the bilingual psychiatric worker, which is sometimes employed in places where there are communities of refugees from the same country or cultures. In this case, attention must be given to boundaries and countertransference. Patients tend to try to recreate the doctor–patient relationship from their country, which often may be different than the accepted model in the US. Some examples include total trust and obedience in the provider (which can translate into a passive attitude or lack of participation), a desire to compensate the provider with gifts, or asking the provider for a letter of reference for a job application. A sensitive but firm delineation of boundaries will help the refugee in learning and adjusting to the US health care system and will promote a healthy societal integration in general. For all clinicians evaluating or treating refugees, but especially for those clinicians who are themselves prior refugees, special attention must be given to counter-transference, and additional peer supervision should be sought if necessary.

Another factor that can affect the attendance of mental health programs and the evaluation of the prevalence of psychiatric disorders in refugees and immigrants is the use of alternative or complementary medicine. Traditionally it was believed that use of alternative medicine is associated with avoidance of Western medicine in immigrants. A study of Cambodian refugees showed that 34 % of them relied on alternative medicine in the past year; however, only 5 % used the alternative medicine exclusively. Surprisingly, using alternative medicine was positively associated with seeking Western sources for mental health care [24].

In addition to the above challenges, given that the phenomenology of mental illness can be very different across cultures, Western diagnoses are not universally accepted as valid for these populations. However, most studies of prevalence utilize Western psychiatric diagnoses as outlined in the Diagnostic and Statistical Manual (DSM). See Chap. 12 for a discussion of standardized assessment scales validated in refugee populations.

PTSD and Depression are by far the most common diagnoses encountered in refugee populations. Table 11.1 presents a summary of the most illustrative studies regarding prevalence of mental health problems in refugees.

Other Psychiatric Disorders

In addition to depression and anxiety, other psychiatric disorders have been described in refugees: *traumatic brain injury* [37], *suicide* (rates were 4–5 times higher in Ethiopian immigrants than in the national population in one study) [38]. *Postnatal depression* has been reported as high as 42 % in migrant women (including immigrants, asylum seekers, and refugees) as opposed to 10–15 % in native-born women [39]. *Pathological gambling* was initially thought to be very common in Cambodian refugees (70 % prevalence [40]); however, a later study, considered to be more representative of Cambodian refugee communities in the US, showed a prevalence of only 13.9 % [41]. *Substance abuse* has been reported as well: 45 % of Indo-Chinese refugees had problems with alcohol or tobacco, while 13.9 % of the same had problems with drugs [42].

Influence of acculturation may vary with gender—in Somali girls for instance, greater Somali acculturation was associated with better mental health, while for Somali boys, greater American acculturation was associated with better mental health [43].

Domestic violence is considered to be underreported due to cultural factors, fear of stigma, but also fear of losing children to the child protection agencies if abuse is reported. Victimized women have a lower tendency to receive psychological support from the family; on a positive note, they were also less likely to use tranquilizers, to smoke, to think of suicide, and to attempt suicide [42].

Finally, comorbidities are extremely frequent; in a clinical sample of 61 refugee outpatients from psychiatric clinics in Norway, 80 % of those who had PTSD had three or more additional psychiatric diagnosis [9].

Resilience and Posttraumatic Growth

Although the prevalence of psychiatric problems is relatively high compared to the general population, many of the refugees succeed in integrating in the receiving society and achieving a good quality of life. The concept of posttraumatic growth, which summarizes the positive personal changes one makes in reaction to traumatic events, has received recent attention from researchers. Posttraumatic growth is

Table 11.1 Prevalence of Depression, Anxiety, and Posttraumatic Stress disorder in refugees

Year	Author	Population	Prevalence (lifetime prevalence, unless specified otherwise)	Assessment
2012	Lopes Cardozo [25]	Cambodian (landmine survivors)	Anxiety 62 % Depression 74 % PTSD 34 %	Harvard Trauma Questionnaire Hopkins Symptom Checklist SF36 Health Survey
2012	Slewa-Younan [26]	Iraqi refugees in Australia	PTSD 48 % MDD 36 % Dysthymia 36 %	Descriptive/clinical
2011	Hussain [27]	Sri Lankan (internally displaced)	PTSD 7 % Anxiety 32.6 % Depression 22.2 %	Harvard Trauma Questionnaire Hopkins Symptoms Checklist
2011	Kroll [8]	Somali men in an inner-city community clinic (*non-Somali men in the same clinic—13.7 % prevalence of psychosis*)	Psychosis 80 %	Clinical evaluation DSM IV based
2011	Schweitzer [19]	Burmese refugees in Australia	PTSD 9 % Anxiety 20 % Depression 36 % Somatization 37 %	Harvard Trauma Questionnaire Post-migration Living Difficulties checklist Hopkins Symptoms Checklist
2009	Fawzi [14]	Haitian refugees	PTSD 11.6 % Depression 14 % PTSD+depression 7.9 %	Interview via standardized questionnaire
2007	Jamil [28]	Iraqi refugees in the US	Anxiety 80 % Depression 80 % PTSD 54.3 % in men 11.4 % in Women	Posttraumatic Stress Diagnostic Scale Hopkins Symptom Checklist
2006	Sabin [29]	Mayan refugees to Guatemala	PTSD 8.9 % Anxiety 17.3 % Depression 47.8 %	Harvard Trauma Questionnaire Hopkins Symptom Checklist 25

(continued)

Table 11.1 (continued)

Year	Author	Population	Prevalence (lifetime prevalence, unless specified otherwise)	Assessment
2005	Basoglu [30]	Refugees from Yugoslavia	PTSD 33 % MDD 10 %	Trauma Survivors Questionnaire (RTSQ) 48-item Emotions and Beliefs After War (EBAW) Semi-Structured Interview for Survivors of War (SISOW) Diagnostic and Statistical Manual of Mental Disorders (DSM-IV) (SCID-I/NP, version 2)
2005	Steel [31]	Vietnamese refugees in Australia	Anxiety 6/1 % Depression 6.1 % Substance dependence 6.1 % (12 months prevalence)	Composite International Diagnostic Interview (CIDI 2.1)
2005	Marshall [13]	Cambodian refugees (99 % had experienced near—death situations, 90 % had a family member of a friend killed)	PTSD 62 % MDD 51 % Alcohol use disorders 4 %	Harvard Trauma Questionnaire
2004	Karunakara [32]	Sudanese	PTSD 46 % in refugees (48 % in stayees and 18 % in Uganda nationals)	Posttraumatic Stress Diagnostic Scale (PDS)
2004	Fenta [5]	Ethiopian refugees and immigrants in Toronto	Depression 9.8 %	Composite International Diagnostic Interview (CIDI)
2004	Van Ommeren [33]	Bhutanese refugees in Nepal	Somatoform pain disorders 31 % PTSD 85 %	Diagnostic interview ICD 10 based
1998	D'Avanzo [34]	Cambodian refugee women	87 % depression (France) 65 % depression (USA)	Hopkins Symptom Checklist
1999	Peltzer [35]	Tibetan refugees	PTSD 32 % Depression 30 %	Hopkins Symptom Checklist
1999	Holtz [36]	Tibetan refugees	Anxiety 41.4 % Depression 14.4 %	Hopkins Symptom Checklist

related to a higher quality of life in general; in addition, it explained more of the variance in quality of life than did posttraumatic stress symptoms, depressive symptoms, or unemployment [45].

Cultural Factors

Each culture has specific syndromes that in the Westerner's eye are classified as psychiatric diseases or specific presentations of more common psychiatric diseases. Various populations can present with specific syndromes, but at the same time, the same syndrome can be seen in different cultures located in different geographic regions. For instance, women who jump into wells in suicide attempts have been described in Pakistan, Punjab, Bangladesh, Sri Lanka [46]. *Koro* (the penis shrinking syndrome) is a classic example of a culture-bound syndrome seen in different ethnic and geographic groups [47]. Survivors of the Rwanda genocide divided mental health symptoms into a mental trauma syndrome (a PTSD like presentation plus some depression symptoms plus "local" symptoms) and a grief syndrome (other depression symptoms plus "local" symptoms) [48]. Multiple culture specific syndromes have been described in the Cambodian population; among them, *Khya^l* attacks (a variant of panic attack, characterized by physical symptoms and fear of heart arrest) or *khmaoch sangot* ("the spirit pushes you down"—a form of sleep paralysis) [49].

Transcultural Psychiatry, which, in part, focuses on the study of these syndromes, is a rapidly growing discipline. Even in the absence of clearly defined cultural syndromes, there are many subtle cultural variations in illness manifestations. In working with refugees, one must not only become familiar with the specific culture to which the patients belong, but also consider local and individual specifics and avoid premature labeling. Many areas of conflict are extremely multicultural or multireligious. As in any clinical setting, maintaining an attitude of inquiry and curiosity will facilitate breaking transcultural barriers.

References

1. Center for Diesease Control. Guidelines for mental health screening during the domestic medical examination for newly arrived refugees. 2013. http://www.cdc.gov/immigrantrefugeehealth/guidelines/domestic/mental-health-screening-guidelines.html; Accessed 3 Apr 2013
2. Harvard Program in Refugee and Trauma, Measuring Trauma, Measuring Torture manual on CD-ROM. http://hprt-cambridge.org/?page_id=420, Accessed 20 Aug 2013.
3. Swinkels H, Pottie K, Tugwell P, et al. Canadian Collaboration for Immigrant and Refugee Health (CCIRH). Development of guidelines for recently arrived immigrants and refugees to Canada: Delphi consensus on selecting preventable and treatable conditions. Can Med Assoc J. 2011;183(12):E928–32.

4. Sondergaard HP, Ekblad S, Theorell T. Screening for post-traumatic stress disorder among refugees in Stockholm. Nord J Psychiatry. 2003;57(3):185–9.
5. Fenta H, Hyman I, Noh S. Determinants of depression among Ethiopian immigrants and refugees in Toronto. J Nerv Ment Dis. 2004;192(5):363–72.
6. Porter M, Haslam N. Predisplacement and postdisplacement factors associated with mental health of refugees and internally displaced persons: a meta-analysis. JAMA. 2005;294(5):602–12.
7. Schubert CC, Punamaki RL. Mental health among torture survivors: cultural background, refugee status and gender. Nord J Psychiatry. 2011;65(3):175–82.
8. Kroll J, Yusuf AI, Fujiwara K. Psychoses, PTSD, and depression in somali refugees in minnesota. Soc Psychiatr Psychiatri Epidemiol. 2011;46(6):481–93.
9. Teodorescu DS, Heir T, Hauff E, et al. Mental health problems and post-migration stress among multi-traumatized refugees attending outpatient clinics upon resettlement to Norway. Scand J Psychol. 2012;53(4):316–32.
10. Mills E, Singh S, Roach B, et al. Prevalence of mental disorders and torture among Bhutanese refugees in Nepal: a systemic review and its policy implications. Med Conflict Surviv. 2008;24(1):5–15.
11. Mollica RF, McInnes K, Poole C, et al. Dose-effect relationships of trauma to symptoms of depression and post-traumatic stress disorder among Cambodian survivors of mass violence. Br J Psychiatry. 1998;173:482–8.
12. Tang SS, Fox SH. Traumatic experiences and the mental health of Senegalese refugees. J Nerv Ment Dis. 2001;189(8):507–12.
13. Marshall GN, Schell TL, Elliott MN, et al. Mental health of Cambodian refugees 2 decades after resettlement in the United States. JAMA. 2005;294(5):571–9.
14. Fawzi MC, Betancourt TS, Marcelin L, et al. Depression and post-traumatic stress disorder among Haitian immigrant students: implications for access to mental health services and educational programming. BMC Public Health. 2009;9:482.
15. Ichikawa M, Nakahara S, Wakai S. Effect of post-migration detention on mental health among Afghan asylum seekers in Japan. Aust New Zeal J Psychiatr. 2006;40(4):341–6.
16. Silove D, Steel Z, Susljik I, et al. The impact of the refugee decision on the trajectory of PTSD, anxiety, and depressive symptoms among asylum seekers: a longitudinal study. Am J Disaster Med. 2007;2(6):321–9.
17. Montgomery E. Long-term effects of organized violence on young middle eastern refugees' mental health. Soc Sci Med. 2008;67(10):1596–603.
18. Warfa N, Bhui K, Craig T, et al. Post-migration geographical mobility, mental health and health service utilisation among Somali refugees in the UK: a qualitative study. Health Place. 2006;12(4):503–15.
19. Schweitzer RD, Brough M, Vromans L, et al. Mental health of newly arrived Burmese refugees in Australia: contributions of pre-migration and post-migration experience. Aust New Zeal J Psychiatr. 2011;45(4):299–307.
20. Nickerson A, Bryant RA, Steel Z, et al. The impact of fear for family on mental health in a resettled Iraqi refugee community. J Psychiatr Res. 2010;44(4):229–35.
21. Hollifield M, Warner TD, Lian N, et al. Measuring trauma and health status in refugees: a critical review. JAMA. 2002;288(5):611–21.
22. Kirmayer LJ, Narasiah L, Munoz M, et al. Canadian Collaboration for Immigrant and Refugee Health (CCIRH). Common mental health problems in immigrants and refugees: general approach in primary care. Can Med Assoc J. 2011;183(12):E959–67.
23. Westermeyer J. Working with an interpreter in psychiatric assessment and treatment. J Nerv Ment Dis. 1990;178(12):745–9.
24. Berthold SM, Wong EC, Schell TL, et al. U.S. Cambodian refugees' use of complementary and alternative medicine for mental health problems. Psychiatr Serv. 2007;58(9):1212–8.
25. Lopes Cardozo B, Blanton C, Zalewski T, et al. Mental health survey among landmine survivors in Siem Reap province, Cambodia. Med Conflict Surviv. 2012;28(2):161–81.

26. Slewa-Younan S, Chippendale K, Heriseanu A, et al. Measures of psychophysiological arousal among resettled traumatized Iraqi refugees seeking psychological treatment. J Trauma Stress. 2012;25(3):348–52.
27. Husain F, Anderson M, Lopes Cardozo B, et al. Prevalence of war-related mental health conditions and association with displacement status in postwar Jaffna district, Sri Lanka. JAMA. 2011;306(5):522–31.
28. Jamil H, Farrag M, Hakim-Larson J, et al. Mental health symptoms in Iraqi refugees: post-traumatic stress disorder, anxiety, and depression. J Cult Divers. 2007;14(1):19–25.
29. Sabin M, Sabin K, Kim HY, et al. The mental health status of Mayan refugees after repatriation to Guatemala. Pan Am J Publ Health. 2006;19(3):163–71.
30. Basoglu M, Livanou M, Crnobaric C, et al. Psychiatric and cognitive effects of war in former Yugoslavia: association of lack of redress for trauma and posttraumatic stress reactions. JAMA. 2005;294(5):580–90.
31. Steel Z, Silove D, Chey T, et al. Mental disorders, disability and health service use amongst Vietnamese refugees and the host Australian population. Acta Psychiatr Scand. 2005;111(4):300–9.
32. Karunakara UK, Neuner F, Schauer M, et al. Traumatic events and symptoms of post-traumatic stress disorder amongst Sudanese nationals, refugees and Ugandans in the west Nile. Afr Health Sci. 2004;4(2):83–93.
33. Van Ommeren M, de Jong JT, Sharma B, et al. Psychiatric disorders among tortured Bhutanese refugees in Nepal. Arch Gen Psychiatry. 2001;58:475–82.
34. D'Avanzo CE, Barab SA. Depression and anxiety among Cambodian refugee women in France and the United States. Issues Ment Health Nurs. 1998;19(6):541–56.
35. Peltzer K. Trauma and mental health problems of Sudanese refugees in Uganda. Cent Afr J Med. 1999;45(5):110–4.
36. Holtz TH. Refugee trauma versus torture trauma: a retrospective controlled cohort study of Tibetan refugees. J Nerv Ment Dis. 1998;186(1):24–34.
37. Mollica RF, Lyoo IK, Chernoff MC, et al. Brain structural abnormalities and mental health sequelae in South Vietnamese ex-political detainees who survived traumatic head injury and torture. Arch Gen Psychiatry. 2009;66(11):1221–32.
38. Arieli A, Gilat I, Aycheh S. Suicide by Ethiopian immigrants in Israel. Harefuah. 1994;127(3–4):65–70.
39. Collins CH, Zimmerman C, Howard LM, et al. Refugee, asylum seeker, immigrant women and postnatal depression: rates and risk factors. Arch Womens Ment Health. 2011;14(1):3–11.
40. Petry NM, Armentano C, Kuoch T, et al. Gambling participation and problems among South East Asian refugees to the United States. Psychiatr Serv. 2003;54:1142–8.
41. Marshall GN, Elliott MN, Schell TL, et al. Prevalence and correlates of lifetime disordered gambling in Cambodian refugees residing in Long Beach, CA. J Immigr Minor Health. 2009;11(1):35–40.
42. Yee BW, Nguyen DT. Correlates of drug use and abuse among Indochinese refugees: mental health implications. J Psychoactive Drugs. 1987;19(1):77–83.
43. Ellis BH, MacDonald HZ, Klunk-Gillis J, et al. Discrimination and mental health among Somali refugee adolescents: the role of acculturation and gender. Am J Orthopsychiatr. 2010;80(4):564–75.
44. Al-Modallal H. Patterns of coping with partner violence: experiences of refugee women in Jordan. Public Health Nurs. 2012;29(5):403–11.
45. Teodorescu DS, Siqveland J, Heir T, et al. Posttraumatic growth, depressive symptoms, post-traumatic stress symptoms, post-migration stressors and quality of life in multi-traumatized psychiatric outpatients with a refugee background in Norway. Health Qual Life Outcome. 2012;10:84.
46. Guzder J. Women who jump into wells: reflections on suicidality in women from conflict regions of the Indian subcontinent. Transcult Psychiatry. 2011;48(5):585–603.

47. Crozier I. Making up koro: multiplicity, psychiatry, culture, and penis-shrinking anxieties. J Hist Med Allied Sci. 2012;67(1):36–70.
48. Bolton P. Local perceptions of the mental health effects of the Rwandan genocide. J Nerv Ment Dis. 2001;189(4):243–8.
49. Hinton DE, Hinton AL, Eng KT, et al. PTSD and key somatic complaints and cultural syndromes among rural Cambodians: the results of a needs assessment survey. Med Anthropol Q. 2012;26(3):383–407.

Chapter 12
Mental Health Screening

Susan Heffner Rhema, Amber Gray, Sasha Verbillis-Kolp, Beth Farmer, and Michael Hollifield

Introduction

There has been a long-standing discussion amongst scholars about the role and use of early mental health screening to detect common mental disorders in refugees. In the development of a health screening protocol for refugees arriving to the US, models were deemed inadequate, in part at least, due to the lack of mental health screening [1]. The wide variance in reported prevalence of symptoms among refugees may be in part due to the lack of empirically developed instruments for use [2]. In encouraging the practice of mental health screening with refugees, authors have discussed both the value of self-report questionnaires to help normalize symptoms

S.H. Rhema, L.C.S.W., A.B.D. (✉)
Kent School, University of Louisville, 212 West Ormsby Avenue,
Louisville, KY 40203, USA
e-mail: susan@susanrhema.com

A. Gray, M.P.H., M.A.
New Mexico Department of Health, 118 Temblon St, Santa Fe, NM 87501, USA
e-mail: amber@ecentral.com

S. Verbillis-Kolp, M.S.W.
Lutheran Community Services Northwest, 605 S.E. Ceasar E. Chavez Blvd.,
Portland, OR 97214, USA
e-mail: sverbilliskolp@lcsnw.org

B. Farmer, M.S.W.
International Counseling and Community Services Program, Lutheran Community Services
Northwest, 4040 S 188th Street, Suite #200, SeaTac, WA 98188, USA
e-mail: bfarmer@lcsnw.org

M. Hollifield, M.D.
Program for Traumatic Stress, VA Long Beach, 5901 E 7th St, Long Beach, CA 90822, USA

Pacific Institute for Research and Evaluation, Albuquerque, NM, USA
e-mail: mhollifield@pire.org

A. Annamalai (ed.), *Refugee Health Care: An Essential Medical Guide*,
DOI 10.1007/978-1-4939-0271-2_12, © Springer Science+Business Media New York 2014

in refugees [3] and the use of structured interviews to enable the collection of important details relevant to mental health [4]. While this debate continues, some suggest that early detection of mental health symptoms in refugees is believed to improve long-term functioning [4, 5].

The Office of Refugee Resettlement guidelines require a health screening in the first 90 days; however, there has been a lack of procedural or financial support for mental health screening for refugees [6]. Technical instructions provided to resettlement agencies by the Centers for Disease Control dated 2012 stated that a mental health screen "may be performed according to resources available for intervention for conditions identified" [7].

State refugee health coordinators surveyed in 2010 reported that only 4 of the 44 states surveyed used a formal screening instrument and 68 % used informal conversation [8]. Refugees endure a high burden of distress and illness with its concomitant impairment; best estimates are that up to 10 % of refugees suffer diagnostic levels of PTSD and depression [9] and approximately 30 % have high levels of distress that might require treatment [10]. This may suggest that routine screening for mental health during resettlement be conducted, as is done for infectious diseases.

The Need for Specialized Instruments

Understanding a refugee's expression of distress requires careful consideration of a variety of factors including language, culture, the individual traumatic history, and the client's medical worldview [11, 12]. Outlined below is research conducted over a period of years leading to the development of screening instruments by a number of authors considering these complex issues. The human biological system response to stress includes a series of common physiological changes [13] which might predict core symptoms, yet the language used to express these varies based on social and cultural factors. For the purpose of screening, identifying the central symptoms that arise from the neurological process and less on the complex communication of them avoids being distracted by cultural and medical frameworks. Assessment after screening contributes to understanding the complex symptoms, comorbidities, and explanatory models that help define treatment needs.

While most refugees anticipate an end to the long-term suffering and uncertainty when they arrive to the city of resettlement, the initial weeks and months is a period of emotional adjustment that can fluctuate between relief and distress, even, in some cases reactivating symptoms of trauma. For others, emotional distress can appear years after arrival. Therefore, mental health screening, at any time, can play a vital role in identifying refugee mental health needs.

The role of a screener requires understanding of the unique challenges related to refugee mental health and refugee trauma [1]. This chapter begins by presenting several issues to be considered when screening refugee clients and continues with an overview of research related to screening instruments. Screening is best thought of as a distinct process from diagnosis or assessment with the intent to efficiently detect common mental disorders and distress with reasonably high sensitivity and specificity.

It is important to note that refugees are a diverse group and represent a broad variety of ethnic, language, and people groups, and this chapter can only present generalizations of the issues affecting them.

Considerations for the Screening Process

Refugees, by definition, have endured experiences of harm, persecution, and loss of security, all of which can reduce an individual's level of trust. Therefore, careful engagement of a refugee and consideration of their need for safety are important. Based on past experience, many refugees hesitate to speak openly or disclose too much information for fear of retaliation, persecution or that the information will be used against them. Establishing a feeling of security is necessary for an accurate measure of health symptoms of any kind [14].

The period of adaptation in the preliminary months of resettlement adds another layer of physical, social and psychological stress, and some refugees may find the process of adjustment to be overwhelming. Emotional responses during this period vary widely, and while some individuals experience an initial "honeymoon" period that masks symptoms, others may find that specific events trigger symptoms even years after arrival. Ongoing challenges of adjustment referred as acculturation can induce significant stress. Language and cultural adjustments, changes in family roles, and social expectations can manifest in a variety of medical or psychological complaints for many years after arrival to the country of resettlement.

Refugee descriptions of symptoms and emotional distress are communicated using language that reflects their medical worldview. Many refugees come from naturalistic or personalistic medical models both of which understand the nature of illness and the body differently than Western medicine [10, 14–16]. A significant number of refugees come from worldviews that do not differentiate between mind and body symptoms [17]. Research has demonstrated that experiences of extreme stress effect a variety of changes in the body [18] and refugees will often report physical symptoms of distress.

Another issue affecting communication is the respect awarded to people in authority. In many cases, refugees will not initiate communication but will only respond to specific questions, and in some cases will avoid any appearance of disagreement even when a provider's advice goes counter to the refugee's belief or understanding.

Language and cultural barriers make using trained interpreters and translated instruments a requirement. Providers working with refugees must have knowledge of and follow proper interpreter protocol. It is important that providers do not ask interpreters to answer questions or "fill in the blanks." Providers should have sufficient knowledge of the cultural context to ensure that an interpreter being used is not representative of a tribe, clan, or ethnic group that had previously persecuted the patient's refugee group. It is important to watch for signs of discomfort, to ask clarifying questions, and to ask the interpreter to follow protocol.

Even with the best tools at hand, understanding what the refugee intends to communicate can, at times, be a challenge. Screening that includes both standardized instruments and an interview is best, as refugee literacy (in their primary language) and comprehension of scale formats may interfere with accurate conclusions [4].

Providers can help overcome some of the challenges of communication by using concrete simple language, and focusing on symptoms, rather than diagnosis. Also, a provider can never assume that a refugee understands the context of the medical encounter and should take time to provide clarity about their role and intention [11]. Careful explanation of the use of any paperwork or documentation the refugee has to sign is warranted, as many may have signed stacks of papers they did not understand either in the context of traumatic experience or in the resettlement process.

Most of all, the refugee experience is one of disempowerment. Refugees are best served when provided with education about procedures and services that include opportunities for choice. Refugees who are protective of information or reluctant to participate in activities that might improve their health are often mislabeled as noncompliant or suffering from a stigma. Explanations and instructions that allow refugees to have control over choices are more effective. When referring refugees for follow up assessment or mental health services, rather than using diagnostic or psychological language, it is useful to describe the services as an opportunity to meet with another provider who can help them to manage the symptoms and increase their comfort.

Besides PTSD and depression, mental health issues that should be considered in a mental health screening include traumatic or acquired brain injuries, forms of psychosis, and conditions previously undiagnosed in adults, including developmental delays, autism spectrum disorders, and similar diagnoses [5]. According to screening guidelines from the CDC, physicians should screen for undiagnosed psychosis and traumatic or acquired brain injury. These conditions are often more complex and may require additional visits or evaluations after primary mental health screening.

Primary care physicians are an important source to identify survivors of torture, and to help them obtain necessary medical and psychiatric care. Statistics for survivors of torture vary widely but according to the International Rehabilitation Council for Torture Victims, up to 35 % of the refugee population is survivors. The best approach to establish whether a refugee is a survivor of torture is to ask several direct questions such as: What led you to become a refugee? or Were you ever held against your will? For more information on evaluating torture survivors see Chap. 14.

Some instruments for screening are discussed below. Providers are also encouraged to familiarize themselves with diagnostic criteria as set forth by the Diagnostic and Statistical Manual—fifth edition (DSM-V) [19].

Instruments for Screening

In a recent survey, respondents composed of refugee health coordinators identified the need for short, culturally appropriate mental health screening tools to identify refugees who need assessment and treatment services [7]. Depending on the clinic environment, and for a busy practitioner, only a primary screening and referral process may be feasible. However, in clinics with additional resources, a second tier clinical assessment that allows for a more comprehensive narrative by the refugee(s), an in-depth history, and diagnostic formulation may be possible.

The primary challenge to developing a screening instrument is that refugees are heterogeneous groups who collectively experience many psychological and somatic symptoms of distress. Theoretically, a screening instrument should include symptoms that optimally predict common disorders in multiple refugee groups with high efficiency. A few instruments have been developed in refugees for specific diagnostic identification.

The Vietnamese Depression Scale (VDS) consists of 15-items that effectively identify depression in Vietnamese refugees [20]. The Harvard Trauma Questionnaire (HTQ) has a 30-item section assessing symptoms that have been used as a proxy for PTSD [21]. Both instruments were developed by expert consensus methods for use in the clinical setting.

The 15-item Health Leaflet (HL) developed to screen for PTSD in two Iraqi language groups reported that the HL was 0.70 sensitive and specific to diagnosis, with two items (difficulty concentrating and exposure to torture), accounting for the discriminatory performance [4]. A Diagnostic and Statistical Methods (DSM-IV) based symptom checklist developed by an expert consensus process identified a psychiatric disorder in nearly 14 % of the 1,058 adult refugees in the Colorado Refugee Program [5].

More recent work on developing a screening instrument has been done by the *Pathways to Wellness* project. The Refugee Health Screener-15 (RHS-15) was designed to be short (15 questions) with neutral language that does not directly address violence, torture, or trauma. The RHS-15 was empirically developed to be a valid, efficient and effective screener for common mental disorders in refugees. The RHS-15 has been integrated into standard physical health screenings for newly arrived refugees at Public Health Seattle & King County and in a number of other places across the country.

Symptoms that form the validated RHS-15 were derived from twenty-seven New Mexico Refugee Symptom Checklist-121 items (NMRSCL-121), the Hopkins Symptom Checklist-25, and the Posttraumatic Stress Symptom Scale Self-Report that were found to be most predictive of anxiety, depression, and PTSD across the target sample of Iraqi, Nepali, Bhutanese, and Burmese refugees. Multiple exploratory methods were used during analysis, including correlations and general linear models using t-tests and analysis of variance to establish the most useful and efficient set of symptom items. The RHS-15 is composed of fourteen symptom items and a distress thermometer that predict each of three diagnostic proxies with sensitivity ranging between 0.81 and 0.95 and specificity ranging from 0.86 to 0.89.

Strengths of the RHS-15 are its metric properties, the efficiency of administration, and its demonstrated preliminary effectiveness and desirability in meeting a clear need. The RHS-15 grew from initial work utilizing empirical multi-method participatory research. Initial items came from qualitative work respecting the voice of Vietnamese and Kurdish refugees used in the development of the NMRSCL-121 which assesses the broad range of persistently distressing symptoms and is a reliable and valid predictor of traumatic experiences, PTSD, anxiety, and depression in Kurdish and Vietnamese refugees [22]. Because developers of the RHS-15 were sensitive to the cultural beliefs and expressions regarding symptoms of mental health, participatory community translation helped ensure cultural equivalence for important words and phrases of distress. The RHS-15 is available in Amharic, Arabic, Burmese, Farsi, French, Karen, Nepali, Russian, Somali, Spanish, Swahili, and Tigrinya. Limitations of the RHS-15 are that prospective efficacy and effectiveness testing is yet to be reported, and generalizability to other refugee groups is still pending.

The RHS-15 has open access and may be obtained through Lutheran Community Services Northwest (LCSNW) at *http://www.lcsnw.org/pathways/index.html*

There are a few instruments developed for refugees that assess symptoms as diagnostic proxies (DPs). None are definitive diagnostic equivalents. The Hopkins Symptom Checklist-25 (HSCL-25) is a valid indicator of anxiety and depression for the general US population and for Indochinese refugees and demonstrates transcultural validity. Item-average scores ≥ 1.75 predict clinically significant anxiety and depression on the scale in general US and refugee samples and are considered valid DPs [23].

The Posttraumatic Symptom Scale Self-Report (PSS-SR) predicts PTSD diagnosis in US populations. Cronbach alpha is 0.91, and 1-month test–retest reliability is 0.74. The 17 items on the scale, each scored from 0 to 3 for symptom frequency, are DSM-IV PTSD diagnostic items. The PSS-SR that may be scored as continuous or a dichotomous DP was found to be highly correlated with war-related trauma, symptoms, and impairment in Kurdish and Vietnamese refugees [24].

Finally, it should be noted that for some refugees post-migration living difficulties may be an equal or stronger predictor of emotional distress than war and migration stress. These factors, such as poverty and unemployment, may be a source of distress either immediately or months after arrival in the new country. The authors recommend that providers remain aware of this issue when screening for mental disorders.

Conclusion

One concern expressed by primary care physicians about mental health screening with a refugee is that it may cause a strong emotional reaction. There is no evidence to suggest that physicians need to be concerned with this and following the guidelines above will increase refugee comfort. Screening for symptoms using an instrument such as the VDS for depression or the RHS-15 for PTSD, anxiety or depression and not initially discussing trauma, torture, or other emotionally laden issues, will mitigate immediate distress. Effective screening of refugees in the primary care setting may increase visit time and does require a focused effort. However, the need for services is great and outcomes have shown that there is value for refugees in receiving services [25]. Ultimately, providers can support the healing process by creating a safe and engaged connection that allows refugees to improve their understanding of the medical system and have power over their own medical care.

Appendix 1

Mental Health SCREENING of Refugees

Sample Screening Questions

Diagnostic criteria	Suggested questions
Hypervigilance	Do you feel you are waiting for something bad to happen?
Intense fear	Do you feel that your body is out of your control?
General anxiety	What do you worry about? Or are you always thinking?
Heart palpitations	Does your heart ever suddenly beat quickly?
Distressing recollections flashbacks	Do you sometimes remember bad things that happened in the past?
Isolation/detachment	Who do you spend time with? How do you spend your time?
Nightmares/sleep disturbance	When do you fall asleep and when do you wake? What keeps you awake or wakes you?
Dissociative periods	Does your mind sometimes go far away?
Startle	Do you jump at loud noises?
Avoidance	Do you visit friends or neighbors? What do you do when you are not at work or school?
Lack of concentration	Do you have trouble learning new things?
Poor memory	Do you forget things?
Anger	Do you get angry?
Lack of affect	Do you feel you do not care about anything?
Depression	Do you get sad? How often do you cry?
Poor future imagining	Can you imagine a happy future in America?
Loss of appetite	How many times in a day do you eat?

Tips for Effective Screening

Reminders	
To Dos	Cautions
Establish connection/safety	Do not assume that you understand
Check understanding with directed questions	Avoid medical jargon and acronyms
Learn something of the social/political context of events faced by the refugee groups in your area	Be aware of ethnic rivals and relationships in your area
Normalize the trauma response and educate in simple terms	Talk in symptoms, not diagnosis
Know and follow interpreter use protocol!!	DO NOT use interpreters to diagnose
Use trained interpreters	Use simple non-colloquial language. Avoid technical medical language
Ask the refugee what is their first language and what is their level of literacy in that language	Clarify understanding by asking specific questions that cannot be answered with yes/no
Ask the refugee what they think is the problem	Do not assume that the refugee understands the purpose of the appointment

References

1. Kennedy J, Seymour D, Hummel B. A comprehensive refugee health screening program. Public Health Rep. 1999;144:469–77.
2. Hollifield M, Warner T, Lian N, et al. Measuring trauma and health status in refugees. JAMA. 2002;288:611–21.
3. Mollica RF, Mcinnes K, Sarajlic N, et al. Disability associated with psychiatric comorbidity and health status in Bosnian refugees living in Croatia. JAMA. 1999;282:433–9.
4. Sondergaard HP, Ekblad S, Theorell T. Screening for post-traumatic stress disorder among refugees in Stockholm. Nord J Psychiatry. 2003;57(3):185–9.
5. Savin D, Seymour DJ, Littleford LN, et al. Findings from mental health screening of newly arrived refugees in Colorado. Public Health Rep. 2005;120(3):224–9.
6. Weine S. Developing preventive mental health interventions for refugee families in resettlement. Fam Process. 2011;50(3):410–30.
7. Center for Disease Control and Prevention. Guidelines for mental health screening during the domestic medical examination for newly arrived refugees. 2012. http://www.cdc.gov/immigrantrefugeehealth/guidelines/domestic/mental-health-screening-guidelines.html
8. Shannon P, Im H, Becher E, et al. Screening for war trauma, torture and mental health symptoms among newly arrived refugees: a National survey of U. S. refugee health coordinators. J Immigr Refug Stud. 2012;10:380–94.
9. Fazel M, Wheeler J, Danesh J. Prevalence of serious mental disorder in 7000 refugees resettled in Western countries: a systematic review. Lancet. 2005;365(9467):1309–14.
10. Hollifield M, Verbillis-Kolp S, Farmer B, et al. The refugee health screener-15 (RHS-15): development and validation of an instrument for anxiety, depression, and PTSD in refugees. Gen Hosp Psychiatry. 2013;35(2):202–9.
11. Codrington R, Iqbal A, Segal J. Lost in translation? Embracing the challenges of working with families from a refugee background. Aust New Zeal J Fam Ther. 2011;32(2):129–43.
12. Kirmayer L. The refugee's predicament. L' Evol Psychiatr. 2002;67:724–42.

13. Bremner J. Does stress damage the brain? Understanding trauma related disorders from a mind body perspective. New York, NY: W. W. Norton and Company; 2005.
14. Lacroix M, Sabbah C. Posttraumatic psychological distress and resettlement: the need for a different practice in assisting refugee families. J Fam Soc Work. 2011;14:43–53.
15. Bolton P, Bentancourt T. Mental health in postwar Afghanistan. JAMA. 2004;292(5):626–8.
16. Geertz C. Anti-anti-relativism. 1983 distinguished lecture. Am Anthropol. 1984;82:263–78.
17. Kohrt B, Harper I. Navigating diagnoses: understanding mind-body relations, mental health, and stigma in Nepal. Cult Med Psychiatr. 2008;32:462–91. doi:10.1007/s11013-008-9110-6.
18. Yehuda R. Biology of posttraumatic stress disorder. J Clin Psychiatr. 2001;62:41–6.
19. American Psychiatric Association. Diagnostic and statistical manual of mental disorders (5th ed). Washington DC: American Psychiatric Publishing; 2013.
20. Kinzie J, Manson SM, Vinh DT, et al. Development and validation of a Vietnamese-language depression rating scale. Am J Psychiatr. 1982;139(10):1276–81.
21. Mollica RF, Caspi-Yavin Y, Bollini P, et al. The Harvard trauma questionnaire: validating a cross-cultural instrument for measuring torture, trauma and posttraumatic stress disorder in Indochinese refugees. J Nerv Ment Dis. 1992;180(2):111–6.
22. Hollifield M, Warner T, Krakow B, et al. The range of symptoms in refugees of war. J Nerv Ment Dis. 2009;197(2):1–9.
23. Derogatis L, Lipman R, Rickels K, et al. The Hopkins symptom checklist, (HSCL): a self-report symptom inventory. Behav Sci. 1974;19:1–15.
24. Foa E, Riggs D, Dancu C, et al. Reliability and validity of a brief instrument for assessing post-traumatic stress disorder. J Trauma Stress. 1993;6:459–73.
25. Vaage AB, Thomsen PH, Silove D, et al. Long-term mental health of Vietnamese refugees in the aftermath of trauma. Br J Psychiatry. 2010;196:122–5.

Chapter 13
Treatment of Mental Illness

Aniyizhai Annamalai and Maya Prabhu

Introduction

As has been outlined in Chaps. 11 and 12, estimates of the prevalence of mental illness in refugees are varied depending on their home countries, their experience, torture, and the process by which they made their way to the US [1]. However, numerous existing studies confirm that several risk factors put refugees at high risk of developing mental illness, While posttraumatic stress disorder (PTSD) and depression are among the commonly reported mental illnesses, several culture specific syndromes are also described [2, 3] (see also Chap. 11). In addition, refugees manifest mental and physical symptoms that result from emotional distress but cannot be classified into any particular disorder or syndrome.

The same challenges that are inherent in assessing mental illness apply to formulating and designing treatment interventions for these illnesses. A major barrier to delivering optimal care is language. Qualified medical interpreters are critical as the efficacy of psychotherapeutic interventions is dependent on effective communication. Subtle differences in meanings particularly of idiomatic speech, if not interpreted correctly, can contribute to a poor understanding of cultural factors in the manifestation of emotional distress or even a misdiagnosis of a frank psychiatric illness.

A. Annamalai, M.D. (✉)
Yale University School of Medicine, 34 Park St., New Haven, CT 06519, USA
e-mail: aniyizhai.annamalai@yale.edu

M. Prabhu, M.D., L.L.B.
Law and Psychiatry Division, Department of Psychiatry, Yale School of Medicine,
34 Park St., New Haven, CT 06519, USA
e-mail: maya.prabhu@yale.edu

A. Annamalai (ed.), *Refugee Health Care: An Essential Medical Guide*,
DOI 10.1007/978-1-4939-0271-2_13, © Springer Science+Business Media New York 2014

Example

An Iraqi man, in his mid-30s, with a history of sexual assault and physical abuse while imprisoned, presented to our refugee clinic. He reported symptoms consistent with PTSD related to his assault including nightmares, intrusive thoughts and intense ongoing fear such that he avoided leaving the house. He also reported seeing images of a "black cat" and "shadows" which the medical interpreter translated as colorful descriptions of the patient's sadness and distress. Several weeks later, the patient was brought to the emergency room grossly psychotic and a different interpreter elicited that the previous symptoms were visual hallucinations.

As described in Chap. 10, many refugees present with physical symptoms such as back pain. Other symptoms such as dizziness, fatigue, dyspepsia are also described [4], and often these symptoms are predictors of anxiety, depression, or PTSD [5]. Management of these medical conditions should include addressing psychiatric issues, if present. Examples of specific physical manifestations in traumatized refugees in certain cultural groups, such as tinnitus related to PTSD [6] and "gastrointestinal focused panic" [7] have been described. The importance of including physical symptoms in psychiatric screening is underscored in the development and use of the Refugee Health Screener (RHS 15) in refugee populations (see Chap. 12).

When there is suspicion for significant psychological distress or psychiatric illness based on history, physical exam, and use of other screening tools, the refugee should be referred to mental health services, if available. Regions greatly vary in availability of local resources and capacity to provide mental health care. Mental health agencies typically have limited capacity to provide specialized care for refugees. Finding adequately qualified interpreters is one of the biggest barriers to delivering appropriate mental health care to refugees [8, 9].

Treatment strategies for refugees should be multidisciplinary. An array of approaches including pharmacological, psychotherapeutic, psychosocial, and community-based interventions should be considered. Refugees are often reluctant to accept mental health treatment even when it is indicated. It may be useful to frame it as support to cope with their past traumas as well as ease their transition to a new society. Refugees also often come from societies where medications are infrequently used to treat anxiety and depression and are viewed as unnecessary.

Psychoeducation is important as the first step in engaging patients in treatment. This would not only include education on any undiagnosed mental illness but should provide an understanding of psychological distress in the context of acculturation and previous traumatic experiences. Refugees may need support in dealing with difficulties of adaptation as well as separation and loss of family, culture, and home. Focus should not just be on past trauma but also on adjustment to living in the new country. Changing of gender roles and intergenerational conflicts may emerge during transition. It is also important for providers to recognize that their approach to mental illness may be very different from that of the refugee and Western treatment modalities should not be applied uniformly to all patients. Supportive therapy based on a person-centered counseling paradigm and empathic understanding should be provided in a non-challenging environment.

Example

A recently resettled Iraqi man, in his late 40s, presented to clinic with passive suicidal ideation. His four sons ranging in ages from teens to early 20s had resettled nearly 2 years earlier and were quicker than the patient to learn English and adapt to the US. The patient reported considerable unhappiness that he was now without employment and status and was unnerved by his children's newfound "lack of respect" for his authority. In addition, he had been physically threatening towards his wife during an argument which led his sons to warn him that they would call the police if he did so in the future, a marked departure from how such a matter would have been handled in Iraq. The patient was not only depressed but demoralized and anxious too. Efforts were made to provide him with supportive therapy but the patient was reluctant to discuss "personal" matters with an "outsider."

Psychopharmacology

There are very few studies evaluating psychotropic treatment for refugees. Most were studies of PTSD and depression and measured symptom change with pharmacological treatment in specific refugee groups without any control groups. Agents used were Selective Serotonergic Reuptake Inhibitors (SSRIs), Serotonergic and Noradrenergic Reuptake Inhibitors (SNRIs), Mirtazapine, and Bupropion. There was improvement in PTSD and depression symptoms [10–12] and in associated somatic symptoms in at least one study [11]. Other medications that have shown efficacy in refugees are Clonidine [13] and Prazosin [14] for PTSD. In a group of Cambodian refugees with PTSD, combination therapy with an SSRI and Cognitive Behavioral Therapy (CBT) was more efficacious than medication alone [15].

Some clinical studies have reported marked sensitivity to side effects of psychotropic medications among refugee groups [16]. Since many refugees are medication naïve, it is recommended that lower doses are initiated to minimize side effects. We have also found that many refugees are unaccustomed to participating in treatment decisions with their physicians so extra efforts to describe patient options and even their right to refuse as part of informed consent are worthwhile.

Psychotherapy

Most research on mental health treatment in refugees has been on trauma-focused therapies and interventions have targeted posttraumatic stress. Outcomes measured are usually symptoms of PTSD or depression. It is important to remember that PTSD in refugees is complex with repetitive and cumulative trauma. This chronic PTSD is compounded by post-migratory living difficulties. Alternative conceptualizations to include a broader range of symptoms, such as Disorders of Extreme

Stress Not Otherwise Specified (DESNOS) have been proposed [17–20]. In spite of the fact that PTSD in its pure form may not be applicable to refugees, it remains the most common diagnosis studied in this population. Since traditional treatment modalities for PTSD that focus on one traumatic event may not be effective, other adaptions have been tried in refugees.

CBT is a contemporary treatment model used widely for PTSD [21] It is based on a PTSD framework that extreme fear at the time of the traumatic event is associated with other stimuli related to the trauma and this results in a conditioned response. Each time any of these stimuli are encountered, a fear response is triggered. One of the CBT techniques is via extinction learning where the person learns that those stimuli are no longer paired with the traumatic event and over time anxiety is diminished. CBT also is useful for altering maladaptive cognitions. Disturbances in processing memories and distorted thinking are responsible for the intrusive and avoidance symptoms of PTSD.

CBT is a common modality of treatment studied in refugees [22]. In addition to traditional CBT methods, the studies adapted culturally appropriate imagery and specialized techniques such as mindfulness and meditation [23, 24]. The focus in these culturally adapted therapies is more on regulating affect rather than exposure. These therapies showed effectiveness for PTSD, depression, and anxiety though dropout rates can be high for a variety of reasons [25].

Although some authors caution against exposure therapy in an already hypervigilant retraumatized refugee population, exposure therapy continues to be a mainstay treatment used for extinction conditioning. In this type of therapy, a person is confronted with or exposed to thoughts or situations that evoke fear and taught to address the fear with relaxation or other techniques. Schauer et al. describe Narrative Exposure Therapy (NET) for traumatic stress after war or torture [26]. It is an adaptation of exposure therapy originally applied to war survivors and also tested in comparison with other modes of therapy in refugees with PTSD [27, 28]. It is a form of testimony psychotherapy, which involves the recounting of the patient's life story focusing on traumatic experiences that led to PTSD. The goal is to integrate the memory of repetitive traumatic experiences into the refugee's life story, so a coherent chronological narrative is formed. The narrative is recorded in written form with both therapist and patient reviewing it, and at the end of the treatment the patient keeps the record.

Culturally sensitive CBT (in South Asians) and NET are two forms of therapy that are relatively well documented in refugees. Following are less well-documented forms of therapy that have been studied in refugees. A non-manualized, psychodynamically oriented trauma focused therapy has been tested and found effective in a small group of refugee patients [29]. Skills training incorporating emotion regulation and interpersonal relationship skills, in addition to trauma related cognitive therapy, was also proven to be effective, reducing PTSD symptom in a group of 70 refugees [30]. Behavioral biofeedback therapy showed modest benefits on chronic pain but not on PTSD or depression [31]. A specific form of nontraditional therapy, the Eye Movement Desensitization and Reprocessing (EMDR) developed for PTSD, has also been tested in refugee children [32].

Various multidisciplinary treatments have been tried in refugees and usually include some combination of psychotherapy, social support, medications, and target PTSD, depression, anxiety and overall functioning. Group psychosocial treatments have also been tried. The efficacy of any of these treatments over the long term has not been well established. Also, treatment of somatic symptoms in traumatized refugees is not well researched. For a review of psychotherapeutic treatment modalities studied in refugees, see Nickerson et al. and Palic et al. [33, 34].

Community-Based Interventions

Post-migration stressors such as under or unemployment, limited finances, language barriers, coupled with the demands of acculturation, decreased social support, possible role changes, combine to increase the psychological distress faced by refugees. Resettlement agencies generally try to incorporate assistance with the resettlement process (residency status, family union, housing, social services, language classes, education, and employment opportunities) and accessing medical care including psychiatric treatment, when necessary. They may also strive to provide some form of psychological support, either direct professional counseling or problem solving at the individual and family level.

Community-based health interventions are also a way to empower local refugee groups to participate in solving their social and health problems. Suggested formats of community-based interventions primarily focus on outreach, workshops, train-the-trainer models, employment of refugees and mentoring programs. There is a focus on self-help, inclusion, empowerment, and advocacy. Examples of activities for refugees can range from professional roles (e.g., advice from medically trained refugees), leadership (e.g., group facilitators), liaison roles (e.g., more established refugees assisting with case management services), to mentoring and individualized support [35]. Using refugees as peer facilitators can be effective in improving social integration. Creating peer support groups matched by gender and ethnicity was found to be successful as a culturally congruent intervention to meet support needs of refugees [36].

Many community-based interventions have been tested in internally displaced refugees and in refugee camps before resettlement. A psychosocial intervention in a refugee camp in Guinea incorporated training of refugee paraprofessional counselors and community leaders, community awareness campaigns as well as clinical group therapy sessions. The clinical group sessions reduced trauma symptoms and improved social functioning [37]. A group interpersonal psychotherapy intervention in displaced adolescents and adults in Uganda led to reductions in depressive symptoms [38, 39].

In the US, a community-based mental health program providing comprehensive services to children, adolescents, and their families was developed as an outreach oriented model for refugees from different backgrounds to overcome obstacles to accessing care. The emphasis was on creating culturally sensitive, individualized services to participants at the level of intensity necessary for each participant. In this sense, it was a comprehensive treatment program; however, the quantity of services did not correlate with clinical improvement [40].

In a school-based intervention in the UK, teachers were responsible for screening, assessment and referral of children and adolescent refugees to clinical services. Teachers and mental health professionals worked closely to make treatment decisions for the refugee children. The teachers either referred the student to a mental health professional, or met with parents to identify local resources, or met directly with the student to discuss issues. Some clinical improvement was seen and attributed to the teacher's increased awareness, parental involvement, and local resources. But direct clinical intervention was also important in reducing other symptom scores [41].

Many child and youth mentoring programs that provide one-on-one educational and social support are being developed around the country. Two examples are http://www.cultureconnectinc.org/gbmp.html and http://oregonmentors.org/programs/detail/466/. The Bridging Refugee Youth and Children's Services (BRYCS) program (http://www.brycs.org/aboutBrycs/index.cfm), which used to be the technical assistance provider for the Office of Refugee Resettlement (ORR), still remains a valuable resource for health care providers on child welfare and schools.

Other interventions such as creative expression therapy (music, dance, drama) as well as other family group interventions are reviewed and summarized by Murray et al. [42].

Summary

Working with refugees can be a most enriching and rewarding experience for physicians and trainees, offering opportunities for exposure to cross-cultural complexities, unusual medical illnesses, and experience in thinking about the relationship between political and social events abroad and health conditions more locally. The key is thinking broadly across a range of modalities of treatment—and incorporating a team of providers, informally and formally. For most refugees whose distress is vast and often inchoate and who are unable to identify specific needs and problem-solve towards meeting them, even the practical guidance physicians can give is invaluable.

On a final note, work with highly traumatized populations may also take a toll on their providers (including medical interpreters) [43] especially in the context of limited resources and services to offer distressed individuals. A growing literature on caregivers working on refugees especially those who are victims of torture suggest that caregivers too are at risk for burnout and vicarious traumatization as well as depression, anxiety, and substance problems [44]. We strongly encourage providers to engage in personal and professional self-care which may include ongoing professional supervision and collaboration, ongoing training and management of caseloads, and, as necessary, ongoing counseling and debriefing.

References

1. Johnson H, Thompson A. The development and maintenance of posttraumatic stress disorder (PTSD) in civilian adult survivors of war trauma and torture: a review. Clin Psychol Rev. 2008;28:36–47.
2. Bodegård G. Depression-withdrawal reaction in refugee children. An epidemic of a cultural-bound syndrome or an endemic of re-traumatized refugees? Acta Paediatr. 2010;99(7):959.
3. Chhim S. Baksbat (broken courage): a trauma-based cultural syndrome in Cambodia. Med Anthropol. 2013;32(2):160–73.
4. Van Ommeren VM, Sharma B, Sharma GK, et al. The relationship between somatic and PTSD symptoms among Bhutanese refugee torture survivors: examination of comorbidity with anxiety and depression. J Trauma Stress. 2002;15(5):415–21.
5. Jamil H, Hakim-Larson J, Farrag M, et al. Medical complaints among Iraqi American refugees with mental health. J Immigr Health. 2006;7(3):145–52.
6. Hinton DE, Chhean D, Pich V, et al. Tinnitus among Cambodian refugees: relationship to PTSD severity. J Trauma Stress. 2006;19(4):541–6.
7. Hinton DE, Chhean D, Fama JM, et al. Gastrointestinal-focused panic attacks among Cambodian refugees: associated psychopathology, flashbacks, and catastrophic cognitions. J Anxiety Disord. 2007;21(1):42–58.
8. Asgary R, Segar N. Barriers to health care access among refugee asylum seekers. J Health Care Poor Underserved. 2011;22(2):506–22.
9. Meghan D, et al. Healthcare barriers of refugees post-resettlement. J Community Health. 2009;34(6):529–38.
10. Mollica RF, Wyshak G, Lavelle J, et al. Assessing symptom change in Southeast Asian refugee survivors of mass violence and torture. Am J Psychiatry. 1990;147:83–8.
11. Hinton DE, Kredlow MA, Bui E, et al. Treatment change of somatic symptoms and cultural syndromes among Cambodian refugees with PTSD. Depress Anxiety. 2012;29(2):148–55.
12. Smajkić A, Weine S, Durić-Bijedić Z, et al. Sertraline, paroxetine and venlafaxine in refugee post traumatic stress disorder with depression symptoms. Med Arh. 2001;55(1 Suppl 1):35–8.
13. Kinzie JD, Leung P. Clonidine in Cambodian patients with post traumatic stress disorder. J Nerv Ment Dis. 1989;177(9):546–50.
14. Boynton L, Bentley J, Strachan E, et al. Preliminary findings concerning the use of prazosin for the treatment of posttraumatic nightmares in a refugee population. J Psychiatr Pract. 2009;15(6):454–9.
15. Otto MW, Hinton D, Korbly NB, et al. Treatment of pharmacotherapy-refractory posttraumatic stress disorder among Cambodian refugees: a pilot study of combination treatment with cognitive-behavior therapy vs sertraline alone. Behav Res Ther. 2003;41(11):1271–6.
16. Moore LJ, Boehnlein JK. Posttraumatic stress disorder, depression, and somatic symptoms in U.S. Mien patients. J Nerv Ment Dis. 1991;179(12):728–33.
17. Rasmussen A, Katoni B, Keller AS, Wilkinson J. Posttraumatic idioms of distress among Darfur refugees: Hozun and Majnun. Transcult Psychiatry. 2011;48(4):392–415.
18. Hinton DE, Lewis-Fernández R. The cross-cultural validity of posttraumatic stress disorder: implications for DSM-5. Depress Anxiety. 2011;28(9):783–801.
19. Miller KE, Omidian P, Kulkarni M, Yaqubi A, Daudzai H, Rasmussen A. The validity and clinical utility of post-traumatic stress disorder in Afghanistan. Transcult Psychiatry. 2009;46(2):219–37.
20. van der Kolk BA, et al. Disorders of extreme stress: the empirical foundation of a complex adaptation to trauma. J Trauma Stress. 2005;18(5):389–99.
21. Koucky EM, Dickstein BD, Chard KM. Cognitive behavioral treatments for posttraumatic stress disorder: empirical foundation and new directions. CNS Spectr. 2013;18(2):73–81.
22. Hinton DE, Rivera EI, Hofmann SG, Barlow DH, Otto MW. Adapting CBT for traumatized refugees and ethnic minority patients: examples from culturally adapted CBT (CA-CBT). Transcult Psychiatry. 2012;49(2):340–65.

23. Hinton DE, Pham T, Tran M, et al. CBT for Vietnamese refugees with treatment resistant PTSD and panic attacks: a pilot study. J Trauma Stress. 2004;17(5):429–33.
24. Hinton DE, Chhean D, Pich V, et al. A randomized controlled trial of cognitive-behavior therapy for Cambodian refugees with treatment-resistant PTSD and panic attacks: a cross-over design. J Trauma Stress. 2005;18(6):617–29.
25. Bomyea J, Lang AJ. Emerging interventions for PTSD: future directions for clinical care and research. Neuropharmacology. 2012;62(2):607–16.
26. Schauer M, Neuner F, Elbert T. Narrative exposure therapy: a short-term intervention for traumatic stress disorders after war, terror or torture. Cambridge, MA: Hogrefe & Huber; 2005.
27. Neuner F, Schauer M, Klaschik C, et al. A comparison of narrative exposure therapy, supportive counseling, and psychoeducation for treating posttraumatic stress disorder in an African refugee settlement. J Consult Clin Psychol. 2004;72:579–87.
28. Neuner F, Onyut PL, Ertl V, et al. Treatment of posttraumatic stress disorder by trained lay counselors in an African refugee settlement: a randomized controlled trial. J Consult Clin Psychol. 2008;76:686–94.
29. Holmqvist R, Andersen K, Anju T, et al. Change in self-image and PTSD symptoms in short-term therapies with traumatized refugees. Psychoanal Psychother. 2006;20:251–65.
30. Kruse J, Joksimovic L, Cavka M, et al. Effects of trauma-focused psychotherapy upon war refugees. J Trauma Stress. 2009;22:585–92.
31. Muller J, Karl A, Denke C, et al. Biofeedback for pain management in traumatised refugees. Cogn Behav Ther. 2009;38(3):184–90.
32. Oras R, de Ezpeleta SC, Ahmad A. Treatment of traumatized refugee children with eye movement desensitization and reprocessing in a psychodynamic context. Nord J Psychiatry. 2004;58:199–203.
33. Nickerson A, Bryant RA, Silove D, et al. A critical review of psychological treatments of posttraumatic stress disorder in refugees. Clin Psychol Rev. 2011;31(3):399–417.
34. Palic S, Elklit A. Psychosocial treatment of posttraumatic stress disorder in adult refugees: a systematic review of prospective treatment outcome studies and a critique. J Affect Disord. 2011;131(1–3):8–23.
35. Williams ME, Thompson SC. The use of community-based interventions in reducing morbidity from the psychological impact of conflict-related trauma among refugee populations: a systematic review of the literature. J Immigr Minor Health. 2011;13(4):780–94.
36. Stewart M, Simich L, Shizha E, et al. Supporting African refugees in Canada: insights from a support intervention. Health Soc Care Community. 2012;20(5):516–27.
37. Stepakoff S, Hubbard J, Katoh M, et al. Trauma healing in refugee camps in Guinea: a psychosocial program for Liberian and Sierra Leonean survivors of torture and war. Am Psychol. 2006;61:921–31.
38. Bolton P, Bass J, Betancourt T, et al. Interventions for depression symptoms among adolescent survivors of war and displacement in Northern Uganda: a randomized controlled trial. JAMA. 2007;298(5):519–27.
39. Bolton P, Bass J, Neugebauer R, et al. Group interpersonal psychotherapy for depression in rural Uganda: a randomized controlled trial. JAMA. 2003;289(23):3117–24.
40. Birman D, Beehler S, Merrill Harris E, et al. International family, adult and child enhancement services (FACES): a community-based comprehensive services model for refugee children in resettlement. Am J Orthopsychiatry. 2008;78(1):121–32.
41. Fazel M, Doll H, Stein A. A school-based mental health intervention for refugee children: an exploratory study. Clin Child Psychol Psychiatry. 2009;14(2):297–309.
42. Murray KE, Davidson GR, Schweitzer RD. Review of refugee mental health interventions following resettlement: best practices and recommendations. Am J Orthopsychiatry. 2010;80(4):576–85.
43. Splevins KA, Cohen K, Joseph S, Murray C, Bowley J. Vicarious posttraumatic growth among interpreters. Qual Health Res. 2010;20(12):1705–16.
44. Pross C. Burnout, vicarious traumatization and its prevention. Torture. 2006;16(1):1–9.

Chapter 14
Torture and Refugees

Mara Rabin and Cynthia Willard

Introduction

The nature of war has shifted dramatically over the past 100 years. War now claims the lives of more civilians than previously. In World War I and II, an estimated 10 % and 50 % of casualties respectively were civilians. In armed conflicts since 1945, up to 90 % of casualties are civilians [1]. As a result, it is now common for a refugee to have witnessed or experienced mass atrocities, violence, and state sponsored torture in their journey to safety.

Torture is defined by the World Medical Association as "the deliberate, systematic or wanton infliction of physical or mental suffering by one or more persons acting alone or on the orders of any authority, to force another person to yield information, to make a confession, or for any other reason" [2]. At its core, torture destroys trust between two individuals: the perpetrator and the victim, and can lead to lifelong impaired mental, physical, and spiritual health of the survivor. The impact of torture is also far reaching: it not only has the power to destroy individuals but also their families and the greater community. Torture is a worldwide public health epidemic, and is an important consideration in the primary health care of refugees. Torture is perpetrated in nearly 100 countries [3, 4]. In every conflict that has generated refugees, torture exists. As a result, many refugees are torture survivors.

M. Rabin, M.D. (✉)
Utah Health and Human Rights, 225 South 200 East, Suite 250,
Salt Lake City, UT 84111, USA
e-mail: mara.rabin@uhhr.org

C. Willard, M.D., M.P.H.
Department of Community and Family Medicine, Keck School of Medicine,
Chapcare Health Center, University of Southern California, 3160 Del Mar Blvd.,
Pasadena, CA 91107, USA

A. Annamalai (ed.), *Refugee Health Care: An Essential Medical Guide*,
DOI 10.1007/978-1-4939-0271-2_14, © Springer Science+Business Media New York 2014

There are two classifications of torture survivors: primary and secondary. Primary torture survivors are individuals who were tortured or who witnessed the torture of another. Secondary torture survivors are closely related family members or partners of primary survivors. Secondary survivors were not present during the torture and may not know the extent of the torture. Secondary survivors may also be symptomatic, but tend to be less symptomatic than primary survivors [5].

The common methods of physical torture include these:

- Beatings to the head
- Beatings, kicking, striking body with objects: falanga—beating the soles of the feet with cudgels and whips; telefono—beating both ears simultaneously with cupped hands causing tympanic membrane rupture and hearing loss
- Being placed in a small box, hole, sack, or cell
- Burning
- Electric shocks to genitals and other body parts
- Exposure to heat, sun, strong light, and cold
- Stretching—suspension or forced abduction of limbs
- Starvation
- Unhygienic conditions that can lead to disease
- Near drowning, repeated submersion underwater
- Sexual torture—rape, insertion of objects in vagina, rectum
- Forcing consumption of urine or feces; having urine or feces thrown at one

The common methods of mental torture include these:

- Threats of pain, torture, execution
- Sensory deprivation or overload (forced darkness, excessive noise)
- Mock executions
- Sleep deprivation
- Prolonged interrogation
- Isolation
- Uncertainty about release
- Threats of harm to family members
- Harm to family members

Torture Prevalence

There are a limited number of studies that document torture prevalence in refugee populations living in the US. The most commonly cited study estimates that 5–35 % of the world's refugees are torture survivors [6]. By this count, there may be up to 630,000 torture survivors living in the US. Refugees resettling in the US are an extraordinarily diverse group. As a result of this diversity, torture prevalence varies greatly by country of origin, ethnicity, and gender. Only a handful of studies document torture prevalence in specific refugee subgroups: 5 % among Bhutanese refugees; 13 % among refugees from Burma (including ethnic minority groups) [5]; 21 % among Tibetan refugees [7]; 36 % among Somali refugees, 55 % among

Ethiopian Oromo refugees [8]; 54 % among Cambodians who survived the Khmer Rouge reign [9]; and 57 % in Iraqis resettled post-2006 [10]. Only one study on torture prevalence has been conducted in a complete set of refugees arriving for resettlement in a single US state. This study found an overall torture prevalence of 19 %, but when looking at specific populations found a prevalence that ranged from 5–57 % [5]. Gender differences are found in torture prevalence, but this also varies by ethnicity and country. Some recent studies show a gender difference in primary torture prevalence: 25 % and 47 % respectively among Somali men and women [8] and 59.3 % and 55.1 % among Iraqi men and women respectively [10]. An estimated 4–7 % of child refugees are torture survivors [10–12].

Health Effects of Torture

Regardless of the type of torture experienced, survivors are often left with physical, sexual, and psychological sequelae including chronic pain, depression, and posttraumatic stress disorder (PTSD) that can present acutely, or years later. Once torture has been identified as a possible cause of physical or psychological symptoms, it is important to consider contacting a specialized torture treatment program that may provide integrated rehabilitation with a comprehensive bio-psycho-social model [13]. The ethical protection of torture survivors and their need for comprehensive medical and psychiatric care has been well established in the Istanbul Protocol [14]. Treatment programs in the US can be located by contacting the National Consortium of Torture Treatment Programs (www.ncttp.org). However, access to these programs can be limited, and many torture-related health issues can be addressed in the primary care setting with specialty assistance if needed. Recently, there has been a move to identify the "best practices" in the care of torture survivors so that the highest quality of care can take place in most medical settings [15].

Physical Effects

The most common physical consequence of torture is pain, both acute and chronic. Literature shows that survivors of torture have a very high prevalence of persistent pain [16]. For a survivor, daily pain resulting from torture is a constant reminder of the past and can impact an individual's ability to heal. One of the most common forms of torture is beating, but most other torture methods can also lead to either localized or somatic pain. Some studies suggest that the focus of pain is often related to the location of torture, but not always. For example: beatings around the head can give rise to chronic headaches, suspension can lead to lower back pain, falanga or beating to the feet leads to foot pain, and sexual torture can result in both lower back pain, and genital pain [17, 18]. Survivors also experience somatic symptoms such as atypical chest pain, irritable bowel syndrome, myalgias, and fatigue.

Specific types of torture can result in characteristic signs and symptoms, depending on the severity of the torture method. Suspension can lead to brachial plexus injuries, lumbo-sacral plexus injuries, neuropathic pain, and polyarthritis in the wrist and ankle joint commonly referred to as "stretch arthritis" [19]. In addition to severe foot pain, falanga can lead to sensory dysfunction such as neuropathy and connective tissue disorders both of which affect mobility [20]. Telefono can lead to tympanic membrane rupture, tinnitus, vertigo, and hearing loss [21]. Asphyxiation techniques including water-boarding or submarino can lead to severe psychological consequences such as a fear of drowning or nightmares. Scars can be found on the body from electrical shock, chemical, cigarette, or other heat burns, and lacerations. Sexual torture can lead to intestinal damage from insertion of foreign objects into the rectum, genital trauma, sexual dysfunction, and chronic genital or pelvic pain [22–24]. Torture survivors may also have been verbally humiliated, threatened with death, or told that they would be permanently "damaged" or made infertile during their torture. As clinicians, our medical evaluation and care can be reassuring and enormously healing for the patient. Finally, the comprehensive documentation of torture sequelae is sometimes needed for forensic reasons. Several comprehensive reference sources provide guidance in this area [14, 25]. Please refer to Chap. 17 for a review of forensic evaluation of asylum seekers.

Traumatic Brain Injury

Closed head injuries have been reported by nearly 70 % of torture survivors [26, 27] many times accompanied by loss of consciousness. Head injuries may be a result of asphyxiation, direct blows to the head, poisoning, nutritional deprivation, or water-boarding/submarino. These injuries can lead to traumatic brain injury (TBI), with resulting symptoms including: chronic headaches, dizziness, cognitive dysfunction, memory loss, and sleep disturbance. A study of South Vietnamese torture survivors showed that those with TBI were more likely to suffer symptoms of depression, PTSD, and anxiety. Structural changes in the brain also showed thinner prefrontal and temporal cortices among Vietnamese torture survivors with TBI [28]. TBI sequelae can be difficult to treat and are likely to have an adverse impact on resettlement. Cognitive dysfunction, in particular, poses challenges to learning English and new job skills, which can negatively impact a survivor's ability to gain employment and citizenship. Diagnostic testing for TBI includes brain imaging and neuropsychiatric testing. These tests can be helpful in differentiating TBI symptoms from PTSD [29]. Challenges in conducting neuropsychiatric testing include a lack of culturally and linguistically validated measures [29].

Mental Health Effects

The mental health sequelae of torture are often the most frequent, long-lasting, and disabling consequences. Mental health issues can manifest in somatic complaints, difficulties with successful resettlement, cognitive deficits, sleep disorders, PTSD, anxiety, and depression. Usually there is an overlay of several of these issues. PTSD is one of the most common mental health conditions noted in survivors of torture with observed prevalence rates of 30–90 %, even years after the torture experience [30, 31]. Mental health issues can manifest in varying ways among cultures, and torture survivors may not readily describe their symptoms. Torture can make survivors distrustful of others and their own experiences. In addition, torture experience can impact memory often making it difficult for survivors to concisely convey their experiences.

Certain aspects of a medical visit can re-traumatize survivors of torture and it is important to minimize these triggers including: prolonged wait times; crying babies; uncompassionate staff; unfamiliar forms; multiple questions; and small, windowless exam rooms. In addition, some procedures including venipuncture, opthalmic exam, and an electrocardiogram may all remind a survivor of their torture experience. Re-traumatization can trigger flashbacks, fear, anger, or panic, which may prevent survivors from accessing care and following their clinician's recommendations.

The stressors of exile and resettlement can also exacerbate mental health symptoms in torture survivors. Many refugees experience a symptom-free honeymoon period immediately after resettlement with symptoms appearing later. Screening for mental health issues in refugees is discussed in Chap. 12.

Chronic Disease and Torture

Torture survivors are at an increased risk of chronic disease development [32]. Longitudinal health studies in Cambodians show that Cambodian torture survivors have a 20 % increased risk of diabetes mellitus compared to their age matched, non-torture survivor peers [33]. Physicians should also consider pre-migration stressors including food insecurity, malnourishment, and micronutrient deficiencies that can occur more often in torture survivors, as other risks for chronic disease development due to compromised organ development and function [34]. For torture survivors from developed countries where the prevalence of obesity and chronic disease is already significantly elevated, the risk for an individual may be even higher. In a recent study of refugees 8 months after arrival, over half were found to have at least one chronic, non-communicable disease diagnosis [35]. Due to possible increased risks, clinicians should consider screening torture survivors for chronic diseases although the literature does not currently support this.

Children

Even very young, pre-verbal children may be significantly impacted by witnessing or hearing the sounds of torture. Younger children may be more traumatized than older children who are able to articulate their fears and horrors surrounding the events experienced. The Adverse Childhood Events (ACE) study of 17,000 children showed that those who experienced childhood trauma have an increased risk of developing chronic physical and mental health conditions, as well as substance abuse as adults [36]. Although the ACE study does not focus specifically on torture, these findings strongly support the theories that childhood trauma can lead to significant health issues in adulthood. Child survivors of torture may be at an increased risk of chronic disease development.

Mediators

A group of studies have shown that some characteristics in refugees provide protection from the consequences of torture while others may exacerbate sequelae. Survivors with higher levels of political activism, better social support networks, and male gender may suffer less psychological effects. A strong belief system has been found to be both protective and a risk factor in various studies [37, 38].

Screening for Torture

The Centers for Disease Control (CDC) Refugee Health guidelines recommend screening refugees for mental health symptoms and a history of violence within the first 90 days of resettlement [39]. However, less than half of states follow these recommendations [40]. Even fewer screen for a history of war trauma and/or torture. Other experts recommend screening refugees for a torture history if they exhibit signs of depression, PTSD, or unexplained pain [41]. Torture is arguably the most severe form of violence. If refugees are not identified as torture survivors during the refugee health screening, they are unlikely to be asked this history by their primary care clinician. Studies indicate that even in high risk clinical settings—community health centers in Boston, New York, and Los Angeles, primary care clinicians rarely asked their patients about a history of political violence or torture [42, 43]. Only 3 % of survivors shared their trauma history with a primary care clinician without being asked [42]. Therefore, the most common barrier to identifying torture survivors is a clinician's failure to ask the patient about a past history of trauma [44, 45]. Other barriers include the survivor's lack of trust in the clinician, fear of authority (medical personnel participate in up to 20 % of torture cases worldwide) [46] and re-traumatization. The purpose of a screening test is to identify individuals at risk and provide an intervention that will improve health. Torture increases the risk of acute and chronic mental and physical health conditions [47–51]. Torture survivors appear no different than other refugees, but may present to their primary care clinicians more often with complaints of anxiety, chronic pain, cognitive dysfunction, depression, headaches, insomnia, and PTSD, than non-tortured refugees.

The following validated question was developed by Dr. David Eisenman to screen for torture and violence:

> "In this clinic we see many patients who have been forced to flee their homes because of violence or threats to the health and safety of patients and their families. I'm going to ask you a question about this now. Were you [or any of your family members] victims of violence and/or torture in your home country?" [52]

This question destigmatizes the experience of torture/violence, and reassures the patient that the clinician is comfortable with this issue and prepared to help. If an individual responds "yes," it is helpful to ask further questions in order to understand the scope of a patient's traumatic experiences and possible sequelae. This may be done over a few visits to insure the comfort and trust of the patient. However, it is not necessary to have a patient recount their entire trauma story, and doing so may be destabilizing for the individual [53]. Many torture survivors report that their physician is the first person with whom they have shared their torture history. Although it can be difficult to hear about these experiences, acknowledging these atrocities can be therapeutic to a survivor of torture. It is important that a clinician allow adequate time for the patient to share their experience, and to never doubt or deny a survivor's story no matter how unbelievable.

The screening question seeks to identify secondary survivors through its inclusion of "or any of your family members." Secondary survivors are at an increased risk of adverse health outcomes because of their vicarious exposure to the torture through the survivor.

Another reason to consider screening refugees for torture early in the resettlement process is that it allows referral to appropriate specialists while the patient is still covered by Refugee Medical Assistance (up to 8 months after resettlement in most states.) This may be less urgent if most states opt to implement the Affordable Care Act, which includes a Medicaid expansion. A recent study found that 46.5 % of refugees with chronic health conditions did not have health insurance beyond the initial resettlement period [54].

Some physicians may be uncomfortable or fearful about asking a patient about torture. Clinicians are asked to address many difficult issues. However, identifying this history will allow more effective treatment for refugees' health conditions. Tragically, most of the 3 million refugees living in the US have suffered human rights violations in their journeys to safety. Within these refugee communities, many torture survivors live and continue to suffer from their past histories of severe trauma. By bringing a survivor's history to light and not shying away from this darkness, we can help our patients regain their health. If we do not screen for torture, we will never know our patient's past. By not understanding our patient within the context of torture, we perpetuate the vast injustices that a survivor has already suffered.

Women and Violence

Unfortunately, women and girls across the world face many types of violence regardless of socioeconomic strata, age, or ethnicity. One in three women across the world have been beaten, coerced into sex, or otherwise abused in her lifetime [55]. The largest worldwide study on the prevalence of violence in women and girls was conducted by the World Health Organization (WHO) in 2005. The WHO Multi-Country Study of Women's Health and Domestic Violence Against Women included

24,000 women across ten countries and assessed their experience with intimate partner violence as well as non-partner violence including physical abuse and sexual assault. Thirteen to sixty-one percent of women experienced intimate partner violence (IPV), while 5–65 % of women experienced non-partner violence combining physical and sexual assault [56].

Violence against women is largely based in unequal power relations, which perpetuate and condone violence within the family, community and state [56, 57]. Refugee women, depending on their country of origin and migration pattern, may be particularly vulnerable to gender-based violence during armed conflict, flight from conflict, and in refugee camps [58, 59]. Rape has been used as a weapon of war throughout history, and has been widely documented in recent conflicts including Bosnia, Cambodia, Congo, Liberia, Peru, Somalia, and Uganda [60, 61].

Intimate Partner Violence

IPV is defined as a pattern of assaultive and coercive behaviors designed to establish control by a person who is, was, or wishes to be involved in an intimate or dating relationship with an adult or adolescent. Assaultive and coercive behaviors can include physical, psychological, emotional and sexual abuse, stalking, threats, social isolation. Intimate partners include current and former spouses, common-law spouses, and dating partners of either sex. Intimate partners may or may not be cohabitating [62]. IPV can affect all women regardless of socioeconomic status, educational background, and culture. It can carry serious and long lasting consequences in that it tends to be repetitive and accompanied by psychological and sexual violence as well [63]. While recent reviews of the current literature did not find the prevalence of IPV higher in refugee communities [64, 65], the data is very limited, and most agree that refugees may be particularly vulnerable to IPV. Some studies suggest that lifetime rates of IPV in women living in refugee camps are close to 50 % [66, 67].

In the US, nearly one-third of American women experience physical or sexual abuse by a husband or boyfriend at some point in their lives [68]. In addition to possible IPV before arrival, refugee women may be more vulnerable to IPV once in the US for several reasons. Refugee women experience limited English proficiency (LEP), which may limit their ability to seek help. While most refugees have official refugee legal status in the US, women may still have fears about jeopardizing their immigration status or that of their partner-perpetrator by reporting IPV. Many refugee women lack social networks that would encourage help-seeking, despite attempts by the US State Department to resettle refugees as families and even communities. Many refugee women are impoverished and possibly dependent on the perpetrator for economic survival. Refugee women may lack an understanding of US laws around IPV [65].

Screening

Some recent studies have failed to show benefits from universal IPV screening, and the US Preventive Task Force neither supports nor rejects the concept [69]. However, The US Department of Health and Human Services has endorsed the Institute of Medicine's recommendations that IPV screening and counseling be a core part of women's health visits [70]. The American Congress of Obstetricians and Gynecologists (ACOG) also recommends that all women be screened at periodic intervals [71]. Screening may be particularly important in refugees due to their numerous barriers to seeking help. A number of IPV screening tools are used in clinical practice [72]. To our knowledge, none have been validated for use across cultures and languages, or specifically in refugee populations [73]. It is critical that screening take place privately in the context of a trusting relationship, in a culturally and linguistically appropriate way. Clinicians should be familiar with IPV reporting laws in their state, and be prepared to provide immediate assistance and safety planning for victims of IPV.

Resources

National Domestic Violence Hotline
1-800-799-SAFE (7233)
www.thehotline.org
Futures Without Violence
www.futureswithoutviolence.org
National Coalition Against Domestic Violence
www.ncadv.org
National Resource Center on Domestic Violence
www.nrcdv.org
Office on Violence Against Women
www.usdoj.gov/ovw

References

1. Rupesinghe K, Anderlini SN. Civil wars. Civil peace. An introduction to conflict resolution. London: Pluto Press; 1998.
2. WMA Declaration of Tokyo. Guidelines for physicians concerning torture and other cruel, inhuman or degrading treatment or punishment in relation to detention and imprisonment adopted by the 29th world medical assembly. Tokyo, Japan. October 1975; editorially revised by the 170th WMA Council Session. Divonne-les-Bains, France. May 2005 and the 173rd WMA Council Session. Divonne-les-Bains, France. May 2006.
3. Rejali D. Torture and democracy. 1st ed. Princeton, NJ: Princeton University Press; 2007.

4. Amnesty International Annual Report. 2012. http://files.amnesty.org/air12/air_2012_full_en.pdf. Accessed Aug 2013.
5. Rabin M, Willard C. Retrospective review of Utah refugee health screenings. Unpublished data. 2011.
6. Baker R. Psychological consequences for tortured refugees seeking asylum and refugee status in Europe. In: Basoglu M, editor. Torture and its consequences: current treatment approaches. Cambridge: Cambridge University Press; 1992. p. 83–101.
7. Mills E, Singh S, Holtz T, et al. Prevalence of mental disorders and torture among Tibetan refugees: a systematic review. BMC Int Health Hum Right. 2005;9(5):7.
8. Jaranson J, Butcher J, Halcon L, et al. Somali and Oromo refugees: correlates of torture and trauma history. Am J Public Health. 2004;94(4):591–8.
9. Marshall GN, Schell TL, Elliott MN, et al. Mental health of Cambodian refugees 2 decades after resettlement in the United States. JAMA. 2005;294(5):571–9.
10. Willard C, Rabin M, Lawless M. The prevalence of torture and associated symptoms in United States Iraqi refugees. J Immigr Minor Health. 2013. DOI: 10.1007/s10903-013-9817-5.
11. Fazel M, Wheeler J, Danesh J. Prevalence of serious mental disorder in 7000 refugees resettled in western countries: a systematic review. Lancet. 2005;365(9467):1309–14.
12. Quiroga J. Torture in children. Torture. 2009;19(2):66–87.
13. Keller AS. Caring and advocating for victims of torture. Lancet. 2002;360(Suppl):s55–6.
14. Allden K, Baykal T, Iacopino V, et al., editors. Office of high commissioner for human rights. Istanbul protocol: manual on the effective investigation and documentation of torture and other cruel and degrading treatment or punishment. Geneva: United Nations; 2001.
15. Mollica R. Medical best practices for the treatment of torture survivors. Torture. 2011;21(1):8–17.
16. Williams AC, Amris K. Pain from torture. Pain. 2007;133:5–8.
17. Olsen DR, Mongomery E, Bojholm S, et al. Prevalence of pain in the head, back, and feet in refugees previously exposed to torture: a ten year follow-up study. Disabil Rehabil. 2007;29(2):163–71.
18. Carinici AJ, Pankaj M, Christo P. Chronic pain in torture survivors. Curr Pain Headache Rep. 2010;14(2):73–9.
19. Elliott GB, Elliott KA. The torture of stretch arthritis syndrome. Clin Radiol. 1979;30(3):313–5.
20. Prip K, Persson AL, Sjolund BH. Self- reported activity in torture survivors with long-term sequelae including pain and the impact of foot pain from falanga - a cross-sectional study. Disabil Rehabil. 2011;33(7):569–78.
21. Crosby SS, Mohan S, Di Loreto C, et al. Head and neck sequelae of torture. Laryngoscope. 2010;120(2):414–9.
22. Norredam M, Crosby S, Munarriz R, et al. Urological complications of sexual trauma among male survivors of torture. Urology. 2005;65(1):28–32.
23. Ortman J, Lunde I. Prevalence and sequelae of sexual torture. Lancet. 1990;336(8710):289–91.
24. Oosterhoff P, Zwanikken P, Ketting E. Sexual torture of men in Croatia and other conflict situations: an open secret. Reprod Health Matters. 2004;12(23):68–77.
25. Goldfield AE, Mollica RF, Pesavento BH, et al. The physical and psychological sequelae of torture. Symptomatology and diagnosis. JAMA. 1988;259(18):2725–9.
26. Keatley E, Ashman T, Im B, et al. Self-reported head injury among refugee survivors of torture. J Head Trauma Rehabil. 2013;28(6):E8–13.
27. McColl H, Higson-Smith C, Gjerding S, et al. Rehabilitation of torture survivors in five countries: common themes and challenges. Int J Ment Health Syst. 2010;18(4):16.
28. Mollica R, Lyoo K, Chernoff M, et al. Brain structural abnormalities and mental health sequelae in South Vietnamese ex-political detainees who survived traumatic brain injury and torture. Arch Gen Psychiatry. 2009;66(11):1221–32.
29. Jacobs U, Iacopino V. Torture and its consequences: a challenge to clinical neuropsychology. Prof Psychol Res Pract. 2001;32:458–64.
30. Quiroga J, Jaranson J. Politically motivated torture and its survivors. Torture. 2005;15:2–3.

31. Atwoli L, Kathuku DM, Ndetei DM. Post traumatic stress disorder among Mau Mau concentration camp survivors in Kenya. East Afr Med J. 2006;83(7):352–9.
32. Sledjeski EM, Speisman B, Dierker LC. Does number of lifetime traumas explain the relationship between PTSD and chronic medical conditions? Answers from the national comorbidity survey-replication (NCS-R). J Behav Med. 2008;31(4):341–9.
33. Mollica R. Health promotion for torture and trauma survivors. Webinar. http://gulfcoastjewish-familyandcommunityservices.org/refugee/2011/09/15/register-for-the-npct-webinar-on-health-promotion-on-92811/. Accessed Aug 2013.
34. Barker DJ. The fetal and infant origins of adult disease. Br Med J. 1990;301(6761):1111.
35. Yun K, Hebrank K, Graber LK, et al. High prevalence of chronic non-communicable conditions among adult refugees: implications for practice and policy. J Community Health. 2012;37(5):1110–8.
36. Felitti V, Anda R, Nordenberg D, et al. Relationship of childhood abuse and household dysfunction to many of the leading causes of death in adults: the adverse childhood experiences study. Am J Prev Med. 1998;14(4):245–58.
37. Halvorsen J, Kagee A. Predictors of psychological sequelae of torture among South African former political prisoners. J Interpers Violence. 2010;25(6):989–1005.
38. Shrestha NM, Sharma B, Van Ommeren M, et al. Impact of torture on refugees displaced within the developing world: symptomatology among Bhutanese refugees in Nepal. JAMA. 1998;280(5):443–8.
39. Centers for Disease Control. Domestic guidelines for mental health screening during the domestic medical examination for newly arrived refugees. http://www.cdc.gov/immigrantrefugeehealth/guidelines/domestic/mental-health-screening-guidelines.html#resources. Accessed Aug 2013.
40. Shannon P, Hyojin IM, Becher E, et al. Screening for war trauma, torture, and mental health symptoms among newly arrived refugees: a national survey of US refugee health coordinators. J Immigr Refug Stud. 2012;10:380–94.
41. Miles S, Garcia-Peltoniemi R. Torture survivors: what to ask, how to document. J Fam Pract. 2012;61(4):E1–5.
42. Eisenman DP, Gelberg L, Liu H, et al. Mental health and health-related quality of life among adult Latino primary care patients living in the United States with previous exposure to political violence. JAMA. 2003;290(5):627–34.
43. Crosby S, Norredam M, Paasche-Orlow MK, et al. Prevalence of torture survivors among foreign-born patients presenting to an urban ambulatory care practice. J Gen Intern Med. 2006;21(7):764–8.
44. Shannon P, O'Dougherty M, Mehta E. Refugees' perspectives on barriers to communication about trauma histories in primary care. Ment Health Fam Med. 2012;9(1):47–55.
45. Mollica R. Surviving torture. New Engl J Med. 2004;351(1):5–7.
46. British Medical Association. Medical involvement in torture. In: Medicine betrayed the participation of doctors in human rights abuses. Atlantic-Highlands, NJ: Zed Books, Ltd; 1992. p. 33–63.
47. Mollica RF, Brooks R, Tor S et al. The enduring mental health impact of mass violence: a community comparison study of Cambodian civilians living in Cambodia and Thailand. Int J Soc Psychiatry. 2014;60(1):6–20.
48. Rees S, Silove D. Sakit Hati: a state of chronic mental distress related to resentment and anger amongst West Papuan refugees exposed to persecution. Soc Sci Med. 2011;73(1):103–10.
49. Rasmussen A, Rosenfeld B, Reeves K, et al. The effects of torture-related injuries on long-term psychological distress in a Punjabi Sikh sample. J Abnorm Psychiatr. 2007;116(4):734–40.
50. Carinci AJ, Mehta P, Christo PJ. Chronic pain in torture victims. Curr Pain Headache Rep. 2010;14(2):73–9.
51. Weinstein HM, Dansky L, Iacopino V. Torture and war trauma survivors in primary care practice. West J Med. 1996;165(3):112–8.
52. Eisenman D. Screening for mental health problems and history of torture. In: Walker P, Barnett E, editors. Immigrant medicine, chapter 48. Philadelphia, PA: Saunders Elsevier; 2007.
53. Moreno A, Grodin M. Torture and its neurological sequelae. Spinal Cord. 2002;40(5):215.

54. Yun K, Fuentes-Afflick E, Desai MM. Prevalence of chronic disease and insurance coverage among refugees in the United States. J Immigr Minor Health. 2012;14(6):933–40.
55. UNICEF. United Nations high commissioner for refugees. Sexual and gender-based violence against refugees, returnees and internally displaced persons. Chapter 1. Overview of Sexual and gender based violence. www.unhcr.org/3f696bcc4.pdf. May 2003. Accessed Aug 2013.
56. UNHCR. Sexual violence against refugees. Guidelines on prevention and response. Geneva. http://www.unhcr.org/3b9cc26c4.html. 1995. Accessed Aug 2013.
57. UN Data. United Nations. The world's women 2010: trends and statistics. Chapter 6: Violence against women. http://unstats.un.org/unsd/demographic/products/Worldswomen/wwVaw2010. htm. 2012. Accessed Aug 2013.
58. Hynes M, Lopes CB. Sexual violence against refugee women. J Womens Health Gend Based Med. 2000;9(8):819–23.
59. US Department of Health and Human Services, Centers for disease Control and Prevention, National Center for Emerging and Zoonotic Infectious Diseases, Division of Global migration and Quarantine, Bhutanese Refugee Health Profile, January 28, 2013.
60. Brown C. Rape as a weapon of war in the democratic republic of Congo. Torture. 2012;22(1): 24–37.
61. Swiss S, Giller JE. Rape as a crime of war. A medical perspective. JAMA. 1993;270(5): 616–20.
62. Family Violence Prevention Fund. Family preventing domestic violence: clinical guidelines on routine screening. San Francisco, CA: Family Violence Prevention Fund; 1999.
63. Campbell JC. Health consequences of intimate partner violence. Lancet. 2002;359(9314): 1331–6.
64. Rees S, Pease B. Refugee settlement, safety, and wellbeing: exploring domestic and family violence in refugee communities. Immigrant Women's Domestic Violence Service. VicHealth Report. 2006.
65. Yoshihama M. Intimate partner violence in immigrant and refugee communities: challenges, promising practices, and recommendations. Princeton, NJ: Family Violence Prevention Fund for the Robert Wood Johnson Fund; 2009.
66. Khawaja M, Barazi R. Prevalence of wife beating in Jordanian refugee camps: reports by men and women. J Epid Comm Health. 2005;59(10):840–1.
67. Khawaja M, Tewtel-Salem M. Agreement between husband and wife reports of domestic violence: evidence from poor refugee communities in Lebanon. Int J Epidemiol. 2004;33(3): 526–33.
68. The Commonwealth Fund. Health Concerns Across Women's Lifespan: 1998 survey of women's health. Washington, DC: The Commonwealth Fund; 1999.
69. MacMillan HL, Wathen CN, Jamieson E, et al. Screening for intimate partner violence in the health care settings: a randomized trial. JAMA. 2009;302(5):493–501.
70. Institute of Medicine. Recommendations. In: Clinical preventive services for women: closing the gaps. Washington DC: National Academies Press; 2011. p. 71–141.
71. The American College of Obstetricians and Gynecologists. Committee Opinion. Number 518. February 2012.
72. Cronholm PF, Fogarty CT, Ambuel B, et al. Intimate partner violence. Am Fam Physician. 2011;83(10):1165–72.
73. Nelson H, Bougatsos C. Screening woman for intimate partner violence: a systemic review to update the U.S. preventive services task force recommendation. Ann Intern Med. 2012;156(11): 798–808.

Part IV
Special Groups

Chapter 15
Refugee Women's Health

Geetha Fink, Tara Helm, Kaya Belknap, and Crista E. Johnson-Agbakwu

Introduction

Women's health encompasses care provided to women across their reproductive life course and involves not only their reproductive health but also sexual function, cancer screening, and overall psychosocial health. The emphasis placed on women's health is a reflection of available resources and the value placed on women in society. In many war-torn countries, where medical care is limited, women's health hardly exists. In discussing refugee women's health it is prudent to recognize that there are a host of pre-migratory and post-migratory stressors that may impact a woman's health throughout her process of resettlement from conflict regions around the world [1]. Beyond the psychosocial challenges of immigration and assimilation, these women have suffered traumatic experiences, often have been abused as victims of war, and have not received appropriate medical care in their country of origin.

G. Fink, M.D., M.P.H. (✉)
Obstetrics and Gynecology, Phoenix Integrated Residency in Obstetrics and Gynecology,
2601 E. Roosevelt, Phoenix, AZ 85008, USA
e-mail: geetha.fink@mihs.org

T. Helm, M.P.H., B.S.N.
Family Nurse Practitioner Program, Frontier Nursing University,
195 School Street, Hyden, KY 41749, USA
e-mail: tara.helm@frontier.edu

K. Belknap
College of Medicine - Phoenix, University of Arizona,
1624 W. Burgess Ln, Phoenix, AZ 85041, USA
e-mail: kayab@email.arizona.edu

C.E. Johnson-Agbakwu, M.D., M.Sc., F.A.C.O.G.
Obstetrics & Gynecology, Maricopa Integrated Health System,
2601 E Roosevelt Street, Phoenix, AZ 85008, USA
e-mail: crista_johnson@dmgaz.org

A. Annamalai (ed.), *Refugee Health Care: An Essential Medical Guide*,
DOI 10.1007/978-1-4939-0271-2_15, © Springer Science+Business Media New York 2014

Many refugees have lived in refugee camps for years prior to emigration. In these camps they have suffered physical violence, malnutrition, and unsanitary living conditions, as well as rape, sexual abuse, extortion, and physical insecurity [2]. Consequently, there is a high incidence of post-traumatic stress disorder (PTSD) [3].

Post-migration, refugees suffer from increased barriers to care including poverty, insurance status, transportation, language barriers, and lack of understanding of its importance [4]. Additionally there are social differences that may impact health-seeking behavior, such as conservative cultures in which a pelvic exam is unacceptable, or the belief that only the sick need to seek care [5]. Refugees underutilize preventive and primary care, as these facets of health care may not exist in developing countries [6]. Moreover, this lack of familiarity with navigating the health care system increases patient anxiety when faced with accessing care in the hospital setting.

Sweeping generalizations can be made regarding refugee health because of the shared experience of war and immigration. However, it is important to distinguish that refugees come from many different countries, ethnic and cultural backgrounds, have highly varied experiences in their host countries of resettlement, and have widely varying beliefs on reproductive health. The following list delineates important risk factors that may impact women's health and should be identified when caring for refugee women:

- Identify a patient's host country and endemic risks.
- What was her path to immigration? Was she imprisoned in a refugee camp prior to reaching the US?
- Was she a victim of violence or rape?
- Has she lost family in the war (specifically children or her husband)?
- How many children has she already had and how many more does she want? Is she interested in contraception?
- How is her mental health? Is she suffering from PTSD or depression?
- What kind of psychosocial support does she have?
- Does she have religious beliefs that may impact her health or health-seeking behavior?
- Has she been screened for cervical cancer or breast cancer in the past?
- Has she undergone Female Genital Cutting (FGC)? Is she interested in defibulation, if indicated?
- Has she utilized preventive care in the past? Does she have a primary care provider?

Identifying these key factors will guide patient care. Additionally, a keen understanding of her psychosocial background and risk factors can facilitate in providing culturally sensitive and medically complete care.

Preventive Health

Pelvic Exams

Pelvic exams can be stress-inducing for any woman. For refugee women, pelvic exams can be even more anxiety-provoking due to histories of sexual violence or abuse, FGC, and cultural backgrounds that demand modesty and deem such an exam inappropriate. Some cultures view a pelvic exam as a violation of virginity [7]. A history of sexual trauma has been shown to decrease cervical cancer screening due to an aversion to pelvic examination [8]. Suggestions to improve the experience include fostering appropriate communication, safety, trust, and patient control of the situation [8]. A professional interpreter is highly recommended when needed. It is standard practice to have a chaperone present for patient comfort and liability concerns. Female health care providers are preferred when possible. While a pelvic exam may be deferred on the initial visit if the patient is uncomfortable, if indicated, it should still be performed once trust has been established between the patient and her provider. A pelvic exam is essential in identifying pathology, classifying cultural practices such as FGC, performing a Pap test, and testing for sexually transmitted infections. At the time of a pelvic exam, providers should also educate the patient on the value of preventive care [9]. Although a pelvic exam is standard in the female physical exam, patient autonomy and the right to refuse should be respected, provided the patient is appropriately counseled on its importance.

Sexually Transmitted Infection Screening

Screening for Human Immunodeficiency Virus (HIV) is not mandated except in prenatal care. Prior to January 2010 refugees were required to be screened for HIV prior to entry into the US [10]. Current practice is to offer such screening; a potential diagnosis may be missed due to stigma, cultural taboos, and lack of awareness [11]. Given the prevalence of HIV and rape as a weapon of war in refugees' native countries, they are considered a high-risk and vulnerable population. Thus, patients should be screened for these risk factors and tested when indicated. However, there is minimal data in regard to incidence of gonorrhea, chlamydia, and syphilis in refugee populations. A recent study in Minnesota of 18,000 refugees showed very low incidence of these STIs. Thus, routine screening may not be indicated [12]. For a discussion on STI testing in refugees, see Chap. 9.

Cancer Screening

Female cancer screening is primarily composed of pap tests for evidence of cervical dysplasia and mammography for breast cancer. Many refugee women have never had any screening prior to immigration, primarily due to lack of access to care. There is limited data on screening rates in the refugee population. However, immigrants in general tend to be under-screened post-migration due to secondary barriers to care [13]. These barriers include fatalistic attitudes regarding cancer, lack of knowledge about cancer itself and the screening modalities available, fear of Pap tests threatening one's virginity, as well as beliefs that a Pap test is not indicated unless one is ill [7]. Access to a regular source of primary care and, ideally, access to a female health professional have been advocated as a means to increase screening rates [14]. Moreover, patient education about the importance of cancer screening can promote regular health-seeking behavior and reduce the stigma of such screening [15]. Pap tests are regularly performed as part of prenatal screening. Breast cancer screening is less taboo than cervical cancer screening. However, refugee women are still under-screened [16, 17].

Mental Health

Refugee women are at increased risk for depression, anxiety, and PTSD [18]. Given the additional obstacles refugee women face in maintaining their health and well-being [19], high rates of violence and trauma persist post-migration [20]. When appropriate, women should be referred for psychiatric services and/or therapy [21]. There is lack of a valid screening measure for common mental health conditions across multiple refugee populations; however, a new validated screening modality holds promise for utility across varied ethnic and linguistic refugee populations in primary health care settings [22].

Reproductive Health

Nutrition

For pregnant refugee women, malnutrition may be observed due to lack of access to food in war-torn areas and refugee camps. These women are at high risk for nutritional deficiencies such as folic acid, iron, and vitamin D. Iron-deficiency anemia is also commonly seen among Sub-Saharan African refugees arriving in host countries [23]. Anemia is of specific concern during pregnancy and could result from chronic blood loss due to intestinal parasites, menstruation, malabsorption, high parity, prolonged breastfeeding, sickle cell anemia, and malaria [24].

Lower amounts of physical activity and poor diet are commonly seen among refugee populations as they adjust to a "westernized" lifestyle and diet [25], and may give rise to obesity. A lack of familiarity with or knowledge of healthy foods and food preparation techniques are also concerns [26]. Providing nutritional support, counseling, and early intervention will promote healthy diet choices and physical activity, which could prevent obesity and diabetes as well as fetal macrosomia [27].

Cultural and religious practices may create challenges for pregnant women. During Ramadan, providers should assess for any medical and pregnancy-related conditions that may be contraindicated for safe fasting. Education regarding proper nutrition and hydration during fasting periods is also important [28]. Other dietary factors such as vegetarianism or food restrictions during the antepartum, intrapartum, and postpartum period should also be discussed to determine any risk for poor outcomes.

Prenatal Care/Antepartum

An opportunity arises to improve maternal and neonatal health outcomes prior to pregnancy with preconceptional care. Infectious disease is an important area to assess prior to pregnancy with refugee populations as infections in the preconceptional period can affect fertility. Spontaneous abortions and fetal congenital birth defects due to infections can also occur [29]. In some cultures, marriage and child-bearing begins at an early age [30, 31]. Higher rates of teenage pregnancy among recent arrivals have been seen among refugee populations from Africa and Asia [32]. High parity may also be common as societal importance is placed on women's ability to have many children [5, 23].

Due to the lack of health care infrastructure and preventative care in some developing countries, refugee women may not understand the importance of prenatal care. Refugee women may have had prior pregnancies without prenatal care with good outcomes in their countries of origin. Some women may also delay or avoid prenatal care due to a fear of unnecessary tests or interventions that will cause problems during pregnancy and adverse birth outcomes. Providers should also be aware of the fear that women may have in regard to cesarean delivery causing severe complications, even death. This fear leads some women to avoid and/or delay seeking care as well as refuse interventions that could involve cesarean delivery [33].

During prenatal visits, providers should assess patient expectations and provide education and counseling on topics such as the importance of prenatal visits, the delivery room experience, pain medication options, interpreter services, and the possible indications for cesarean sections, as well as the risks and benefits of this surgical procedure. Tours of the hospital should be organized and highly encouraged as well [34]. Prenatal care visits are also an appropriate time for providers to discuss mental health and nutrition practices. Attention should be given to obtaining information regarding complications with prior pregnancies and deliveries, abortions, or issues with menstruation [24]. Providers can also begin to discuss postpartum issues such as postpartum depression, contraceptive options, and breastfeeding.

Pelvic and cervical examinations can cause extreme shame and embarrassment for some refugee women and there may be confusion regarding the necessity of these exams [5]. A pelvic examination may need to be deferred, particularly in women who have undergone infibulation (the most extensive form of FGC) as use of a speculum exam may not be possible or may cause extreme pain to the patient [27].

Routine laboratory tests according to the American College of Obstetricians and Gynecologists standards should be performed [35]. Additional tests recommended for refugee populations include: [27]

- Domestic violence/intimate partner violence or other forms of gender-based violence (see Appendix).
- Immunization history including verification of vaccines for influenza (seasonal vaccine administration is safe during pregnancy), measles/mumps/rubella (MMR), varicella, and tetanus/diphtheria/pertussis (TDaP). If there is no evidence of vaccination or immunity, provide all of the above mentioned vaccines except MMR and varicella, which are live vaccines and thus should be given postpartum.
- Hemoglobin Electrophoresis (for women of African, Southeast Asian, and Mediterranean ancestry) to screen for thalassemia or sickle cell anemia.
- Tuberculin skin test (TST) or Interferon-Gamma Release Assay (IGRA), as indicated, and screening for symptoms. Any patient suspected of having TB disease should receive a complete evaluation that includes medical history, physical examination and chest X-ray. Pregnant women with a positive TST or IGRA should have a shielded posterior–anterior chest X-ray. If asymptomatic and in the first trimester of pregnancy, the chest X-ray may be postponed until the second trimester [36].
- Malaria screening if patient recently emigrated from malaria-endemic region and displays clinical signs and symptoms such as fever.
- Substance use including exposure to tobacco, alcohol, and illicit drugs. Also check for exposure to herbal and other traditional/alternative medications or substances.

Intrapartum

The experience of delivering in a hospital can be extremely overwhelming for refugee women who may be experiencing childbirth in a Western health care setting for the first time. Refugee women who have had successful deliveries at home in their countries of origin with very little to no assistance may find this experience unnecessary or overwhelming. Multiple pelvic examinations, intravenous lines, fetal monitoring equipment, and blood pressure cuffs may be considered disruptive and cause major distress during the birthing process. Aversion to interventions such as labor induction and augmentation, epidural placement, and cesarean delivery procedures may be expressed. A growing number of studies demonstrate that refugee women have a profound fear of cesarean delivery [33, 34, 37]. There is also a common misconception that epidurals will cause paralysis or chronic back pain. Providers should strive to provide anticipatory guidance, education, counseling, and appropriate language interpretation, while empowering refugee women to incorporate traditional health behaviors and/or practices such as walking during labor or specific delivery positions as long as it is deemed safe for both the mother and fetus [27].

Verbal informed consent for procedures in lieu of written consent should be allowed through the assistance of a trained medical interpreter for those patients who have low literacy in English or in their native language [27].

The presence of family and social support should be encouraged. Evidence also suggests that the support of labor coaches or doulas may be beneficial to some refugee women in terms of increasing a positive attitude and experience with labor while decreasing the likelihood of obstetrical interventions [38]. Special attention should be paid to the role of men as it may or may not be culturally appropriate for men to be present during delivery [39, 40].

Decision-making in some cultures may be very different than in US. Health care decisions affect the patient, the family, and the community. Gender roles in some cultures also dictate that men are the decision-makers for the family. During labor, health care providers should assess the level of autonomy of the patient in decision-making and the role that a pregnant woman's spouse and/or matriarchal familial support may play in decision-making [20].

Maternal and Infant Outcomes

While there is conflicting evidence regarding maternal and infant outcomes among refugee populations, some studies have demonstrated poorer maternal and infant outcomes for certain refugee populations [1, 41]. For example, evidence shows that Somali women may be at increased risk for adverse maternal obstetrical outcomes including emergency cesarean delivery for fetal distress, failed induction of labor, post-dates delivery, oligohydramnios, perineal lacerations, and gestational diabetes [34, 42–44].

Adverse neonatal outcomes have been reported including prolonged hospitalization, lower 5-min Apgar scores, meconium aspiration, and assisted ventilation [41, 43, 44]. Low birth weight has been seen among neonates born to some refugee groups, and this trend has continued among refugees following immigration possibly due to psychosocial factors and social determinants of health [41, 45].

Higher infant morbidity and mortality are also seen among certain refugee populations [46]. While the reasons for this association are unclear, differences in mortality are not described solely by maternal risk factors [47]. The association between poor neonatal outcomes, poor access to care, and late prenatal care may explain some of these higher rates among refugees [23, 48].

Postpartum

Refugee women may bring postpartum customs, rituals, and remedies from their home countries. In some cases this dictates when women may leave home, when the infant may be exposed to the sun (40 days for some cultures in Africa and 28 for some Asian cultures), and when it is appropriate to resume intercourse [28]. This period may be disrupted due to economic strains or medical appointments [28]. Speaking with women regarding their cultural rituals and having some flexibility and/or explaining why the appointment timeline is important can go a long way towards enhancing compliance with follow-up care.

Recovering from c-sections may be a new experience for many refugees as they may have neither personal experience nor historical social traditions. Educating women on what to expect during recovery from a c-section is important. A decrease in fertility has been noted after c-sections in Somali women [49]. It is postulated that this may be attributed to the considerable fear of death from c-section in Somali women, but the data to substantiate this is inconclusive [33].

Inquiring about certain variables that put women at risk for poor infant health outcomes (i.e., worry about their infant's health, a mother's educational level, pre-natal class attendance, marital status and their comprehension of the host country's official language) may result in effective use of postnatal home visits [50]. Having an open discussion with patients both in the prenatal period and the postpartum period, and providing anticipatory guidance about expectations and worries can help to dissuade fears or misinformation [51].

Postpartum Depression

Underlying mental health issues are relatively high in refugee women in relation to traumatic events in their home country or on their journey to their host country. They may also be under considerable stress to acculturate and adapt to the customs, language, culture, and daily life of their adopted new home [52]. In addition, social isolation and domestic violence may trigger significant distress [52]. The addition of an infant to this environment, without the familiar assistance and social support from family and community members, and the cultural rituals surrounding child-birth, may precipitate a crisis or significantly increase stress levels. However, deeply religious perspectives among some refugees may facilitate greater resiliency and decrease the risk of harming the infant [53].

It is important to note that refugee women with distress or psychosocial disorders may often present with somatization and physical findings rather than complaints of affective or psychological symptoms [52, 54]. Cultural and religious stigma towards mental health issues may adversely affect women's access to therapy or medication. Providers should be aware of this and provide a comfortable place for communication of stressors and incorporate stress-relieving strategies realizing that they may be the patient's only source of intervention [53, 55].

Breastfeeding

In general, breastfeeding is more common among refugee women than among American women. Depending on the region of origin, women may be accustomed to breastfeeding for up to two and a half years [53]. However, there is a noted decrease in the percentage and length of breastfeeding in relation to how long women have been in US [5, 56]. This has been related to changing economic activity and sociocultural values, the need to return to work, and the discomfort refugee women may experience with pumping. Newly arrived refugee women may believe that formula is better for their infant because they see American children as larger than infants born in their countries of origin, while refugees who have been in the host country for a period of time may feel that breastfeeding is socially unacceptable and thus minimize the practice in order to acculturate [53].

Women may be accustomed to using breastfeeding as a form of natural family planning. However, they should be educated on its failure rate and the availability of additional contraceptive methods. This is especially true for women who are supplementing with formula [28]. Muslim women will often continue to breastfeed during the fasting period of Ramadan and providers should monitor the nutritional status of both the mother and child and encourage women to consume extra liquids before and after fasting [57]. Inquiring about breastfeeding practices with previous children, expectations for breastfeeding and assessing progress at visits will yield valuable information.

Contraception

Refugee women have variable exposure to contraceptive methods which may vary based on their region of origin and previous access to health care. Some women may have religious objections to manipulating their fertility, while for others fertility may be a sign of pride and wealth in a community [28]. Furthermore, it may be necessary for women to consult their husbands regarding contraception in order to conform to cultural ideals in decision-making and gender norms [20]. Providers should offer time and space for this to occur and reengage the conversation on subsequent visits.

Women may be more open to discussing contraception if "family spacing" or "family planning" is used instead of "birth control." However, many women, due to cultural or religious beliefs, may still have an extreme aversion to any form of birth control. Refugee women have been shown to be more successful in using the calendar rhythm method and keeping track of their menstrual cycles very closely [5]. Offering support for this method and providing cycle beads or calendars for women to use can be helpful. However, it is still important to educate women on the failure rate of natural family planning methods.

If women are interested in initiating a hormonal method of birth control and have never previously used one, making sure to outline potential side effects and expected changes in menstruation is important. Unwelcome changes may perpetuate the fear and misinformation surrounding contraception use and side effects, and lead to non-compliance [28, 58].

Intimate Partner Violence

Violence against women is a global public health phenomenon that affects millions of women across racial, ethnic, social, economic, religious, and cultural lines [59, 60]. There are many different kinds of violent acts against women [61]. IPV is the most prevalent form of violence among women, and comprises a pattern of assaultive and coercive behaviors which may include physical assault, psychological or emotional abuse, sexual assault, progressive social isolation, stalking, deprivation, intimidation, and threats. There is some evidence showing high prevalence of IPV among refugee populations, and it often occurs within the context of immigration, acculturation, and rapid changes in family and social structures [62]. Refugee women are distinctly vulnerable in having survived pre-migratory experiences of sexual violence during war/armed conflicts. Upon resettlement in host countries, refugee women may continue to face risks of IPV within the context of language barriers, confusion over their legal rights, and the stress of acculturation to new cultural and social norms.

Beyond the immediate trauma of violence, IPV can have a profound impact on a woman's overall health and well-being. Women who have survived IPV may display psychological symptoms of fear, anxiety, depression, PTSD, insomnia, feelings of hopelessness, and somatization, while physical symptoms may manifest as chronic pelvic pain, menstrual irregularities, sexual dysfunction, musculoskeletal symptoms, and distorted body image. Providers may face difficulty managing chronic illnesses such as diabetes and hypertension, and alcohol and substance abuse issues may become apparent. General perceptions of poor health and worsened health status are also common [61]. While maintaining cultural beliefs and norms may confer protective coping mechanisms through community-centered values, resiliency, and social support, cultural context may also exacerbate the consequences of violence by imbuing psychosocial conflicts in traditional gender roles. Moreover, cultural values and practices may constrain women from seeking help, which when compounded by stigma and shame, may limit women's health-seeking behavior and health care utilization. Institutional racism, sexism, and socioeconomic barriers may further contribute to disparities in refugee women's health.

Hence developing trust with refugee communities is critical. Survivors of IPV need culturally appropriate interventions and programs that address the many challenges specific to refugee communities. Female providers and female interpreters are often at the front lines in being able to help identify concerns for IPV [63]. Culturally tailored interventional programs should support women's self-sufficiency, offer comprehensive services including shelter, safety planning, coordination with police and the judicial system, medical as well as social support (including employment, housing, and services for children) [64].

There are many challenges encountered by health care systems, service organizations, and programs addressing IPV in refugee communities including difficulty getting victims to talk about personal and shameful experiences and convincing them of availability of support and safety if they confront their abusers. Some strategies include changing cultural norms regarding IPV and using advocates who can provide leadership and raise awareness in the community [65].

A growing body of evidence supports the efficacy of routine screening in identifying women who are victims of or at risk for IPV, which provides a primary starting point for early identification of IPV in order to reach women regardless of whether symptoms are immediately apparent. In addition, screening for IPV provides an opportunity for disclosure and provides a woman and her health care provider the chance to develop a plan to protect her safety and improve her health. The Family Violence Prevention Fund has developed National Consensus Guidelines on Identifying and Responding to Domestic Violence Victimization in Health Care Settings [66]. Health care providers and health systems should be aware of and have collaborative relationships with culturally competent resources in the community that are specific to patients' cultural groups and countries of origin [61].

Female Genital Cutting

Female genital cutting (FGC), otherwise known as Female Genital Mutilation (FGM) or Female Circumcision (FC), is an ancient cultural practice that has gained global attention due to immigration from FGC-affected regions of the world. FGC is defined as any procedure that involves partial or total removal of external female genitalia or other injury to female genital organs whether for cultural or nontherapeutic reasons [67]. FGC is often performed as a ritual initiation into womanhood: ensuring one's chastity and eligibility for marriage and instilling pride, honor, value, and aesthetics. FGC affects up to 140 million women worldwide. Each year three million girls are at risk of undergoing this practice [67]. FGC is documented in 28 countries throughout sub-Saharan Africa, and in regions of Southeast Asia and the Middle East. Prevalence rates vary between and within nations, with some regions possessing rates higher than 90 %.

Table 15.1 2007 WHO classification of female genital cutting

Type	Definition
I	Partial or total removal of the clitoris and/or the prepuce *(clitoridectomy)*
	Type Ia—removal of the clitoral hood or prepuce only
	Type Ib—removal of the clitoris with the prepuce
II	Partial or total removal of the clitoris and the labia minora, with or without excision of the labia majora *(excision)*
	Type IIa—removal of the labia minora only
	Type IIb—partial or total removal of the clitoris and the labia minora
	Type IIc—partial or total removal of the clitoris, the labia minora, and the labia majora
III	Narrowing of the vaginal orifice with creation of a covering seal by cutting and appositioning the labia minora and/or the labia majora, with or without excision of the clitoris *(infibulation)*
	Type IIIa—removal and apposition of the labia minora
	Type IIIb—removal and apposition of the labia majora
IV	Unclassified: All other harmful procedures to the female genitalia for nonmedical purposes (i.e., pricking, piercing, incising, scraping, and cauterization)

World Health Organization. *Eliminating Female Genital Mutilation: An Interagency Statement.* Geneva, Switzerland. 2008. Accessed 2/12/13: https://docs.google.com/a/asu.edu/viewer?url=http://www.unifem.org/attachments/products/fgm_statement_2008_eng.pdf

FGC is divided into four categories (Table 15.1; Fig. 15.1). Type I is the partial or total removal of the prepuce or clitoris (clitoridectomy). Type II is the partial or total removal of the clitoris and the labia minora, with or without excision of the labia majora (excision). Type III involves cutting and appositioning the labia minora and/or majora to create a covering that restricts the vaginal introitus (infibulation). This is the most extreme category, but only comprises 10 % of all cases of FGC [68]. However, recent immigration and refugee resettlement from countries where Type III FGC predominates (e.g., Somalia) have resulted in an increased prevalence of females with Type III FGC throughout North America and Europe. Type IV includes other alterations to the genitals that do not remove tissue, such as piercing, pricking, or cauterization [67].

Women who have undergone FGC may experience short and long-term complications. Immediate complications may include pain, infection, laceration of adjacent structures (i.e., the bladder, urethra, vagina, or rectum), and uncontrolled hemorrhage. Long-term complications, seen mostly in women with type III FGC, include chronic urinary tract infections, severe dysmenorrhea, and dyspareunia, which in severe cases may lead to infertility. The extent of long-term morbidity depends on the type, extent, and severity of tissue excised [69–71]. A prospective study across six African countries has demonstrated a trend towards adverse obstetric and neonatal outcomes with increasing severity of FGC when compared to those without FGC; including cesarean delivery, postpartum hemorrhage, extended maternal hospital stay, resuscitation of the infant, and inpatient perinatal death [72]. Sexual function may also be affected [73]. However, more research is needed to further elucidate the impact of varying types of FGC on a woman and her partner's sexual health.

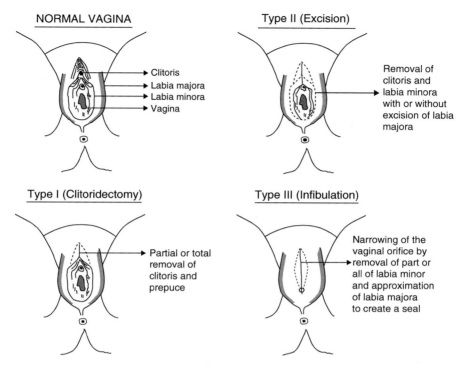

Fig. 15.1 Classification of female genital cutting

For women with Type III FGC, a defibulation procedure can relieve FGC-related morbidity prior to coitus or pregnancy, or during the antepartum or intrapartum period. Defibulation entails the surgical release of the vulvar scar tissue by making a vertical incision along the infibulation to expose the urethral meatus and introitus, followed by approximation of the raw edges on each labia majora. Reconstructive surgery can also be performed to restore clitoral anatomy and function. Local anesthesia should be avoided as this may cause posttraumatic stress symptoms [74, 75]. Excellent postoperative results have been reported with improvement in both sexual function and pain [76].

For pregnant women with type III FGC, cesarean delivery should only be performed for obstetrical indications, and precautions taken to ensure a safe vaginal delivery. Counseling is needed during the antepartum period to discuss what to expect during labor, as well as to determine the most appropriate timing of defibulation (antepartum during the second trimester or intrapartum). Antepartum defibulation avoids excessive blood loss at the time of delivery, facilitates the assessment of cervical dilation, and allows for urethral catheterization and the placement of intrauterine devices, while minimizing patient discomfort.

Counseling should be provided in a nonjudgmental manner; engendering trust and encouraging open dialogue. Women suspected of being at risk for or who have undergone FGC should be asked about their history in a culturally sensitive matter, with careful use of the patient's own terminology [77]. An exploration of the cultural significance ascribed to FGC should ensue along with elicitation of any medical sequela experienced. An interpreter should be available if necessary along with the woman's partner to aid in medical decision-making. During the physical exam, it is important to gain the trust of women who may feel uncomfortable with gynecologic exams. Pelvic exams may pose a challenge in women with a narrowed opening, and a pediatric speculum may be needed. Likewise, performing a bimanual exam may be difficult, and a rectovaginal exam may be required. Visual aids/diagrams illustrating vulvar anatomy should also be incorporated, and sexual health counseling made available for both the woman and her partner.

Legislation and educational campaigns against FGC have led to a significant decline in its prevalence over the last 25 years, although support for its continuation varies widely between and within countries [78]. In December 2012, the United Nations General Assembly passed a resolution banning FGC which is intensifying global efforts to eliminate the practice [79]. Notwithstanding, intense controversy abounds surrounding the medicalization of genital cutting performed on minors (whether male or female) [80]; the confluence of double-standards around female genital cosmetic surgery and an adult woman's ability to choose genital modification procedures [73]; and the Western media's portrayal of FGC without attention to rigorous evidence-based research and balanced public policy debates [81]. Thus, FGC provides a window of opportunity through which health care providers can impart culturally appropriate counseling and education, enabling women to make informed decisions regarding their reproductive health care and circumcision of their daughters.

Appendix: Suggested Assessment Questions and Strategies for Routine Screening of Violence Against Women

The following sample assessment questions can also be used to develop a strategy most comfortable for each individual:

Framing Questions

- "Because violence is so common in many people's lives, I've begun to ask all my patients about it."
- "I am concerned that your symptoms may have been caused by someone hurting you."
- "I don't know if this is (or ever has been) a problem for you, but many of the patients I see are dealing with abusive relationships. Some are too afraid or uncomfortable to bring it up themselves, so I've started asking about it routinely."

Direct Verbal Questions

- "Are you in a relationship with a person who physically hurts or threatens you?"
- "Did someone cause these injuries? Was it your partner/husband?"
- "Has your partner or ex-partner ever hit you or physically hurt you?"
- "Do you (or did you ever) feel controlled or isolated by your partner?"
- "Do you ever feel afraid of your partner? Do you feel you are in danger?"
- "Is it safe for you to go home?"
- "Has your partner ever forced you to have sex when you didn't want to? Has your partner ever refused to practice safe sex?"
- "Has any of this happened to you in previous relationships?"

Effective Assessment Strategies When Working Cross-culturally

It is important to adapt your assessment questions and approach in order to be culturally relevant to individual patients. Listen to patients, pay attention to words that are used in different cultural settings and integrate those into assessment questions. Focusing on actions and behaviors as opposed to culturally specific terminology can also help, or some groups may be more willing to discuss abuse if you use general questions. Be aware of verbal and nonverbal cultural cues (eye contact or not, patterns of silence, spacing, and active listening during the interview).

Some examples include:

- Use your patient's language: "Does your boyfriend disrespect you?"
- Be culturally specific: "Abuse is widespread and can happen even in lesbian relationships.
- Does your partner ever try to hurt you?"
- Focus on behaviors: "Has you partner ever hit, shoved, or threatened to kill you?"
- Begin by being indirect: "If a family member or friend was being hurt or threatened by a partner, do you know of resources that could help them?"

(Adapted from the National Consensus Guidelines on Identifying and Responding to Domestic Violence Victimization in Health Care Settings. The Family Violence Prevention Fund, 2004. Accessed 2/12/2013: http://www.futureswithoutviolence. org/userfiles/file/Consensus.pdf)

References

1. Gagnon AJ, Tuck J, Barkun L. A Systematic review of questionnaires measuring the health of resettling refugee women. Health Care Women Int. 2004;25:111–49.
2. Beyani C. The needs of refugee women: a human-rights perspective. Gend Dev. 1995;3(2):29–35.

3. Momartin S, Silove D, Manicavasagar V, et al. Dimensions of trauma associated with post-traumatic stress disorder (PTSD) caseness, severity and functional impairment: a study of Bosnian refugees resettled in Australia. Soc Sci Med. 2003;57(5):775–81.

4. Asgary R, Segar N. Barriers to health care access among refugee asylum seekers. J Healthcare Poor Underserved. 2011;22(2):506–22.

5. Kornosky J, Peck J, Sweeney A, et al. Reproductive characteristics of Southeast Asian immigrants before and after migration. J Immigr Minor Health. 2008;10:135–43. doi:10.1007/s10903-007-9064-8.

6. Morrison TB, Wieland ML, Cha SS, et al. Disparities in preventive health services among Somali immigrants and refugees. J Immigr Minor Health. 2012;14(6):968–74.

7. Johnson CE, Mues KE, Mayne SL, et al. Cervical cancer screening among immigrants and ethnic minorities: a systematic review using the Health Belief Model. J Low Genit Tract Dis. 2008;12(3):232–41.

8. Cadman L, Waller J, Ashdown-Barr L, et al. Barriers to cervical screening in women who have experienced sexual abuse: an exploratory study. J Fam Plann Reprod Health care. 2012;38(4):214–20.

9. U.S. Center for Disease Control and Prevention. General refugee health guidelines. http://www.cdc.gov/immigrantrefugeehealth/guidelines/general-guidelines.html#cancer_screening. Published 2011. Accessed 2013.

10. U.S. Center for Disease Control and Prevention. Immigrant and refugee health. Screening for HIV infection during the refugee domestic medical examination. http://www.cdc.gov/immigrantrefugeehealth/guidelines/domestic/screening-hiv-infection-domestic.html. Published 2012. Accessed 2013.

11. Lowther SA, Johnson G, Hendel-Paterson B, et al. HIV/AIDS and associated conditions among HIV-infected refugees in Minnesota, 2000–2007. Int J Environ Res Public Health. 2007;9(11):4197–209.

12. Stauffer WM, Painter J, Mamo B, et al. Sexually transmitted infections in newly arrived refugees: is routine screening for *Neisseria gonorrheae* and *Chlamydia trachomatis* infection indicated? Am J Trop Med Hyg. 2012;86(2):292–5.

13. Burnley J, Johnson-Agbakwu CE. Pap tests. In: Loue S, Sajatovic M, editors. Encyclopedia of immigrant health. New York: Springer; 2012. p. 1172–5.

14. Lofters AK, Moineddin R, Hwang SW, et al. Predictors of low cervical cancer screening among immigrant women in Ontario, Canada. BMC Womens Health. 2011;7(11):20.

15. Redwood-Campbell L, Fowler N, Laryea S, et al. 'Before you teach me, I cannot know': immigrant women's barriers and enablers with regard to cervical cancer screening among different ethnolinguistic groups in Canada. Can J Public Health. 2011;102(3):230–4.

16. Percac-Lima S, Milosavljevic B, Oo SA, et al. Patient navigation to improve breast cancer screening in Bosnian refugees and immigrants. J Immigr Minor Health. 2012;14(4):727–30.

17. Saadi A, Bond B, Percac-Lima S. Perspectives on preventive health care and barriers to breast cancer screening among Iraqi women refugees. J Immigr Minor Health. 2011;14(4):633–9.

18. Davidson GR, Murray KE, Schweitzer RD. Review of refugee mental health and well-being: Australian perspectives. Aust Psychol. 2008;43s:160–74.

19. Gagnon AJ, Van Hulst A, Merry L, et al. Cesarean section rate differences by migration indicators. Arch Gynecol Obstet. 2012 [Epub ahead of print] doi: 10.1007/s00404-012-2609-7.

20. Redwood-Campbell L, Thind H, Howard M, et al. Understanding the health of refugee women in host countries: lessons from the Kosovar re-settlement in Canada. Prehosp Disaster Med. 2008;23(4):322–7.

21. Elklit A, Ostergard Kjaer K, Lasgaard M, et al. Social support, coping and posttraumatic stress symptoms in young refugees. Torture. 2012;22(1):11–23.

22. Hollifield M, Verbillis-Kolp S, Farmer B, et al. The refugee health screener-15 (RHS-15): development and validation of an instrument for anxiety, depression, and PTSD in refugees. *General Hospital Psychiatry*. 2013; 35(2):202–9.

23. Harris M, Humphries K, Nabb J. Asylum seekers: delivering care for women seeking refuge. RCM J. 2006;9:190–2.

24. Costa D. Health care of refugee women. Aust Fam Physician. 2007;36(3):151–4.
25. Willis M, Buck J. From Sudan to Nebraska: Dinka and Nuer refugee diet dilemmas. J Nurs Educ Behav. 2007;39:273–80.
26. Barnes D, Almasy N. Refugees' perceptions of healthy behaviors. J Immigr Health. 2005;7(3):185–93. doi:10.1007/s10903-005-3675-8.
27. John Snow Institute. Refugee Health Technical Assistance Center: Pregnancy. http://www.refugeehealthta.org/physical-mental-health/health-conditions/womens-health/pregnancy/. Published 2011. Accessed 2013.
28. Bruce H. Women's health issues. In: Walker PF, Barnett ED, editors. Immigrant medicine. Philadelphia, PA: Saunders Elsevier; 2007. p. 567–96.
29. Coonrod DV. Infectious diseases in preconceptional care. In: Karoshi M, Newbold S, B-Lynch C, Keith L, editors. Textbook of preconceptional medicine. London: Global Library of Women's Medicine; 2011.
30. Gupta N, Mahy M. Sexual initiation among adolescent girls and boys: trends and differentials in Sub-Saharan Africa. Arch Sex Behav. 2003;32(1):41–53.
31. Doyle A, Mavedzenge S, Plummer M, et al. The sexual behaviour of adolescents in sub-Saharan Africa: patterns and trends from national surveys. Trop Med Int Health. 2012;17(7):796–807.
32. Goosen S, Uitenbroek D, Wijsen C, et al. Induced abortions and teenage births among asylum seekers in The Netherlands: analysis of national surveillance data. J Epidemiol Community Health. 2009;63:528–33. doi:10.1136/jech.2008.079368.
33. Brown E, Carroll J, Fogarty C, et al. "They get a C-section…they gonna die": Somali women's fears of obstetrical interventions in the United States. J Transcult Nurs. 2010;21(3):220–7.
34. Herrel N, Olevitch L, DuBois DK, et al. Somali refugee women speak out about their needs for care during pregnancy and delivery. J Midwifery Womens Health. 2004;49(4):345–9. doi:10.1016/j.jmwh.2004.02.008.
35. American College of Obstetricians and Gynecologists. Frequently asked questions: routine tests in pregnancy. http://www.acog.org/~/media/For%20Patients/faq133.pdf?dmc=1&ts=201 20529T1704217092. Published 2011. Accessed 2013.
36. U.S. Center for Disease Control and Prevention. Guidelines for screening for tuberculosis infection and disease during the domestic medical examination for newly arrived refugees. http://www.cdc.gov/immigrantrefugeehealth/pdf/domestic-tuberculosis-refugee-health.pdf. Published 2012. Accessed 2013.
37. Halvorsen T. Pregnancy and birth in Minnesota's Hmong population. Minn Med. 2012;95(5):49–52.
38. Dundek L. Establishment of a Somali doula program at a large metropolitan hospital. J Perinat Neonatal Nurs. 2006;20(2):128–37.
39. Wiklund H, Aden A, Hogberg U, et al. Somalis giving birth in Sweden: a challenge to culture and gender specific values and behaviours. Midwifery. 2000;16:105–15.
40. Erwin A. A physician's guide for understanding Hmong health care beliefs. http://www.d.umn.edu/medweb/Erwin/hmong.html#Pregnancy. Accessed 2013.
41. Cripe SM, O'Brien W, Gellaye B, et al. Maternal morbidity and perinatal outcomes among foreign-born Cambodian, Laotian, and Vietnamese Americans in Washington state, 1993–2006. J Immigr Minor Health. 2011;13(3):417–25.
42. Vangen S, Stoltenberg C, Johansen RE. Perinatal complications among ethnic Somalis in Norway. Acta Obstet Gynecol Scand. 2002;81(4):317–22.
43. Johnson EB, Reed SD, Hitti J, et al. Increased risk of adverse pregnancy outcome among Somali immigrants in Washington State. Am J Obstet Gynecol. 2005;193:475–82.
44. Small R, Gagnon A, Gissler M, et al. Somali women and their pregnancy outcomes postmigration: data from six receiving countries. BJOG. 2008;115:1630–40.
45. Dejin-Karlsson E, Ostergren P. Country of origin, social support and the risk of small for gestational age birth. Scand J Public Health. 2004;32:442–9. doi:10.1080/14034940410028172.
46. Gissler M, Alexander S, Macfarlane A, et al. Stillbirths and infant deaths among migrants in industrialized countries. Acta Obstet Gynecol Scand. 2009;88:134–48.

47. Essen B, Hanson BS, Ostergren PO, et al. Increased perinatal mortality among sub-Saharan immigrants in a city-population in Sweden. Acta Obstet Gynecol Scand. 2000;79:737–43.
48. Treacy A, Byrne P, Collins C. Pregnancy outcome in immigrant women in the Rotunda Hospital. Ir Med J. 2006;99:22–3.
49. Salem W, Flynn P, Weaver A, et al. Fertility after cesarean delivery among Somali-born women resident in the USA. J Immigr Minor Health. 2011;13:494–9.
50. Edwards NC, Boivin JF. Ethnocultural predictors of postpartum infant-care behaviours among immigrants in Canada. Ethn Health. 1997;2(3):163–76.
51. Carroll J, et al. Caring for Somali women: implications for clinician–patient communication. Patient Educ Couns. 2007;66:337–45.
52. Allotey P. Travelling with 'excess Baggage': health problems of refugee women in Western Australia. Women Health. 1998;28(1):63–81.
53. Hill N, Hunt E, Hyrkas K. Somali immigrant women's health care experiences and beliefs regarding pregnancy and birth in the US. J Transcult Nurs. 2012;23(1):72–81.
54. Lin EH, Carter WB, Kleinman AM. An exploration of somatization among Asian refugees and immigrants in primary care. Am J Public Health. 1985;75(9):1080–4.
55. Hammoud M, White C, Fetters M. Opening cultural doors: providing culturally sensitive health care to Arab American and American Muslim patients. Am J Obstet Gynecol. 2005;139:1307–11.
56. Carpenter S, Vaucher Y. Cultural transition and infant-feeding practices among Somali immigrant women in San Diego, California. Pediatr Res. 1999;45:279A.
57. Rakicioglu N, Samur G, Topcu A, et al. The effect of Ramadan on maternal nutrition and composition of breast milk. Pediatr Int. 2006;48:278–83.
58. Skidmore M. Menstrual madness: women's health and well-being in urban Burma. Women Health. 2008;35(4):81–99.
59. Watts C, Zimmerman C. Violence against women: global scope and magnitude. Lancet. 2002;359:1232–7.
60. World Health Organization. Multi-country study on women's health and domestic violence against women: summary report of initial results on prevalence, health outcomes and women's responses. http://www.who.int/gender/violence/who_multicountry_study/summary_report/summary_report_English2.pdf. Published 2005. Accessed 2013.
61. Ekblad S, Kastrup MC, Eisenman DP et al. Interpersonal violence towards women. In: Walker PF, Barnett ED, editors. Immigrant medicine. Philadelphia, PA: Saunders Elsevier; 2007. p. 567–596.
62. Nilsson JE, Brown C, Russell EB, Khamphakdy-Brown S. Acculturation, partner violence, and psychological distress in refugee women from Somalia. J Interpers Violence. 2008;23(11):1654–63.
63. Foster J, Newell B, Kemp C. Women. In: Kemp C, Rasbridge LA, editors. Refugee and immigrant health: a handbook for health professionals. Cambridge, UK: Cambridge University Press. 2004; p. 67–79.
64. Bureau of Justice Statistics, U.S Department of Justice. Intimate partner violence in the United States. https://docs.google.com/a/asu.edu/viewer?url=http://bjs.ojp.usdoj.gov/content/pub/pdf/ipvus.pdf. Published 2007. Accessed 2013.
65. Runner M, Yoshihama M, Novick S. Intimate partner violence in immigrant and refugee communities: challenges, promising practices and recommendations. A report by the family violence prevention fund for the Robert Wood Johnson Foundation. https://docs.google.com/a/asu.edu/viewer?url=http://www.futureswithoutviolence.org/userfiles/file/ImmigrantWomen/IPV_Report_March_2009.pdf. Published 2009. Accessed 2013.
66. National consensus guidelines on identifying and responding to domestic violence victimization in health care settings. The family violence prevention fund. http://www.futureswithoutviolence.org/userfiles/file/Consensus.pdf. Published 2004. Accessed 2013.
67. World Health Organization. Eliminating female genital mutilation: an interagency statement. https://docs.google.com/a/asu.edu/viewer?url=http://www.unifem.org/attachments/products/fgm_statement_2008_eng.pdf. Published 2008. Accessed 2013.

68. Yoder PS, Khan S. Numbers of women circumcised in Africa: the production of a total. Macro International Inc: Calverton; 2007.
69. Fernandez-Aguilar S, Noel JC. Neuroma of the clitoris after female genital cutting. Obstet Gynecol. 2003;101:1053–4.
70. Nour NM. Urinary calculus associated with female genital cutting. Obstet Gynecol. 2007;107:521–3.
71. Almroth L, Elmusharaf S, El Hadi N, et al. Primary infertility after genital mutilation in girlhood in Sudan: a case–control study. Lancet. 2005;366:385–91.
72. World Health Organization. Study group on female genital mutilation and obstetric outcome. WHO collaborative prospective study in six African countries. Lancet. 2006;367(9525): 1835–41.
73. Johnsdotter S, Essén B. Genitals and ethnicity: the politics of genital modifications. Reprod Health Matters. 2010;18(35):29–37.
74. Johnson C, Nour NM. Surgical techniques: defibulation of Type III female genital cutting. J Sex Med. 2007;4(6):1544–7.
75. Foldes P. Reconstructive surgery of the clitoris after ritual excision. J Sex Med. 2006;3: 1091–4.
76. Foldes P. Reconstructive plastic surgery of the clitoris after sexual mutilation. Prog Urol. 2004;14:47–50.
77. Rosenberg LB, Gibson K, Shulman JF. When cultures collide: female genital cutting and U.S. obstetric practice. Obstet Gynecol. 2009;113(4):931–4.
78. Center for Reproductive Rights. Female genital mutilation (FGM): legal prohibitions worldwide.http://reproductiverights.org/en/document/female-genital-mutilation-fgm-legal-prohibitions-worldwide. Published 2000. Accessed 2013.
79. World Health Organization. Female genital mutilation. http://www.who.int/mediacentre/fact-sheets/fs241/en/#. Published 2013. Accessed 2013.
80. Darby R, Svoboda JS. A Rose by any other name? Med Anthropol Q. 2007;21(3):301–23.
81. The Public Policy Advisory Network on Female Genital Surgeries in Africa. Seven things to know about female genital surgeries in Africa. Hastings Cent Rep. 2012;6:19–27.

Chapter 16
Health Issues in Refugee Children

Sural Shah, Meera Siddharth, and Katherine Yun

Introduction

In the past decade, an estimated 200,000 children have come to the US as refugees [1]. Their exposure to health-related risk and protective factors varies by nationality, socioeconomic status, and time period. In 2005, the majority of US-bound refugees originated in Cuba (12 %), Laos (16 %), Russia (11 %), and Somalia (19 %) [2]. In 2011, individuals from Bhutan (27 %), Burma (30 %), and Iraq (17 %) predominated [2]. Even within the same ethnic or national group, children's experiences and exposures vary. For example, access to early childhood nutrition or preventive health services is often different for children born in refugee camps or other transitional settings when compared to their older siblings. Similarly, disease risk for children from the same camp or region may wax and wane over time as outbreaks flare or preventive health programs, such as micronutrient supplementation or presumptive deworming, take root.

After arriving in the US, growth and nutrition, communicable conditions, vaccine catch-up, and entry into primary and specialty care are the focus of health care. Over time, psychosocial needs and chronic disease management may predominate. Psychosocial support is likely to be particularly important for survivors of violence

S. Shah, M.D. (✉)
Internal Medicine and Pediatrics, Children's Hospital of Philadelphia, Hospital of the
University of Pennsylvania, 34th and Civic Center Blvd, Philadelphia, PA 19104, USA
e-mail: sz357@partners.org

M. Siddharth, M.D., F.A.A.P.
Primary Care, Karabots Primary Care Centre, Children's Hospital of Philadelphia,
4865 Market Street, Philadelphia, PA 19139, USA
e-mail: SIDDHARTH@email.chop.edu

K. Yun, M.D.
Pediatrics, Perelman School of Medicine & The Children's Hospital of Philadelphia,
University of Pennsylvania, 3535 Market Street, 15th Floor, Philadelphia, PA 19104, USA
e-mail: yunk@email.chop.edu

A. Annamalai (ed.), *Refugee Health Care: An Essential Medical Guide*,
DOI 10.1007/978-1-4939-0271-2_16, © Springer Science+Business Media New York 2014

and for those who have come to the US without their parents or legal guardians, receiving assistance as unaccompanied refugee minors [3].

This chapter will focus on refugee groups who have arrived in the US in the prior decade. The intent is to review core information and concepts, bearing in mind that children's specific health needs, exposures, and experiences are heterogeneous. Because most studies have focused on children's health during the time immediately following arrival, known as *reception and placement*, the majority of recommendations focus on this period.

Nutrition and Growth

Nutrition and growth are among the most common concerns for health professionals caring for refugee children in the US. The social forces that uproot families can also disrupt access to food; expose children to infectious diseases associated with malnutrition; and limit access to medical care. Children may also come to the US from regions where childhood obesity is an emerging concern.

The prevalence of growth and nutrition problems among refugee children varies by population. In a study of children who resettled in Massachusetts in the late 1990s, *wasting* (low weight-for-height, which is often associated with acute malnutrition. For additional information about anthropometry, see Table 16.1) was present among 8 % of children from developing regions in Africa and Asia but few other children.[1] Similarly, *stunting* (low height-for-age; often associated with chronic malnutrition) was present among a high proportion of children from Africa (13 %), the Near East (19 %), and East Asia (30 %) but very few children from Yugoslavia and the former USSR [4]. These findings are consistent with more recent studies from refugee camps in Africa and Asia. A survey of five long term refugee camps in East and North Africa demonstrated wasting in 9–21 % of children aged 6–59 months [5]. Similarly, a 2007 survey of Bhutanese children aged 6–59 months living in one of seven refugee camps in Nepal found that stunting was present in 27 % of children and wasting in 4 % [6].

Children from other regions may be at higher risk of overweight and obesity. For example, an analysis of pre-departure data from Jordan found that 14 and 11 % of US-bound children from Iraq were overweight and obese, respectively [7]. Children may also experience excessive weight gain subsequent to resettlement, either because of increasing food availability, adoption of an "American" diet, or decreased physical activity [8, 9].

Children of any weight and stature may experience malnutrition in the form of micronutrient deficiencies (Table 16.2). Among refugee children, common micronutrient deficiencies include vitamin A, iron, vitamin B12, and vitamin D

---

[1] In this study, each region predominantly comprised children from one or two national or ethnic groups, as follows: Africa (89 % Somalia), Near East (98 % Iraqi or Kurdish), East Asia (90 % Vietnam), former Yugoslavia (96 % Bosnian), former USSR (41 % Ukrainian, 27 % Russian).

Table 16.1 Selected anthropometric assessment of children's growth and nutritional status

Growth classification[a]	Measurement[b]	Definition	Limitations
Wasting[c]	Weight-for-height	Z-score below −2 on the sex-specific weight-for-height WHO growth chart	
Stunting[c]	Height-for-age	Z-score below −2 on the sex-specific height-for-age WHO growth chart	Requires accurate assessment of age
Stunting[d]	Height-for-age	Below the 5th percentile of the sex-specific height-for-age CDC growth chart	Requires accurate assessment of age Based on US norms
Underweight[c]	Weight-for-age	Z-score below −2 on the sex-specific weight-for-age WHO growth chart	Requires accurate assessment of age
Underweight[d]	Body mass index (weight in kilograms divided by the square of the height in meters; BMI)	Below the 5th percentile of the sex-specific BMI-for-age growth chart	Requires accurate assessment of age Based on US norms Applicable for children 2–19 years
Overweight[d]	Body mass index (BMI)	85th to less than the 95th percentile of the sex-specific BMI-for-age growth chart	Requires accurate assessment of age Based on US norms Applicable for children 2–19 years
Obesity[d]	Body mass index (BMI)	Equal to or greater than the 95th percentile of the sex-specific BMI-for-age growth chart	Requires accurate age assessment Based on US norms Applicable for children 2–19 years

[a]The CDC's Division of Global Migration and Quarantine recommends that clinicians use WHO standardized growth references for children younger than 2 years of age and CDC/NCHS references for older children (CDC 2012)
[b]In children under 2 years of age, recumbent length is measured rather than standing height
[c]WHO (1995) Physical status: the use and interpretation of anthropometry, WHO Technical Report Series #854; WHO (2007); WHO. Child growth standards. http://www.who.int/childgrowth/en/
[d]CDC (2002) CDC growth charts. http://www.cdc.gov/growthcharts/cdc_charts.htm; Barlow SE et al. Expert committee recommendations regarding the prevention, assessment, and treatment of child and adolescent overweight and obesity: summary report. Pediatrics. 2007;120:S164–92

[5, 6, 9–12]. Studies on refugees in Africa and Asia have highlighted the susceptibility of children dependent on long-term food aid [5, 11, 13], demonstrating rates of vitamin A deficiency of 21–62 % and iron deficiency of 23–75 % among young children aged 6–59 months. Vitamin B12 deficiency has been less widely studied. However, data from the CDC Migrant Serum Bank suggest that 32–59 % of adolescents and young adults (15–29 years) from Bhutan may be affected [14].

Table 16.2 Brief overview of micronutrient deficiencies in refugee children

Micronutrient	Clinical presentation	Screening and treatment
Iodine	Risk: residence in mountainous and inland areas with little naturally occurring iodine in the soil Symptoms: thyroid disease, mental retardation (congenital) US-bound refugees: Iodine deficiency has not been reported in children following resettlement in US, but data are limited. Many refugee camps provide iodized salt	Thyroid exam. Laboratory screening is not currently recommended for asymptomatic children
Iron	Risk: one to three quarters of children in refugee camps in Asia, Africa, and the Middle East [5, 6, 11, 80] Symptoms: microcytic anemia, neurocognitive delay US-bound refugees: Iron deficiency is common, with variable risk by age and region of origin. Care should be taken to distinguish iron deficiency from hemoglobinopathies and G6PD deficiency	Screening for iron deficiency begins with assessment of hemoglobin or hematocrit concentrations Deficient children should be treated with oral iron supplementation
Vitamin A	Risk: one in five preschool-aged children worldwide; up to 62 % of young children in some refugee settings [5, 74, 81] Symptoms: infection; vision problems, including irreversible corneal damage and retinal problems, e.g., night blindness. Physical exam findings include dry skin, hair, or eyes, and Bitot spots Prevention: periodic oral supplementation programs US-bound refugees: Vitamin A deficiency has not been reported in children following resettlement in US, but data are limited	Measurement of serum retinol. However, routine screening of asymptomatic children is not currently recommended Oral supplementation is highly effective, but severe eye findings may require parenteral treatment and monitoring for toxicity
Vitamin B1 (Thiamine)	Risk: altered metabolism (e.g., thyroid disease), losses (e.g., chronic diarrhea) Symptoms: dry beriberi, characterized by progressive weakness and peripheral neurologic abnormalities; wet beriberi, a cardiomyopathy that can progress to congestive heart failure; infantile beriberi (congenital), which mimics shock; Wernicke encephalopathy, a triad of ophthalmoplegia, nystagmus, and ataxia US-bound refugees: Vitamin B1 deficiency has not been reported in children following resettlement in US. Data are limited	Measurement of whole blood transketolase activation. Laboratory screening is not currently recommended for asymptomatic children Mild beriberi in older children is treated with oral supplementation (10 mg/day). Severe beriberi and infantile beriberi require parenteral therapy

(continued)

Table 16.2 (continued)

Micronutrient	Clinical presentation	Screening and treatment
Vitamin B3 (Niacin)	Risk: diet dependent on corn or millet Symptoms: pellagra, characterized by "diarrhea, dermatitis, and dementia" or GI symptoms (glossitis, angular stomatitis, cheilitis, diarrhea), skin lesions (beginning as painful erythema on sun-exposed surfaces, skin eventually becomes rough and hard), and neurologic symptoms (e.g., irritability, depression, fatigue, memory impairment) US-bound refugees: Vitamin B3 deficiency has not been reported in children following resettlement in US. Data are limited	Measurement of 24-h urine niacin and N_1-methylnicotinamide excretion. Laboratory screening is not currently recommended for asymptomatic children Treatment with oral nicotin-amide supplementation is effective
Vitamin B12 (Cobalamin)	Risk: one in three adolescents from Bhutan [14], maternal vitamin B12 deficiency (breastfed infants), intrinsic factor deficiency, severe gastritis (e.g., *H pylori*) Symptoms: macrocytic anemia; pancytopenia; peripheral neuropathy; nonspecific neurologic symptoms, e.g., fatigue, irritability; severe congenital cases may lead to profound neurocognitive regression, development delay, or obtundation US-bound refugees: Vitamin B12 deficiency is common among adolescents from Bhutan. Data are limited for other national groups	Presumptive supplementation is recommended for refugees from Bhutan. Many clinicians also screen using serum cobalamin levels In adults, high dose oral treatment (e.g.,1000 mcg/day) is effective. Data on optimal dosing in children are limited. Children with severe neurologic symptoms may require IM or parenteral treatment. High dose therapy has not been associated with toxicity
Vitamin C (Ascorbic acid)	Risk: limited access to fruits and vegetables, as vitamin C is not stored in the body and must be continually replenished Symptoms: early symptoms include fatigue, aching lower extremities, and follicular hyperkeratotic papules (often on the shins); later symptoms include bleeding gums, perifollicular hemorrhage, and frank scurvy US-bound refugees: Outbreaks have been reported in refugee camps. Deficiency has not been reported in children following resettlement in US. Data are limited	Laboratory screening is not currently recommended for asymptomatic children

(continued)

Table 16.2 (continued)

Micronutrient	Clinical presentation	Screening and treatment
Vitamin D	Risk: refugee status, diseases associated with fat malabsorption	Measurement of serum 25-hydroxyvitamin D. Many clinicians screen or provide presumptive supplementation
	Symptoms: bone pain, dental caries and other tooth defects, impaired growth, rickets US-bound refugees: Vitamin D deficiency and insufficiency are highly prevalent, affecting approximately three-quarters of children [12].	Oral supplementation with 2000–5000 IU of ergocalciferol (vitamin D2) is effective. Chronic overuse can result in complications from hypercalcemia
Zinc	Risk: children with limited access to zinc-rich foods (e.g., meats) are believed to be at risk for mild-to-moderate deficiency [82]	Laboratory screening is not currently recommended for asymptomatic children
	Symptoms: zinc deficiency is characterized by immune dysfunction and disruption of mucosal integrity, resulting in acro-orificial skin lesions, diarrhea, susceptibility to infection, and poor growth US-bound refugees: Deficiency has not been reported in children following resettlement in US. Data are limited	Oral supplementation is effective

Younger children are less likely to be vitamin B12 deficient than adolescents. However, infants with vitamin B12 deficiency—most often breastfed infants with vitamin-deficient mothers—are at risk of severe neurocognitive regression and hematologic abnormalities [15–18].

Micronutrient deficiencies are not exclusive to children who arrive in the US after living in refugee camps. In a diverse sample of refugee children who had recently resettled in Massachusetts, nearly 70 % of young children (≤5 years) and 80 % of school-aged children (6–20 years) were vitamin D insufficient or deficient [12]. Vitamin D abnormalities were common even among individuals from the Middle East, Europe or Central Asia, and Latin America or the Caribbean, many of whom move to the US after living in urban areas rather than refugee camps[2]. Table 16.2 demonstrates the significant impact micronutrient deficiencies can have on childhood health and development and emphasizes its importance in evaluations of resettled youth.

---

[2] In this study, demographic data were not disaggregated by age. However, individuals from Iraq (28 %), Burma (20 %), and Bhutan (15 %) were the three largest national groups in the overall sample. The majority of individuals from the Middle East were from Iraq, while individuals from Europe/Central Asia were predominantly from Moldova, Ukraine, and Russia and those from Latin America/Caribbean were predominantly Cuban.

The causes of growth abnormalities and malnutrition are multifactorial. In refugee settings, perishable foods can be difficult to transport and store, and movement or financial restrictions may prevent individual foraging or purchases in food markets. Even when children receive an adequate number of calories, they may lack food diversity or access to outdoor activities. As a result, micronutrient deficiencies may be present even when a child's growth has been normal. Children living in refugee settings are often also at risk of acquiring comorbid communicable conditions associated with poor nutrition and growth. These include tuberculosis and *Helicobacter pylori,* which may impair micronutrient absorption [19, 20]. The relationship between growth and intestinal parasite burden is less clear. Research by Geltman et al. in Massachusetts found no association between intestinal parasite infection and the growth of recently arrived refugee children after taking into account demographic characteristics, such as country of origin [4]. This finding is consistent with a Cochrane review of intermittent de-worming, which found minimal association with growth improvement [21].

Growth is also highly dependent upon heritable factors, although population-level variation between national or ethnic groups remains an area of investigation. Early childhood growth potential appears comparable for all children, provided that they have access to optimal nutrition [22]. Data on adolescent growth are less clear, and it is possible that interpopulation variation explains at least some differences in growth between adolescents from different regions [23, 24]. At present, however, children from all groups are evaluated using standard WHO or CDC growth curves.

The CDC has proposed thorough guidelines for the evaluation of nutritional status in recently arrived refugees, including reviewing past medical history, a detailed dietary family and social history, anthropometry, physical examination, and laboratory screening (Table 16.3). Because most anthropometric references provide age-specific standards, clinicians should use ancillary records (e.g., vaccination cards) and narrative history (e.g., season and location of birth, age in relationship to other children) to try to accurately assess the age of children whose birth date is unknown. Children aged 6–59 months should be prescribed an age-appropriate multivitamin with iron. Practitioners should be alert for signs and symptoms of micronutrient deficiencies among children of any age, including children who have exhibited normal growth.

Infectious Conditions: Consideration for Children

As described in earlier chapters, the diagnosis and treatment of communicable conditions is a core component of primary care for recently resettled refugees. While many aspects of diagnosis and care are similar for adults and children, in this section we highlight issues specific to children.

Table 16.3 Evaluating refugee children for problems of growth and nutrition

History		
	Medical	Birth history (e.g., prematurity, SGA)
		Major infections
		Blood transfusions
		Surgical procedures
		Chronic diarrhea
		Rashes
		Vision problems
		Hearing problems
		Dental or gingival problems
		Fractures
		Developmental milestones
		Prior malnutrition diagnosis and/or treatment
	Dietary	General habits
		Breast-feeding (where age appropriate)
		Dietary restrictions
		Cultural dietary norms
		Food allergies
		Prior micronutrient supplementation
	Social	Food insecurity
		Economic support
	Family	Maternal history of malnutrition or micronutrient deficiency (for breast-fed infants)
Exam		
Growth	Anthropometry[a]	Weight-for-height (wasting)
		Height-for-age (stunting)
		Weight-for-age (underweight)
		Body mass index (underweight, overweight)
Micronutrient Deficiencies	Oral cavity	Caries
		Gingivitis or gingival bleeding
	Eyes	Bitot spots
		Xerophthalmia
	Skin	Dermatitis
		Alopecia
		Stomatitis
		Purpura or petechiae
	Endocrine	Goiter
	Cardiac	Flow murmur
		Stigmata of heart failure
	Musculoskeletal	Bone pain
		Bony deformities (skull, ribs, extremities)
		Muscle weakness
		Tetany
	Neurologic	Cognition/development
		Ataxia
		Peripheral neuropathy

(continued)

Table 16.3 (continued)

Labwork		
	General	Complete blood count with differential
		Iron studies[b]
		Lead[c]
		Vitamin D[d]
	Population specific	Vitamin B12[e]
Supplementation		
	Population specific	Multivitamin with iron (children 6–59 months)
		Vitamin B12 (refugees from Bhutan)[e]
Referral		
	General	National school lunch program
		Supplemental nutrition assistance program (SNAP)
	Population specific	Women, infants, and children (WIC; children <60 months)

Based upon the CDC's Guidelines for evaluation of the nutritional status and growth in refugee children during the domestic medical screening examination (April 16, 2012) unless otherwise noted

[a]The CDC recommends that clinicians use WHO standardized growth references for children younger than 2 years of age and CDC/NCHS references for older children (see Table 16.1 for details)

[b]Evaluation for iron deficiency is recommended as a secondary screening test in children with anemia. Failure to respond to iron therapy should prompt evaluation for other causes of anemia, including hemoglobinopathies and G6PD deficiency

[c]Blood lead levels are recommended for all children 6 months to 16 years at the time of arrival in the US. Follow-up blood lead testing is recommended 3–6 months later (CDC DMQ, Lead screening during the domestic medical examination for newly arrived refugees, April 16, 2012)

[d]Although routine screening for vitamin D deficiency is not currently recommended by the CDC, insufficiency and deficiency are common [12] and clinicians commonly practice routine screening or presumptive supplementation

[e]The CDC recommends oral vitamin B12 supplementation for all refugees from Bhutan (CDC DMQ, Refugee health profile, Bhutanese refugees, nutrition, June 22, 2012). Although routine screening for vitamin B12 is not recommended, some clinicians engage in either targeted screening of infants, adolescents, and adults from Bhutan or universal screening of all newly arrived refugees

Tuberculosis

Although there is variation by country of transit and origin, most studies report tuberculosis prevalence rates of between 14 and 33 % among recently arrived refugee children, the vast majority of whom have latent tuberculosis [25–28]. Tuberculosis is less common among refugee children from Iraq than among refugees from sub-Saharan Africa, where tuberculosis among the general population is also significantly more common [29]. Data are not available on US-bound refugees from Burma or Bhutan. However, studies of tuberculosis treatment programs in camps on the Thai–Burma border and in Nepal suggest that tuberculosis is prevalent amongst refugees arriving from these settings [30, 31].

Tuberculosis screening begins prior to US arrival during the Overseas Medical Examination (OME), and protocols differ for younger and older children [32]. Screening evaluation for those <2 years depends upon history and exam alone. Toddlers and younger children (2–14 years) receive Mantoux tuberculin skin tests (TST) or are tested using interferon gamma release assays (IGRA) (see Chap. 5 for details). Older children (≥15 years) are screened using chest radiograph without TST or IGRA. The use of TST or IGRA to screen younger children was initiated in 2007 and has been implemented on a rolling basis [33]. As a result, there may be increasing concordance between screening conducted overseas and that conducted in the US. Previously, however, children aged 2–14 years were screened using history and exam only. Consequently, many children with normal screening results overseas were diagnosed with tuberculosis after arrival in the US [25]. Thus, the CDC recommends that any child without documented TST or IGRA in their overseas examination should be screened at the domestic evaluation.

Amongst children who undergo screening in the US, diagnosis with latent infection is far more common than active disease [25, 27, 28]. Either TST or IGRA may be used for screening older children, although the latter, which does not cross-react with Bacillus Calmette–Guerin (BCG) vaccine antigens, may be preferred when screening older children who have received BCG. However, the CDC recommends caution in using IGRA for children <5 years, as there are limited data about test performance in this age group and young children may rapidly progress from latent infection to severe forms of active disease, e.g., tuberculosis [34]. TST may be performed in children of any age, though there may be more false negative results in the younger population.

When TST is used, interpretation is the same for children who have and have not received BCG [34, 35].

Although the diagnosis of latent tuberculosis may seem commonplace for clinicians, it is important to remember that even latent tuberculosis can be a source of fear and stigma for families. Adequate explanation about the difference between latent infection and active disease is particularly important, as are assurances about confidentiality and reassurance that tuberculosis is not caused by poor parental care [36–38]. Parents may also be skeptical when children who have received BCG are diagnosed with tuberculosis. However, BCG is effective only in preventing disseminated disease and tuberculosis meningitis in children. It does not prevent primary infection or the reactivation of latent infection.

Parasites

As noted in Chap. 6, pre-departure presumptive treatment for intestinal helminths, schistosoma, and malaria have significantly decreased the risk of infection among children arriving from endemic or holoendemic regions [39, 40]. However, primary care providers should remain alert to signs and symptoms of infection in children. Children with age-based, weight-based, or medical contraindications may receive partial or no pre-departure presumptive treatment[3] [41], or pre-departure treatment may not have been implemented as recommended [42]. Additionally, some common infections, e.g., *Giardia intestinalis,* are not susceptible to single dose Albendazole, currently the most common pre-departure presumptive therapy, and even susceptible organisms may not be eradicated in all children [40]. Similarly, presumptive pre-departure treatment for malaria is not effective against the intrahepatic life-stage of non-*falciparum* species, including *Plasmodium ovale* and *Plasmodium vivax.* Finally, parasitic infections may also be present among children from groups who are not currently recommended to receive pre-departure presumptive treatment. For example, southern Nepal and the Thai–Burma border are both malaria-endemic regions [43], and strongyloides may infect upwards of 10 % of children in endemic areas of Africa [44, 45].

Hepatitis B and C

Hepatitis B prevalence rates for recently arrived refugee children in the US range from <1 to 12 %, with significant variation by age group and region of origin [25, 26, 28, 46, 47]. The addition of hepatitis B vaccination to many national childhood vaccine programs in the 1990s and 2000s has likely led to a decrease in childhood prevalence over time and lower risk relative to adults from the same communities [47]. Regardless, the severe long-term sequelae of childhood infection, risk of household transmission [48], and availability of treatment support routine serologic screening for children from endemic regions [49].

The prevalence of hepatitis C is also believed to be higher in regions of Africa and Asia than US [47, 50]. Relative to children in the US, refugees are at higher risk of having acquired hepatitis C through unsafe medical procedures or maternal-child transmission. However, screening is not routine, and as such data are limited. Although hepatitis C is not currently included in the CDC's recommended screening guidelines for recently arrived refugees, many providers screen children with risk factors, including arrivals from regions where the prevalence exceeds 3 %.

---

[3] Children <1 year of age, pregnant adolescents in the first trimester, and children with known or suspected cysticercosis (e.g., unexplained seizures) do not receive presumptive treatment with single dose Albendazole. Children <4 years and those with known or suspected cysticercosis (e.g., unexplained seizures) do not receive presumptive treatment with Praziquantel. Children <15 kg or measuring <90 cm and pregnant adolescents do not receive presumptive treatment with Ivermectin. (CDC Overseas Guidelines).

HIV and Sexually Transmitted Infections

HIV/AIDS has not been commonly reported among recently arrived refugee children in the US, although data are limited [27]. However, extant data on HIV among adults from Iraq and the Thai–Burma border suggest that the prevalence of HIV among recently arrived children from these regions is relatively low [7, 28, 51]. As noted in Chap. 7, screening for HIV is recommended for all children after arrival in the US [52]. Subsequent to the reception and placement period, screening practices should be in accordance with guidelines for the general population, which recommend routine periodic HIV screening in all adolescents and risk-related screening for other STIs [53].

Psychosocial Issues: Considerations for Children

Refugee children are typically exposed to a broad range of social and emotional stressors both prior to and during the resettlement period [54–56]. The prevalence of traumatic stress reactions and other forms of psychological distress vary considerably by prior exposure to adverse life events [57–59]. Although the best available estimate of the PTSD prevalence among refugee children resettled in Western countries is 11 % (7–17 %) [60], strong lines of evidence suggest that the prevalence of psychological distress differs greatly between different waves of refugee arrivals. Children who have been exposed to violent conflict and unaccompanied refugee minors may be at particularly high risk [54, 57, 58, 61].

Equally remarkable is that the majority of refugee children manifest good psychological adjustment. And while longitudinal data are limited, there is also evidence that the prevalence of distress decreases over time after arrival [59]. Additionally, even those with PTSD, generalized anxiety, somatization, traumatic grief, and generalized behavior problems may be at relatively low risk for engagement in substance abuse, criminal activity, or self-harm [61]. Stable resettlement, family cohesion, and access to social supports may be particularly important as protective factors [54, 62]. As might be expected, perceptions of broader social acceptance, as well as support from peers, are associated with self-esteem and improved psychological functioning. Acculturation is both difficult to define and to measure, but having some degree of alignment with both the host culture and with the child's original culture may be beneficial.

As described by Betancourt and Williams, treatment for children experiencing emotional distress or mental health problems may be conceptualized as psychosocial or psychiatric [63]. Psychosocial interventions are intended to help children get back to "normal" by restoring routines and building/rebuilding a child's social environment. Psychiatric approaches start by identifying children with mental disorders and delivering therapeutic interventions designed to address specific diagnoses.

Access to both psychosocial and psychiatric interventions is often challenging for refugee children. After resettlement, little about a child's setting may be familiar, and even family relationships may undergo changes. For example, parents may become increasingly dependent on their children, who often learn English more quickly, or relationships may shift when children are separated from or reunited with extended family members. Consequently, restoring routines and reconstituting a familiar social environment can be difficult, particularly when parents and caregivers are also under strain.

Accessing psychiatric interventions can be equally challenging. Families may be asked to complete screening intake questionnaires using standardized instruments that have not been translated or validated for a wide variety of languages or cultures [64]. Access to bicultural interpreters or counselors is often limited, and in small communities interpreters and patients may derive from the same social milieu. This may raise concerns about confidentiality or stigma. Increasingly, however, refugee resettlement agencies and primary care providers are collaborating with mental health providers in order to ensure that refugee children are able to access needed care.

At present, the evidence base for both psychosocial and psychiatric approaches is limited but growing. Approaches to mental health care for refugee children are typically based upon the broader evidence base for children's mental health treatment, with special attention to issues of language and culture [55, 56]. Empirically evaluated approaches that show promise among refugee children include school-based mental care and group-based interventions. Data are limited on family and expressive arts approaches. A thorough overview can be found in *Resilience & Recovery After War: Refugee Children and Families in the United States* [56].

General Primary Care

The clinician must take care to address primary care issues as they would with any child. The periodic screenings performed by the primary care physician are of special importance to refugee children, as most often they have not had prior periodic screening. Key components include development, growth/nutrition, lead, and anemia. In infants, it may also include newborn screening for genetic and metabolic disorders.

Developmental screening is important to assess any motor or language delays, as well as any behavioral health issues, including but not limited to autism. Currently, commonly used tools in US, such as the Ages and Stages Questionnaire (ASQ), the Parents' Evaluation of Developmental Status (PEDS), and the Modified-Checklist for Autism in Toddlers (M-CHAT), have been validated in only few languages, e.g., English and Spanish. However, validation efforts for other national and ethnic groups are ongoing, and translations are often available in a wide variety of languages.[4,5,6] These include Arabic (M-CHAT; PEDS), French (ASQ-3, M-CHAT, PEDS), Somali (ASQ-PTI, M-CHAT, PEDS), and Vietnamese (M-CHAT, PEDS).

---

[4] http://www2.gsu.edu/~psydlr/Diana_L._Robins,_Ph.D.html.

[5] http://www.pedstest.com/Translations/PEDSinOtherLanguages.aspx.

[6] http://agesandstages.com/what-is-asq/languages/.

After the initial assessment of growth and nutrition mentioned previously, the primary care provider needs to continue to assess these on an ongoing basis. Children whose charts show wasting upon arrival need to be followed carefully for catch-up growth. For all children, weight gain also needs careful follow up to assure that it does not result in increasing BMI. After arrival in the US, children may adopt a high-calorie, low-nutrient diet as well as a more sedentary lifestyle.

Periodic lead and anemia screenings are also of great importance for refugee children. The prevalence of elevated blood lead levels (defined as >10 mcg/dL in existing studies[7]) ranges from <2 % among children from Iraq to >20 % among children from sub-Saharan Africa [28, 65], with intermediate levels (5 %) observed among children from Burma [66, 67]. A study of refugee children under 7 years of age arriving to Massachusetts between 2000 and 2007 demonstrated that 16 % had elevated lead levels, as compared to 1.4 % of US children between 1995 and 1999 [65]. Using the more recent cut point of 5 mcg/dL [Ref: http://www.cdc.gov/nceh/lead/ACCLPP/Final_Document_030712.pdf], one study from the Thai–Burma border found that 73 % of children had elevated blood lead levels. Sources of environmental lead exposure that may be unique to refugee children include lead-alloy cookware, car batteries used as household generators, and contaminated foods, cosmetics, or traditional medications.

Because children of all ages may be exposed to contaminated products, laboratory screening is recommended for all newly arrived refugee children and adolescents (6 months to 16 years). In urban areas with older housing stock, children may also be exposed to environmental lead after arrival in the US [65, 68]. For this reason, repeated screening is recommended for all children <6 years between 3 and 6 months after arrival [69]. Additionally, children <6 years should receive an age-appropriate multivitamin with iron, as individuals with malnutrition and micronutrient deficiencies are at increased risk for lead poisoning.

The treatment of elevated blood lead levels focuses on removing the source of lead contamination and, in severe cases, chelation and decontamination. Although blood lead levels <10 mcg/dL may impair neurodevelopment [70], acute symptoms are typically present only with levels of 45 mcg/dL or higher. These include headache, abdominal pain, constipation, and neurologic impairment, such as clumsiness or lethargy. Severe acute neurologic effects include ataxia, seizures, coma, and death. Detailed management of elevated blood lead levels is beyond the scope of this chapter, but should be consistent with established guidelines (www.cdc.gov/lead/scientificandeducation.htm; www.cdc.gov/nceh/lead). Educational materials in different languages are available from many state and local childhood lead poisoning prevention programs, including Minnesota (http://www.health.state.mn.us/divs/eh/lead/fs/) and Philadelphia (http://www.phila.gov/health/childhoodlead/EducationOutreach.html), as well as refugee-serving organizations (http://www.refugees.org/resources/for-refugees--immigrants/health/healthy-living-toolkit/).

---

[7]The majority of publications on elevated blood lead levels among refugee children predate the CDC's decision to revise the blood lead level reference value to 5 mcg/dL.

Anemia is also variable among refugee children in the US, affecting 4–43 % of newly arrived children, with significant variability between age groups and regions of origin [4, 27, 28, 65, 68, 71, 72]. Recent data offer limited detail but suggest that the overall prevalence of anemia is 10–20 % among children arriving in the US and may be higher among children from Bhutan and Burma than those from Iraq [28, 65]. Prior population-based studies from refugee camps in Nepal suggest that anemia is more common among infants than older children and, among adolescents, more common among females than males [6, 73, 74].

Causes of anemia include micronutrient deficiencies, for example iron or vitamin B12, and hereditary forms of anemia, such as G6PD deficiency, thalassemia, and sickle cell anemia. Unlike children born in the US, refugee children have not undergone newborn screening, and they may have limited information about their family's medical history. As a result, hereditary anemias may be diagnosed at a later age than might be typical for other primary care patients. Children at risk for hereditary anemias include those from the Middle East (thalassemia, G6PD deficiency, rarely sickle cell anemia) [75, 76]; Burma and other regions of South and South East Asia (thalassemia) [77], and sub-Saharan Africa (G6PD deficiency, thalassemia, sickle cell anemia). For each of these diseases, the prevalence rates differ by population but may be as high as 20 %. As a result, clinicians should have a high index of suspicion for hereditary etiologies when evaluating anemic children from these regions.

Refugee children, like other immigrant children, are especially at risk for dental problems, particularly caries [4, 46, 72, 78]. In a detailed examination of oral health for children who resettled in Massachusetts in 2002, caries were notably common among all refugees, however prevalence varied by region of origin. For example, children from Africa (predominantly Somalia, Liberia, and Sudan) were least likely to have any caries. Nonetheless, one in three African children was affected and 1 in 20 required urgent dental care. Caries were significantly more common (88 %) among children from Europe (predominantly Bosnia), the largest comparator group [78].

Primary care providers should survey a refugee child's teeth as part of routine health surveillance and refer any acute dental issues immediately. They may also apply dental varnish if available, and review the basics of dental hygiene. Most importantly, they should refer all refugee children to a primary pediatric dentist for routine dental care as soon as possible after arrival in the US.

In addition to managing primary care conditions, clinicians for recently resettled children must simultaneously strive to provide linguistically and culturally appropriate care. This is of particular importance when treating adolescents, as some aspects of adolescent health care in the US are not routine components of the patient–doctor relationship in many other regions of the world. Adolescents and their parents often do not expect the physician to complete a breast or genital exam or to ask questions about social functioning, substance use, or sexual and reproductive health. Orienting adolescents and their parents beforehand can help to normalize these experiences, as may giving adolescents the option of having a gender concordant provider.

Similarly, clinicians may collaborate with community leaders and other experts to develop anticipatory guidance that is consistent with a refugee community's frame of reference, opportunities, and expectations (i.e., culturally relevant), as well as parents' literacy level. For example, dietary guidance may be most effective when based upon foods that are both familiar to families and accessible in the US and can often build upon parents' existing beliefs regarding healthy and unhealthy nutritional practices. In contrast, anticipatory guidance regarding home safety, e.g., use of smoke and carbon monoxide detectors, may require that clinicians introduce an entirely new set of concepts and objects for families who have come from refugee camps or agrarian regions with limited access to electricity. Similarly, families with low literacy levels may require visual aids, such as pictograms or marked syringes, to safely administer medication to their children, while those with very high literacy levels may prefer written or even online information in their preferred language.

In general, approaches characterized by cultural humility, defined by Tervalon and Murray-Garcia [79] as a long-term process of engagement and reflection with the intention of learning to work respectfully and effectively with patients from different cultural groups, can help clinicians develop strong therapeutic relationships with children and families. Working with families in this way is a unique learning experience for the provider and a critical point of engagement for children and families who may be intimidated or overwhelmed by the complexity of the US health system. Primary care providers, who are often a child's first point of contact with US health care, play an indispensible and often formative role in determining how children will experience all subsequent care.

References

1. Department of Homeland Security. Yearbook of immigration statistics: Table 15. Washington, DC: Department of Homeland Security; 2005–2011.
2. Department of Homeland Security. Yearbook of immigration statistics: Table 14d. Washington, DC: Department of Homeland Security; 2011.
3. Unaccompanied Refugee Minors (URM). Washington, DC. http://www.acf.hhs.gov/programs/orr/programs/urm, 2013.
4. Geltman PL, Radin M, Zhang Z, et al. Growth status and related medical conditions among refugee children in Massachusetts, 1995–1998. Am J Publ Health. 2001;91:1800–5.
5. Seal AJ, Creeke PI, Mirghani Z, et al. Iron and vitamin A deficiency in long-term African refugees. J Nutr. 2005;135:808–13.
6. CDC. Malnutrition and micronutrient deficiencies among Bhutanese refugee children—Nepal, 2007. MMWR. 2008;57:370–3.
7. Yanni EA, Naoum M, Odeh N, et al. The Health profile and chronic diseases comorbidities of US-bound Iraqi refugees screened by the International Organization for Migration in Jordan: 2007–2009. J Immigr Minor Health. 2013;15:1–9. doi:10.1007/s10903-012-9578-6.
8. AaM S-B, Wiegersma PA, Bijleveld CM, et al. Obesity in asylum seekers' children in The Netherlands–the use of national reference charts. Eur J Publ Health. 2007;17:555–9. doi:10.1093/eurpub/ckm013.
9. Hjern A. Health and nutrition in newly resettled refugee children from Chile and the Middle East. Acta Paediatr Scand. 1991;80:859–67.

10. Banjong O, Menefee A, Sranacharoenpong K, et al. Dietary assessment of refugees living in camps: a case study of Mae La Camp, Thailand. Food Nutr Bull. 2003;24:360–7.
11. Kemmer T, Bovill M. Iron deficiency is unacceptably high in refugee children from Burma. J Nutr. 2003;133:4143–9.
12. Penrose K, Hunter Adams J, Nguyen T, et al. Vitamin d deficiency among newly resettled refugees in massachusetts. J Immigr Minor Health. 2012;14:941–8. doi:10.1007/s10903-012-9603-9.
13. Blanck HM, Ba B, Serdula MK, et al. Angular stomatitis and riboflavin status among adolescent Bhutanese refugees living in southeastern Nepal. Am J Clin Nutr. 2002;76:430–5.
14. CDC. Vitamin B12 deficiency in resettled Bhutanese refugees – United States, 2008–2011. MMWR. 2011;60:343–6.
15. WHO. Physical status: the use and interpretatio of anthropometry – infants and children. Geneva: WHO; 1995.
16. Doyle J. Nutritional vitamin B12 deficiency in infancy: three case reports and a review of the literature. Pediatr Hematol Oncol. 1989;6:161–72.
17. Guez S, Chiarelli G, Menni F, et al. Severe vitamin B12 deficiency in an exclusively breastfed 5-month-old Italian infant born to a mother receiving multivitamin supplementation during pregnancy. BMC Pediatr. 2012;12:85.
18. Kühne T, Bubl R, Baumgartner R. Maternal vegan diet causing a serious infantile neurological disorder due to vitamin B 12 deficiency. Eur J Pediatr. 1991;150:205–8.
19. Benson J, Maldari T, Turnbull T. Vitamin B12 deficiency: why refugee patients are at high risk. Aust Fam Physician. 2010;39:215–7.
20. Kaptan K, Beyan C, Ural A, et al. Helicobacter pylori–is it a novel causative agent in Vitamin B12 deficiency? Arch Intern Med. 2000;160:1349–535.
21. Taylor-Robinson D, Maayan N, Soares-Weiser K, et al. Deworming drugs for soil-transmitted intestinal worms in children: effects on nutritional indicators, haemoglobin and school performance (review). The Cochrane Collaborative. 2012.
22. de Onis M, Garza C, Onyango AW, et al. Comparison of the WHO child growth standards and the CDC 2000 growth charts. J Nutr. 2007;137:144–8.
23. Butte NF, Garza C, de Onis M. Evaluation of the feasibility of international growth standards for school-aged children and adolescents. J Nutr. 2007;137:153–7.
24. Haas J, Campirano F. Interpopulation variation in height among children 7 to 18 years of age. Food Nutr Bull. 2006;27:s212–23.
25. Lifson AR, Thai D, O'Fallon A, et al. Prevalence of tuberculosis, hepatitis B virus, and intestinal parasitic infections among refugees to Minnesota. Public Health Rep. 2002;117:69–77.
26. Sheikh M, Pal A, Wang S, et al. The epidemiology of health conditions of newly arrived refugee children: a review of patients attending a specialist health clinic in Sydney. J Paediatr Child Health. 2009;45:509–13. doi:10.1111/j.1440-1754.2009.01550.x.
27. Watts D-J, Friedman JF, Vivier PM, et al. Health care utilization of refugee children after resettlement. J Immigr Minor Health. 2012;14:583–8. doi:10.1007/s10903-011-9530-1.
28. Ramos M, Orozovich P, Moser K, et al. Health of resettled Iraqi refugees—San Diego County, California, October 2007–September 2009. Morb Mortal Wkly Rep. 2011;59:1614–8.
29. WHO. Global Tuberculosis report. Geneva: WHO; 2012.
30. Bam TS, Da E, Hinderaker SG, et al. High success rate of TB treatment among Bhutanese refugees in Nepal. Int J Tubercul Lung Dis. 2007;11:54–8.
31. Minetti A, Camelique O, Hsa Thaw K, et al. Tuberculosis treatment in a refugee and migrant population: 20 years of experience on the Thai–Burmese border. Int J Tubercul Lung Dis. 2010;14:1589–95.
32. CDC. Technical instructions for tuberculosis screening and treatment. Atlanta: Division of Global Migration and Quarantine; 2009.
33. CDC. Tuberculosis screening and treatment technical instructions using cultures and directly observed therapy implementation. Atlanta: Division of Global Migration and Quarantine; 2012.

34. CDC. Updated guidelines for using interferon gamma release assays to detect mycobacterium tuberculosis infection – United States, 2010. MMWR. 2010; 59:1–26.
35. CDC. Guidelines for screening for tuberculosis infection and disease during the domestic medical examination for newly arrived refugees. Atlanta: Division of Global Migration and Quarantine; 2012.
36. Carey J, Oxtoby M, Nguyen L, et al. Tuberculosis beliefs among recent Vietnamese refugees in New York State. Public Health Rep. 1997;112:66–72.
37. Sheikh M, MacIntyre CR. The impact of intensive health promotion to a targeted refugee population on utilisation of a new refugee paediatric clinic at the children's hospital at Westmead. Ethn Health. 2009;14:393–405. doi:10.1080/13557850802653780.
38. Wieland ML, Ja W, Yawn BP, et al. Perceptions of tuberculosis among immigrants and refugees at an adult education center: a community-based participatory research approach. J Immigr Minor Health. 2012;14:14–22. doi:10.1007/s10903-010-9391-z.
39. Geltman PL, Cochran J, Hedgecock C. Intestinal parasites among African refugees resettled in Massachusetts and the impact of an overseas pre-departure treatment program. Am J Trop Med Hyg. 2003;69:657–62.
40. Swanson SJ, Phares CR, Mamo B, et al. Albendazole therapy and enteric parasites in United States-bound refugees. N Engl J Med. 2012;366:1498–507. doi:10.1056/NEJMoa1103360.
41. CDC. Refugee health guidelines: intestinal parasites overseas recommendations. Atlanta, GA: Division of Global Migration and Quarantine; 2013.
42. Phares CR, Kapella BK, Doney AC, et al. Presumptive treatment to reduce imported malaria among refugees from east Africa resettling in the United States. AmJTrop Med Hyg. 2011;85:612–5.
43. WHO. World malaria report. Geneva: WHO; 2012.
44. Dawson-Hahn EE, Greenberg SLM, Domachowske JB, et al. Eosinophilia and the seroprevalence of schistosomiasis and strongyloidiasis in newly arrived pediatric refugees: an examination of Centers for Disease Control and Prevention screening guidelines. J Pediatr. 2010;156:1016–8. doi:10.1016/j.jpeds.2010.02.043.
45. Olsen A, van Lieshout L, Marti H, et al. Strongyloidiasis–the most neglected of the neglected tropical diseases? Trans R Soc Trop Med Hyg. 2009;103:967–72. doi:10.1016/j.trstmh.2009.02.013.
46. Meropol SB. Health status of pediatric refugees in Buffalo, NY. Arch Pediatr Adolesc Med. 1995;149:887–92.
47. Paxton GA, Sangster KJ, Maxwell EL, et al. Post-arrival health screening in Karen refugees in Australia. PloS One. 2012;7:e38194.
48. Hurie M, Mast E, Davis J. Horizontal transmission of hepatitis B virus infection to United States-born children of Hmong refugees. Pediatrics. 1992;89:269–74.
49. CDC, editor. Evaluating and updating immunizations during the domestic medical examination for newly arrived refugees. Atlanta: Division of Global Migration and Quarantine; 2012
50. Greenaway C, Wong DKH, Assayag D, et al. Screening for hepatitis C infection: evidence review for newly arriving immigrants and refugees. Can J Med. 2011. doi:10.1503/cmaj.090313.
51. Plewes K, Lee T, Kajeechewa L, et al. Low seroprevalence of HIV and syphilis in pregnant women in refugee camps on the Thai-Burma border. Int J STD & AIDS. 2008;19:833–7. doi:10.1258/ijsa.2008.008034.
52. CDC. Screening for sexually transmitted diseases during the domestic medical examination for newly arrived refugees. Atlanta: Division of Global Migration and Quarantine; 2012.
53. CDC. STD treatment guidelines. Atlanta: Division of STD Prevention; 2010.
54. Fazel M, Reed RV, Panter-Brick C, et al. Mental health of displaced and refugee children resettled in high-income countries: risk and protective factors. Lancet. 2012;379:266–82. doi:10.1016/S0140-6736(11)60051-2.

55. Lustig S, Kia-Keating M, Knight W, et al. Review of child and adolescent refugee mental health. J Am Acad Child Adolesc Psychiatr. 2004;43:24–36. doi:10.1097/01. chi.0000096619.64367.37.

56. APA. Resilience & recovery after war: refugee children and families in the United States: task force on the psychosocial effects of war on children and families who are refugees from armed conflict residing in the United States. Washington DC: APA; 2010.

57. Bean T, Derluyn I, Eurelings-Bontekoe E, et al. Comparing psychological distress, traumatic stress reactions, and experiences of unaccompanied refugee minors with experiences of adolescents accompanied by parents. J Nerv Ment Dis. 2007;195:288–97. doi:10.1097/01. nmd.0000243751.49499.93.

58. Bean TM, Eurelings-Bontekoe E, Spinhoven P. Course and predictors of mental health of unaccompanied refugee minors in the Netherlands: one year follow-up. Soc Sci Med. 2007;64:1204–15. doi:10.1016/j.socscimed.2006.11.010.

59. Montgomery E. Trauma and resilience in young refugees: a 9-year follow-up study. Dev Psychopathol. 2010;22:477–89. doi:10.1017/S0954579410000180.

60. Fazel M, Wheeler J, Danesh J. Prevalence of serious mental disorder in 7000 refugees resettled in western countries: a systematic review. Lancet. 2005;365:1309–14. doi:10.1016/ S0140-6736(05)61027-6.

61. Betancourt TS, Newnham EA, Layne CM, et al. Trauma history and psychopathology in war-affected refugee children referred for trauma-related mental health services in the United States. J Trauma Stress. 2012;25:682–90.

62. Porter M, Haslam N. Predisplacement and postdisplacement factors associated with mental health of refugees and internally displaced persons: a meta-analysis. JAMA. 2005;294:602–12. doi:10.1001/jama.294.5.602.

63. Betancourt T, Williams T. Building an evidence base on mental health interventions for children affected by armed conflict. Intervention (Amstelveen). 2008;6:1–15. doi:10.1097/ WTF.0b013e3282f761ff.Building.

64. Davidson G, Murray KE, Schweitzer RD. Review of refugee mental health assessment: best practices and recommendations. J Pacific Rim Psychol. 2010;4:72–85.

65. Eisenberg KW, van Wijngaarden E, Fisher SG, et al. Blood lead levels of refugee children resettled in Massachusetts, 2000 to 2007. A J Pubic Health. 2011;101:48–54. doi:10.2105/ AJPH.2009.184408.

66. Mitchell T, Jentes E, Ortega L, et al. Lead poisoning in United States-bound refugee children: Thailand–Burma border, 2009. Pediatrics. 2012;129:e392–9.

67. Power D, Moody E, Trussell K, et al. Caring for the Karen: a newly arrived refugee group. Minn Med. 2010;93(4):49–53.

68. Geltman P, Brown M, Cochran J. Lead poisoning among refugee children resettled in Massachusetts, 1995 to 1999. Pediatrics. 2001;108:158–62. doi:10.1542/peds.108.1.158.

69. CDC. Lead screening during the domestic medical examination for newly arrived refugees. Atlanta: Division of Global Migration and Quarantine; 2012.

70. Canfield RL, Henderson CR, Cory-Slechta DA, et al. Intellectual impairment in children with blood lead concentrations below 10 mcg per deciliter. N Engl J Med. 2003;348:1517–26.

71. Entzel PP, Fleming LE, Trepka MJ, et al. The health status of newly arrived refugee children in Miami – Dade county, Florida. Am J Public Health. 2003;93:286–8.

72. Hayes E, Talbot S. Health status of pediatric refugees in Portland, ME. Arch Pediatr. 1998;152:564–8.

73. Bilukha O, Howard C, Wilkinson C, et al. Effects of multimicronutrient home fortification on anemia and growth in Bhutanese refugee children. Food Nutr Bull. 2011;32:264–76.

74. CDC. Nutritional assessment of adolescent refugees – Nepal 1999. Morbid Mortal Wkly Rep. 2000;49(38):864–7.

75. Hamamy HA. Genetic diseases in Iraq. In: Teebi AS, editor. Genetic disorders among Arab populations. 2nd ed. New York: Springer; 2010. p. 297–323.

76. Nkhoma ET, Poole C, Vannappagari V, et al. The global prevalence of glucose-6-phosphate dehydrogenase deficiency: a systematic review and meta-analysis. Blood Cells Mol Dis. 2009;42:267–78. doi:10.1016/j.bcmd.2008.12.005.

77. Fucharoen S, Winichagoon P. Haemoglobinopathies in Southeast Asia. Indian J Med Res. 2011;134:498–506.

78. Cote S, Geltman P, Nunn M, et al. Dental caries of refugee children compared with US children. Pediatrics. 2004;114:e733–40. doi:10.1542/peds.2004-0496.

79. Tervalon M, Murray-Garcia J. Cultural humility versus cultural competence: a critical distinction in defining physician training outcomes in multicultural education. J Health Care Poor Underserved. 1998;9:117–25.

80. Khatib IM, Samrah SM, Zghol FM. Nutritional interventions in refugee camps on Jordan's eastern border: assessment of status of vulnerable groups. East Mediterr Health J. 2010 Feb;16(2):187-93.

81. Rice AL, West KP Jr, Black RE. Vitamin A deficiency. In: Ezzati M, Lopez AD, Rogers A, Murray CJL, editors. Comparative quantification of health risks: Global and regional burden of disease due to selected major risk factors (Volume 1). Geneva: World Health Organization; 2004.

82. Caulfield LE, Black RE. Zinc deficiency. In: Ezzati M LA, Rogers A, Murray CJL (ed). Comparative quantification of health risks: global and regional burden of disease attributable to selected major risk factors. Volume 1. Geneva: World Health Organization, 2004:257-79.

Chapter 17
Medical Evaluation of Asylum Seekers

Katherine C. McKenzie

Introduction

An asylum seeker is a refugee who enters the US without legal status, fleeing persecution and torture. Asylum seekers have suffered physical and/or emotional trauma in the country and believe that they will be in danger if they return. Every year, thousands of victims seek refuge in the US, and apply for asylum; in 2011, nearly 25,000 people were granted asylum in the US [1]. A medical forensic report from an expert clinician can provide strong support in immigration court.

Asylum Seekers

As defined by US law, a refugee is an alien in the US "who is unable or unwilling to return to … [his or her] country … because of persecution or… fear of persecution… on account of race, religion, nationality, membership in a particular social group or political opinion [2].

Sometimes torture survivors enter the US with a tourist or student visa. Once they stay beyond the time allowed on the visa, they choose to apply for asylum so that they are not sent back to the countries from which they have come. While asylum seekers are awaiting a court decision, they are not able to work legally and are not eligible for government assistance. Other asylees enter the US through an airport or at a land border, without a visa. Under these circumstances, they are placed in a detention center near this entry point and the evaluation occurs there.

K.C. McKenzie, M.D. (✉)
Department of Medicine, Yale School of Medicine, 800 Howard Avenue,
New Haven, CT 06519, USA
e-mail: Katherine.mckenzie@yale.edu

A. Annamalai (ed.), *Refugee Health Care: An Essential Medical Guide*,
DOI 10.1007/978-1-4939-0271-2_17, © Springer Science+Business Media New York 2014

Torture

Torture is officially condemned by most nations but continues to be carried out in almost 150 countries; it is widespread in more than 70 [3].

In 1984, the United Nations General Assembly Convention Against Torture and Other Cruel, Inhuman or Degrading Treatment and Punishment (CAT) defined torture as:

> "Any act by which severe pain or suffering, whether physical or mental, is intentionally inflicted on a person for such purposes as obtaining from him or a third person information or a confession, punishing him for an act he or a third person has committed or is suspected of having committed, or intimidating or coercing him or a third person, or for any reason based on discrimination of any kind, when such pain and suffering is inflicted by or at the instigation of or with the consent or acquiescence of a public official or other person acting in an official capacity. It does not include pain or suffering arising only from, inherent in or incidental to lawful sanctions" [4].

The CAT also requires that no member UN state "shall expel, return ... or extradite a person to another State where there are substantial grounds for believing that he would be in danger of being subjected to torture" [5].

While torture is the intentional infliction of severe mental or physical pain, persecution covers a wider spectrum of hardships [6]. Torture is a form of persecution, and both are considered valid reasons for granting a client asylum.

Physical and psychological sequelae from common forms of torture are listed in Table 17.1.

Types of psychological torture include deprivation and inhumane conditions during detention, humiliation (especially sexual), proximity to torture of others, threats, blackmail, harassment, and interrogation. Victims subjected to psychological torture can demonstrate anxiety, depression, posttraumatic stress disorder (PTSD), failure to thrive, insomnia, nightmares, and sexual dysfunction.

Female genital mutilation/cutting (FGM) as a form of torture is a manifestation of gender inequality. It most commonly occurs in African countries, but is practiced in India and the Middle East as well. FGM is a practice entrenched in the social, economic, political, and religious institutions of the communities where it occurs.

Table 17.1 Sequelae of torture [7]

Common forms of physical torture	Common physical and psychological sequelae
Burns	Scars
Blunt trauma/beatings	Chronic pain
Genital cutting/skin mutilation	Infertility
Sexual assault and female genital mutilation/cutting	Sexual dysfunction
Forced positioning	Chronic pain; functional neurological symptoms
Suffocation and waterboarding	PTSD and anxiety
Electrical torture	Scars

It is inflicted most commonly on girls between the ages of 0–15 and in some cases is part of a "coming of age" ceremony for girls. Families perceive that the societal benefits outweigh the harm to the girls and their families; families and daughters can be ostracized if they refuse to allow FGM. For example, a girl whose family refuses to allow FGM may never be allowed to marry.

The severity of the cutting varies in each society, but in many cases the practice allows the girl's virginity to be ascertained, decreases her ability to experience sexual pleasure, and enhances male sexual pleasure. FGM is classified into four types [8]. See Chap. 15 for more details.

Role of the Expert Clinician [7]

Asylum seekers present to physicians and other clinicians seeking professional evaluation of emotional and/or physical trauma. Medical care is explicitly not provided during this evaluation; the clinician must gather objective evidence to be used in the legal case for asylum. Consequently asylum seekers are considered clients, not patients. This evaluation requires clinical judgment and medical expertise of the physician or mental health professional.

Clinicians interview the client, determine whether the client's physical and/or psychological sequelae are consistent with the alleged ill treatment, and produce a written report of these findings. The clinician evaluator is not responsible for verifying a client's identity, confirming the veracity of the client's report, determining whether claims of torture meet CAT criteria, predicting what would happen if the client returns to their country, or deciding whether a client qualifies for asylum.

Client Referral

Clinicians of any specialty can be trained by advocacy groups to perform asylum evaluations. These training meetings typically last for a half to a full day. Advocacy groups also provide ongoing mentorship for expert clinicians. Asylees are referred to trained clinicians from private lawyers (some of whom see clients pro bono and some of whom charge a fee), from advocacy groups such as Physicians for Human Rights or HealthRight International or from law schools. An attorney will interview the client and a report that outlines the persecution or torture will be shared with the clinician prior to the medical evaluation. A background report on the country of origin of the asylee may be provided as well, to outline details of the political climate of the country. When necessary, the law office or advocacy group will arrange for a translator to accompany the client.

Interviewing the Client

Meetings with the client usually last 60–90 min and begin with acknowledgement of the alleged trauma the client has experienced. Clinicians must strive to provide the client with a sense of control during the encounter; to this end, a client can be told that the interview can be paused or halted if the discussion becomes too traumatic. Although the client has already been informed that the purpose of the meeting is to gather medical information to provide in court, expectations regarding the interview are reviewed with the client. The client is again informed that medical care will not be provided.

The information that was sent from the attorney is reviewed, with emphasis on the details of the torture and persecution. Note should be made of post-injury treatment as well, including medical care provided, medication given, procedures, hospitalization, or surgery. The client is asked to be as specific as possible when describing the incidents of torture. A detailed account is considered to be more credible in court.

Nevertheless, some survivors of torture have poor recall due to head trauma, sensory deprivation during detention, or post traumatic stress disorder. If the client is nonspecific in describing the trauma, a cause should be elicited and outlined. Although many clients are seen also by a mental health professional, it is appropriate to investigate persistent psychological symptoms during the medical interview.

Examining the Client

The physical exam is focused on areas of the body where there are scars from the trauma. Other scars that are unrelated to trauma are noted, with description of the unrelated injury mentioned in the report.

In some cases, there is no physical evidence on exam. This can happen if torture occurs, but the area of trauma heals entirely. Rape, especially in a parous woman, often leaves no scars. Nevertheless, documentation of the history along with an exam from an internist still has value, and should include commentary from the internist regarding any psychological symptoms related to the torture or rape. Internists usually assess psychological distress based on a client's affect and explicit symptoms. More thorough and objective psychological evaluations occur with mental health professionals.

The Report

After the interview and exam, the clinician writes a report outlining the findings. This report takes the form of a declaration, which does not require notarization, or an affidavit, which does. The attorney determines which form is required.

The clinician begins with a brief outline of the client's life preceding the torture, any medical history and background about country conditions. The clinician then outlines the details of the alleged torture, while providing a detailed history of exactly what the client remembers of the torture or persecution. For example, if a client was detained and tortured, details such as the number of abductors, the type of weapons or instruments of torture that were used, and the number of days in detention are all important.

Physical findings are noted in the report. They can also be documented on body diagrams (see Figs. 17.1 and 17.2) [9], with photos or both. Scar documentation should be as precise as possible, with specific measurements and explicit descriptions. The report outlines any psychological findings as well.

The trained clinician must use medical expertise to determine specificity of physical findings and characterize them as outlined in Table 17.2.

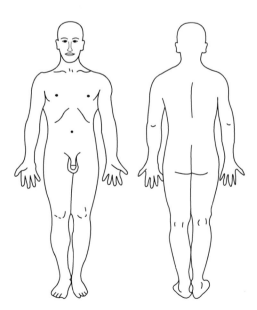

Fig. 17.1 Line drawing, male

Fig. 17.2 Line drawing,
female

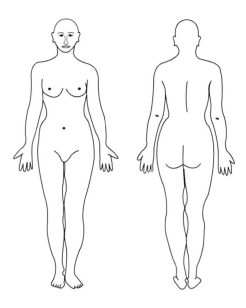

Table 17.2 Expressing degrees of consistency [10]

Not consistent	The lesion could not have been caused by the trauma described
Consistent with	The lesion could have been caused by the trauma described, but it is nonspecific and there are many other possible causes
Highly consistent	The lesion could have been caused by the trauma described, and there are few other possible causes
Typical of	This is an appearance that is usually found with this type of trauma, but there are other possible causes
Diagnostic of	This appearance could not have been caused in any way other than that described

Court Testimony

The client's attorney or the government attorney may request testimony in court from the clinician; this usually lasts less than 30 min and can be provided telephonically in most cases. During testimony, attorneys may review the clinician's credentials. Both the client's attorney as well as the US government attorney can ask questions based on the information in the affidavit or report. The clinician provides an expert opinion regarding whether the history, physical findings and psychological symptoms are consistent with the reported torture.

Summary

An expert forensic medical exam by a trained clinician can be invaluable to an asylee applying for refuge in the US. Objectivity and credibility along with detailed physical descriptions can greatly enhance the chances that a torture victim will be allowed to obtain asylum.

Immigration courts explicitly indicate that clinicians are not responsible for determining whether a client's report of abuse is true, nor are they required to determine if a client meets the requirements for asylum. It is only necessary to use medical expertise to judge how consistent a client's history is with the injuries and emotional state. Most cases referred from law clinics and advocacy groups have been well vetted, and the findings strongly support claims of torture or persecution.

Performing evaluations of torture survivors allows clinician to use their training and medical skills in an unusual manner. It is not often that a clinician can impact a person's life in this unique way. The experience of interviewing and examining people who have suffered such profound trauma is emotionally and intellectually challenging, but deeply rewarding.

References

1. Office of Immigration Statistics, Department of Homeland Security. 2011 Yearbook of immigration statistics. 2012: p. 43. http://www.dhs.gov/immigration-statistics. Accessed Aug 2013.
2. United States Immigration and Nationality Act 101 (a) 42. http://www.uscis.gov/ilink/docView/SLB/HTML/SLB/0-0-0-1/0-0-0-29/0-0-0-101.html. Accessed Aug 2013.
3. Amnesty International. Torture worldwide: an affront to human dignity. New York: Amnesty International; 2000. p. 2–3.
4. United Nations General Assembly. United Nations General Assembly convention against torture and other cruel, inhuman or degrading treatment or punishment, Article 1. 1984. http://www.un.org/documents/ga/res/39/a39r046.htm. Accessed Aug 2013.
5. United Nations General Assembly. United Nations General Assembly convention against torture and other cruel, inhuman or degrading treatment or punishment, Article 3. 1984. http://www.un.org/documents/ga/res/39/a39r046.htm. Accessed Aug 2013.
6. Ark T. Immigration and nationality law handbook: 2002–03 edition, v 1. Washington: American Immigration Lawyers Association; 2002. p. 278.
7. HealthRight International/Human Rights Clinic. Training manual for physicians and mental health professionals. 6th ed. 2012
8. World Health Organization. Eliminating female genital mutilation: an interagency statement. 2008. http://whqlibdoc.who.int/publications/2008/9789241596442_eng.pdf. Accessed Aug 2013.
9. Physicians for Human Rights. Examining asylum seekers: a clinician's guide to physical and psychological evaluations of torture and ill treatment. 2012. http://physiciansforhumanrights.org/asylum. Accessed Aug 2013.
10. Office of the High Commissioner for Human Rights. Istanbul protocol: manual on the effective investigation and documentation of torture and other cruel, inhuman or degrading treatment or punishment. New York/Geneva: United Nations; 2001. p. 34–35.

Index

A. Annamalai (ed.), *Refugee Health Care: An Essential Medical Guide*,
DOI 10.1007/978-1-4939-0271-2, © Springer Science+Business Media New York 2014

Printed in Great Britain
by Amazon